OBSTETRICS ILLUSTRATED

OBSTETRICS ILLUSTRATED

M. M. GARREY
MB DPH FRCOG
Glasgow Royal Maternity Hospital

A. D. T. GOVAN
MD PhD FRCP(G) FRCP(Ed) FRCOG FCPath
Glasgow Royal Maternity Hospital

C. H. HODGE
MB FRCS(Ed) MRCOG
Rankin Memorial Hospital Greenock

R. CALLANDER
FFPh MMAA
Medical Illustration Unit, University of Glasgow

THIRD REPRINT

CHURCHILL LIVINGSTONE

EDINBURGH AND LONDON

1972

E. & S. LIVINGSTONE LIMITED 1969

First Edition 1969

Revised Reprint 1970

Second Reprint 1971

Third Reprint 1972

ISBN 0 443 00627 X

PRINTED IN THE BRITISH COMMONWEALTH

PREFACE

It has been our object to produce a textbook which will be of use to the student both undergraduate and graduate. The provision of visual and other aids has become a necessity if the student is to find time to acquire his all-important practical experience; and it is hoped that by combining a concise and simple text with a very liberal use of illustrations, the information in these pages can be easily assimilated by the busy reader.

Most women have normal confinements, and modern obstetrics has become more and more the practice of preventive medicine. A large part of the book has been given to descriptions of normal physiology and the processes of normal labour, and to antenatal care and the treatment of those diseases which may complicate the antenatal period. Throughout we have tried to adopt a clinical approach and to emphasise the need for constant expectant care if abnormalities are to be avoided. However, as there is no abnormality which the obstetrician may safely assume to be as it were extinct, and as his surgical skill and judgment may be put to the test at any moment, we have described in detail the more common operations, and have referred briefly to some that are becoming obsolete.

We are indebted to many sources of information but have made no attempt to provide references or to indicate further reading on different subjects. We believe that if the student gains a clear understanding of principles he will be able by himself to extend his knowledge from the abundant and increasing literature.

We should like to express our thanks to Messrs. E. & S. Livingstone for their patient and helpful co-operation; to Mrs Elizabeth Callander for her painstaking work on the index; and to Mrs Gillian Skea whose secretarial efficiency made the months of work so easy and agreeable.

Glasgow
January 1969

M. M. Garrey
A. D. T. Govan
C. H. Hodge
R. Callander

CONTENTS

CHAPTER I

PHYSIOLOGY OF REPRODUCTION

OVULATION AND MENSTRUATION

CYCLICAL OVARIAN CHANGES

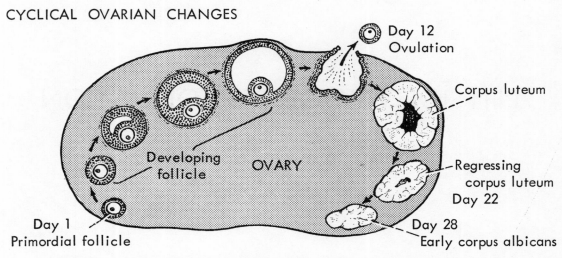

During the normal 28 day cycle a sequence of changes occurs in the ovary aimed at the production of a mature ovum, capable of being fertilized. This sequence also controls the quantity and quality of steroids necessary for the preparation of the uterus for reception of the ovum.

PITUITARY CONTROL of OVARY

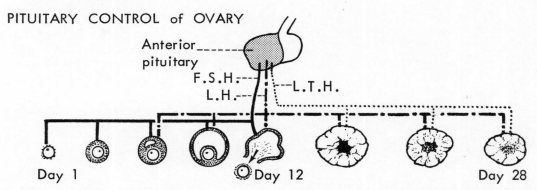

The ovarian changes are to a great extent under the control of the anterior pituitary which produces certainly two and possibly three gonadotrophins – follicle stimulating hormone (F.S.H.) which initiates follicle growth; luteinizing hormone (L.H.) which transforms the lining granulosal cells into luteal cells after escape of the ovum; and possibly a luteotrophic hormone (L.T.H.) responsible for growth and maintenance of the corpus luteum.

OVULATION AND MENSTRUATION

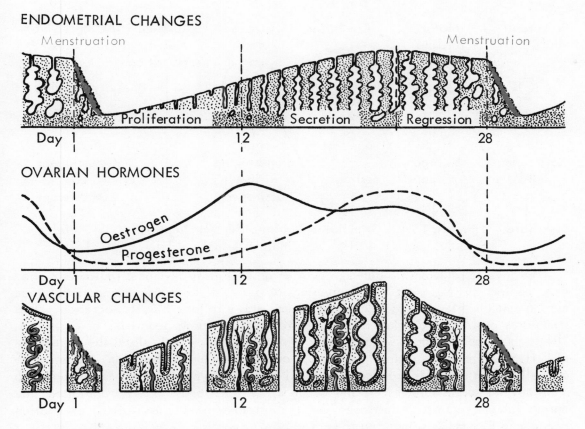

ENDOMETRIAL CHANGES

Menstruation   Menstruation

Proliferation   Secretion   Regression

Day 1   12   28

OVARIAN HORMONES

Oestrogen

Progesterone

Day 1   12   28

VASCULAR CHANGES

Day 1   12   28

PROLIFERATIVE PHASE – Stimulated by oestrogen, the endometrium is reconstructed. Glands are straight and do not secrete.

SECRETORY PHASE – Stimulated mainly by progesterone, the endometrium is highly vascularized. Glands enlarge and become tortuous and secrete or store glycogen, mucin and other substances which can nourish a fertilized ovum. Blood vessels become more coiled.

PREMENSTRUAL (REGRESSIVE) PHASE – Endometrial growth ceases 5 – 6 days before menstruation. Before menstruation it shrinks due to decreased blood flow and discharge of secretion. This increases the tortuosity of glands and blood vessels.

OVULATION AND MENSTRUATION

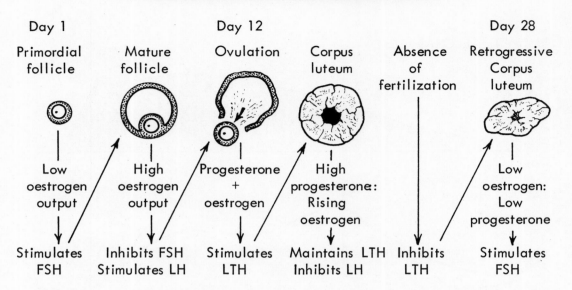

Day 1		Day 12			Day 28
Primordial follicle	Mature follicle	Ovulation	Corpus luteum	Absence of fertilization	Retrogressive Corpus luteum
Low oestrogen output	High oestrogen output	Progesterone + oestrogen	High progesterone: Rising oestrogen		Low oestrogen: Low progesterone
Stimulates FSH	Inhibits FSH Stimulates LH	Stimulates LTH	Maintains LTH Inhibits LH	Inhibits LTH	Stimulates FSH

The inverse relationship between ovarian and pituitary hormones indicates a two-way control system.   At the beginning of a cycle the ovary is inactive.   The consequent low blood level of oestrogen stimulates pituitary F.S.H. secretion.   This stimulates growth of ovarian follicles which secrete large quantities of oestrogen. The high blood oestrogen inhibits production of F.S.H. and initiates the next phase of L.H. production, resulting in ovulation and corpus luteum formation. Progesterone as well as oestrogen is produced by luteal cells.   Pituitary L.T.H. is stimulated to maintain the corpus luteum.   If the ovum is not fertilized L.T.H. is inhibited, the corpus luteum regresses, oestrogen and progesterone production falls, menstruation occurs and F.S.H. is stimulated to start the next cycle.

PITUITARY GONADOTROPHINS   OVARIAN HORMONES

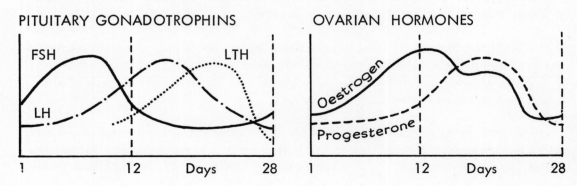

FERTILIZATION AND NIDATION

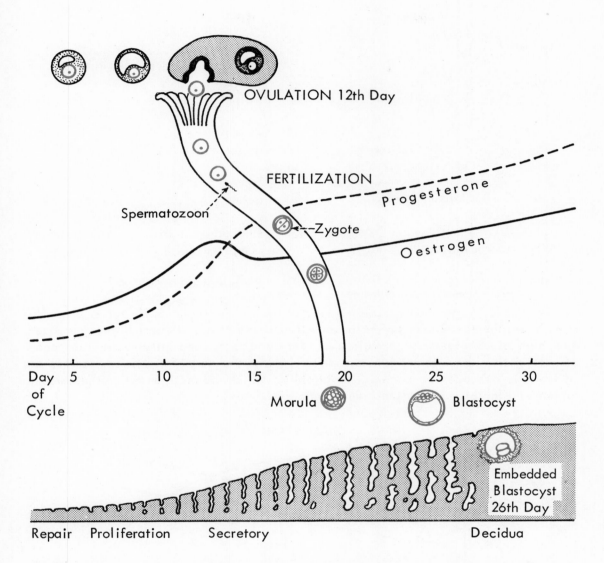

OVULATION 12th Day

FERTILIZATION

Progesterone

Spermatozoon

Zygote

Oestrogen

Day
of
Cycle

5   10   15   20   25   30

Morula   Blastocyst

Embedded
Blastocyst
26th Day

Repair   Proliferation   Secretory   Decidua

After fertilization in the fallopian tube the zygote (fertilized ovum) divides repeatedly to form a solid sphere of cells – the Morula. It reaches the uterine cavity by the 7th day after ovulation and is fully embedded by the 14th day after ovulation.

HORMONAL RELATIONSHIPS IN EARLY PREGNANCY

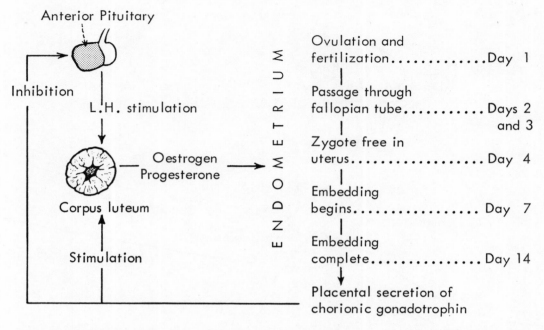

During the first 14 days of pregnancy the growth of the uterus and decidua (the endometrium of pregnancy) is maintained by the corpus luteum under the influence of hypophysial luteinizing hormone. After 14 days the primitive chorion secretes a luteinizing hormone (chorionic gonadotrophin) which assumes control of the corpus luteum and inhibits pituitary gonadotrophic activity.

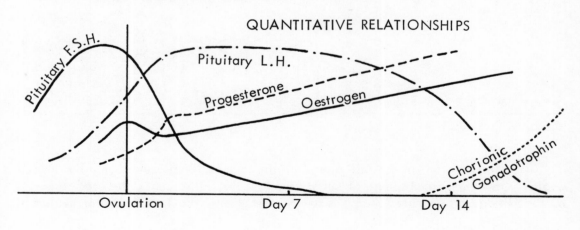

HORMONAL RELATIONSHIPS IN EARLY PREGNANCY

Under the influence of placental luteinizing hormone the corpus luteum continues to grow and secret steroids for the maintenance of uterine decidual growth. Chorionic gonadotrophin output reaches a peak around 10 – 12 weeks and then declines to an almost constant level until term. With this decline the corpus luteum activity fails but placental steroid production commences to replace it so that the output of oestrogens and progesterone rises steadily to term.

OVARIAN and PLACENTAL STEROID OUTPUT

	Progesterone/24 hr	Urinary Oestrogens/24 hr
Peak of Corpus Luteum phase	30 mg	30 ug
Placental phase 20 weeks	75 mg	4 – 5 mg
Placental phase 40 weeks	250 – 300 mg	More than 50 mg

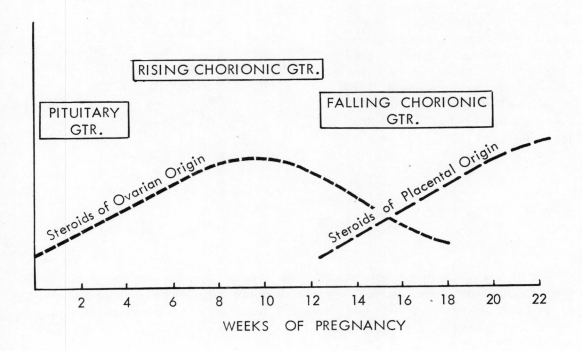

DEVELOPMENT OF THE EMBRYO

While still in the fallopian tube the fertilized ovum divides repeatedly to form a round mass of cells – the morula.

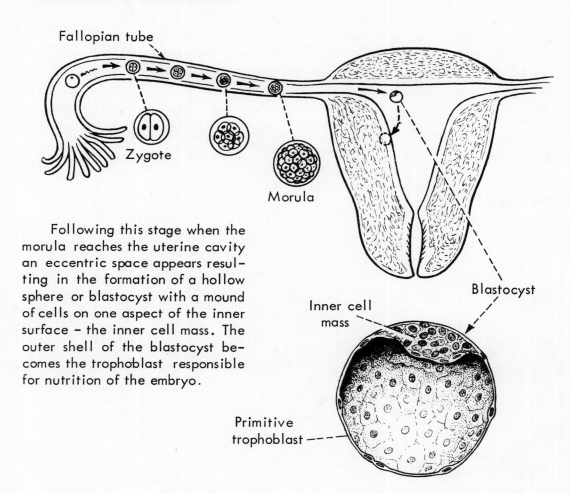

Fallopian tube

Zygote

Morula

Inner cell mass

Blastocyst

Primitive trophoblast

Following this stage when the morula reaches the uterine cavity an eccentric space appears resulting in the formation of a hollow sphere or blastocyst with a mound of cells on one aspect of the inner surface – the inner cell mass. The outer shell of the blastocyst becomes the trophoblast responsible for nutrition of the embryo.

Up to this point the secretions within the tube and uterus have been sufficient for the initial growth of the zygote. Further development demands an increased supply of food and oxygen, and the zygote must gain access to the maternal blood supply by embedding in the decidua.

DEVELOPMENT OF THE EMBRYO

The inner cell mass differentiates and forms two distinct masses, the outer or ectodermal layer and the inner or entodermal. A further differentiation produces a third layer, the mesoderm, between these two. This grows outwards and eventually lines the blastocyst. The combination of trophoblast and primitive mesoderm is termed the chorion.

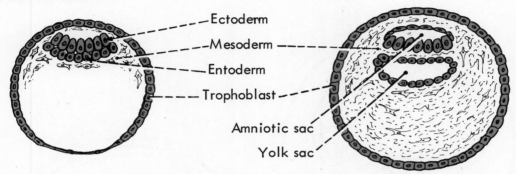

- Ectoderm
- Mesoderm
- Entoderm
- Trophoblast

Amniotic sac

Yolk sac

Two small cavities appear, one in the ectoderm forming the amniotic sac, the other in the entoderm – the yolk sac.

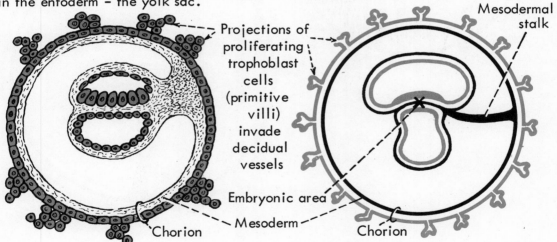

Projections of proliferating trophoblast cells (primitive villi) invade decidual vessels

Mesodermal stalk

Embryonic area

Mesoderm

Chorion

Chorion

The two small spheres, covered by mesoderm, move into the middle of the blastocyst cavity, the mesoderm forming the connecting stalk. The two opposing layers of ectoderm and entoderm together with the interposed mesoderm are destined to form the actual embryo. Expansion of the amniotic sac takes place.

DEVELOPMENT OF THE EMBRYO

Expansion of the amniotic cavity continues until the amnion reaches the wall of the blastocyst. At the same time it enfolds the yolk sac. Part of the yolk sac becomes enclosed within the embryo while the remainder forms a vestigial tube applied to the original mesodermal stalk.

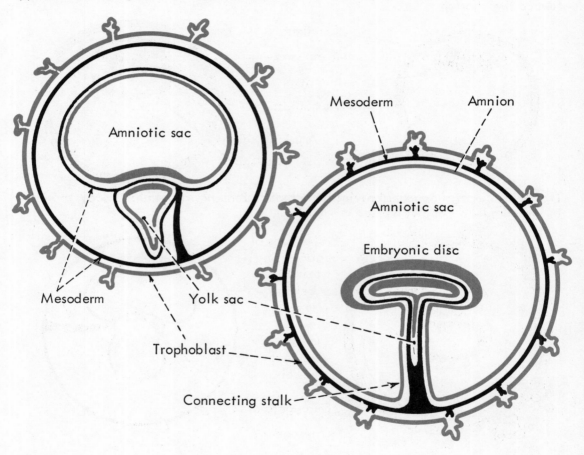

Blood vessels develop in the embryonic mesoderm and in the mesoderm of the trophoblast. Extension of these vessels along the connecting stalk result in the formation of the umbilical arteries and vein.

DEVELOPMENT OF THE EMBRYO

Within the embryo the vessels at the cephalic end differentiate to form the heart. Foetal blood formation occurs within the primitive blood vessels of the trophoblast and foetus. Interchange between mother and foetus is facilitated by the formation of this foeto-trophoblastic circulation. The formation and differentiation of the haemopoietic-vascular system occurs between the third and fourth week of pregnancy. From then on full development of the foetus can take place.

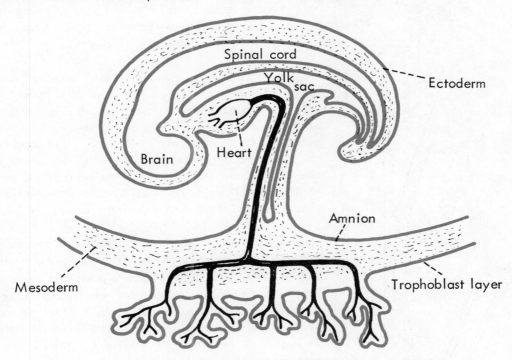

STRUCTURES DERIVED FROM PRIMARY LAYERS

ECTODERM   Skin and appendages, nervous system including medulla of adrenal, glands such as anterior pituitary and salivary.

ENTODERM   Gastro-intestinal tract, liver, gall bladder, biliary tract, pancreas, respiratory tract, germ cells of gonads.

MESODERM   Bone, muscle, cartilage, connective tissue, serous linings, cardio-vascular system, kidneys and most of genital tract.

DEVELOPMENT OF THE FOETUS—CIRCULATION

Head

Foramen ovale

D. arteriosus

S.V.C.

Arm

Aorta

Pulm. A.

L.A.

R.A.

Lung

Lung

L.V.

I.V.C.

R.V.

D. venosus

Liver

Viscera

Placenta

Umbilical vein

Umbilical arteries

Leg   Leg

Oxygenated blood from the placenta returns to the foetus via the umbilical vein. This vessel penetrates the liver and gives off small branches to that organ. Most of the blood is directed via the ductus venosus into the inferior vena cava which is carrying the returning non-oxygenated blood from the lower limbs, kidneys, liver etc.

The mixed oxygenated and reduced blood enters the right atrium. Much of this stream is directed via the foramen ovale into the left atrium and thence to the left ventricle and aorta. This blood which is relatively well oxygenated supplies the head and upper extremities. The remainder of the blood from the superior vena cava mixes with that of the inferior vena cava, passes to the right ventricle and thence to pulmonary artery. A very small amount of blood goes to the lungs. Most of it passes on via the ductus arteriosus into the aorta beyond the vessels supplying the head and upper extremities. Thereafter it passes down the aorta to supply the viscera and lower limbs. Little blood actually goes to the lower limbs. Most at this level passes into the umbilical arteries which arise as branches of the right and left internal iliac arteries.

At birth the umbilical vessels contract. Breathing helps to create a negative thoracic pressure thus sucking more blood from the pulmonary artery into the lungs and diverting it from the ductus arteriosus which gradually closes. The foramen ovale is a valvular opening, the valve functioning from right to left. The left auricular pressure rises and closes this valve.

DEVELOPMENT OF THE ORGANS—TIMETABLE

ORGAN	DIFFERENTIATION	COMPLETE FORMATION
Spinal cord	3 – 4 weeks	20 weeks
Brain	3	28
Eyes	3	20 – 24
Olfactory apparatus	4 – 5	8
Auditory apparatus	3 – 4	24 – 28
Respiratory system	5	24 – 28
Heart	3	6
Gastro–intestinal system	3	24
Liver	3 – 4	12
Renal system	4 – 5	12
Genital system	5	7
Face	3 – 4	8
Limbs	4 – 5	8

OSSIFICATION CENTRES

HEAD	Weeks
Mandible	7
Occipital bone	8 – 10
Maxilla	8
Temporal bone	9
Sphenoid bone	9 – 14
Nasal bone	10
Frontal bone	9 – 10
Bony labyrinth	17 – 20
Teeth	17 – 28
Hyoid bone	28 – 32

BODY	
Clavicle	7
Scapula	8 – 9
Ribs 5,6,7.	8 – 9
2,3,4; 8,9,10,11.	9
1 and 12.	10
Sternum	21 – 24

UPPER LIMB	Weeks
Humerus	8
Radius	8
Ulna	8
Phalanges	9 – 16
Metacarpals	9 – 12

LOWER LIMB	
Femur	9
Tibia	9
Fibula	9
Epiphysis around knee joint	35 – 40
Os calcis	21 – 29
Astragalus	24 – 32
Cuboid	40
Metatarsals	9 – 12
VERTEBRAE	9 – 12

PLACENTA—DEVELOPMENT

The primitive trophoblast erodes the surface of the decidua by enzyme action, destroys glands and stroma, and eventually penetrates the large maternal sinusoids which have formed. The blastocyst now lies in a pool of maternal blood fed by the maternal arterioles and drained by maternal veins. The trophoblast cells proliferate and form pseudopodial-like masses which branch repeatedly. This greatly increases the surface area and facilitates foeto-maternal exchange. The trophoblast anchors the blastocyst by adhering to the intervening decidual stroma.

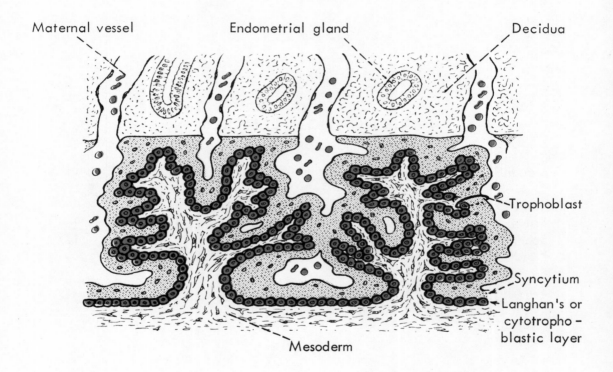

Maternal vessel   Endometrial gland   Decidua

Trophoblast

Syncytium

Langhan's or cytotropho- blastic layer

Mesoderm

The trophoblast differentiates into two layers. The outer or syncytiotrophoblast, in contact with the maternal blood, becomes a multi-nuclear syncytium with no distinct cell boundaries; the inner or cytotrophoblast, also called Langhan's layer, forms a single layer of cuboidal cells.

PLACENTA—DEVELOPMENT

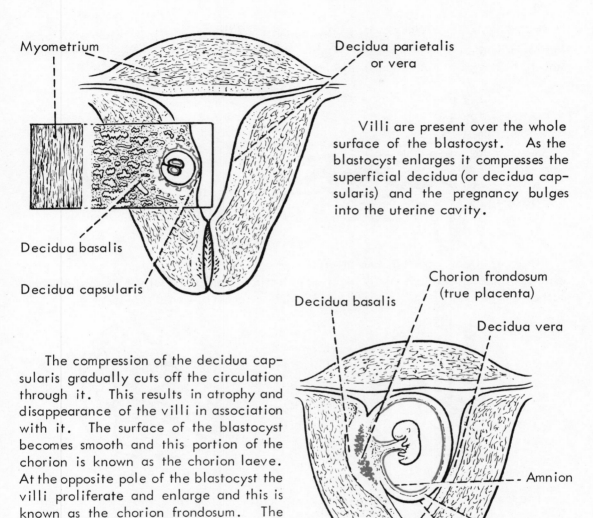

Myometrium

Decidua parietalis
or vera

Decidua basalis

Decidua capsularis

Villi are present over the whole
surface of the blastocyst. As the
blastocyst enlarges it compresses the
superficial decidua (or decidua capsularis) and the pregnancy bulges
into the uterine cavity.

The compression of the decidua capsularis gradually cuts off the circulation
through it. This results in atrophy and
disappearance of the villi in association
with it. The surface of the blastocyst
becomes smooth and this portion of the
chorion is known as the chorion laeve.
At the opposite pole of the blastocyst the
villi proliferate and enlarge and this is
known as the chorion frondosum. The
connecting stalk of the embryo is attached
to the wall of the blastocyst at this point.
Ultimately with the expansion of the
blastocyst the decidua capsularis comes
in contact with the decidua vera and the
uterine cavity is obliterated.

Decidua basalis

Chorion frondosum
(true placenta)

Decidua vera

Amnion

Chorion
laeve

Decidua
capsularis

15

PLACENTA—DEVELOPMENT OF CORD

The fully formed placenta is a disc, approximately one inch in thickness, tapering towards the edges. It weighs roughly 500g and is dark red, the colour being due mainly to the maternal blood in the intervillous spaces.

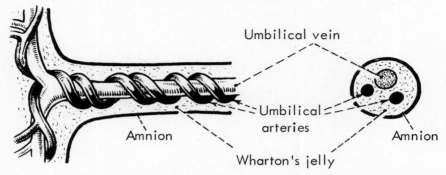

The umbilical cord has two arteries and one vein, embedded in Wharton's jelly which is a loose myxomatous tissue of mesodermal origin. This jelly acts as a physical buffer and prevents kinking of the cord and interference with circulation.

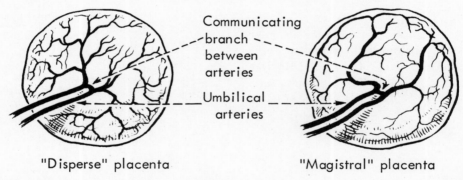

"Disperse" placenta   "Magistral" placenta

The umbilical vessels are generally attached to the placenta near its centre. They immediately divide repeatedly to form branches all over the surface. This is known as the "disperse" type of placenta. Occasionally the main vessels may extend almost to the margins of the placenta before dividing (although they give off small branches in their course). This is the "magistral" type of placenta.

There is a short communicating branch between the two umbilical arteries just as they reach the placental surface. This serves to equalise the pressure and flow to each half of the placenta.

PLACENTA—FUNCTIONS

The functions depend on the structure and health of the placental villi. These villi are bathed in maternal blood but there is no direct connection between foetal and maternal blood. There is a foetal (placental) barrier.

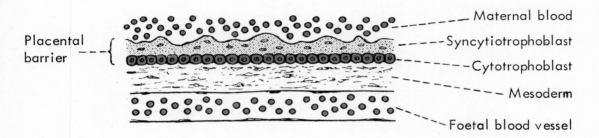

The functions of the placenta are:-

After 16 - 20 weeks the cytotrophoblast regresses. The syncytiotrophoblast is reduced in thickness as pregnancy advances; the foetal blood vessels of villi dilate and the mesoderm is reduced in amount. This reduces the physical barrier between foetal and maternal circulations.

Thickness of placental barrier:-

At 12 weeks.............0.025 mm.;   at term...........0.002 mm.

The functions of the placenta are:-

A. RESPIRATORY

The fall in pressure as the maternal blood enters the placenta and the resulting slow flow aid the foeto-maternal interchange. Maternal blood has a relatively high O_2 and a low CO_2 content. The passage of O_2 to the foetus and of CO_2 to the mother is thus made easy. In addition it is thought that foetal haemoglobin is able to take up O_2 even when the concentration of maternal O_2 is low.

B. EXCRETORY

Little is known of the excretory mechanisms across the placenta. Urea is present in the same concentration in both foetal and maternal bloods.

C. NUTRITIONAL

Active transport mechanisms exist in the placenta to aid the exchange of substances between mother and foetus. For instance, naturally occurring amino acids which are laevo-rotatory are transported across the placental barrier more quickly than synthetic dextro-rotatory forms.

PLACENTA—FUNCTIONS

D. ENDOCRINE

The placenta produces:-
1. Oestrogens
2. Progesterone
3. Chorionic gonadotrophin
4. Growth hormone-like substance
5. Cortico-steroids
6. ? Post-pituitary-like substance

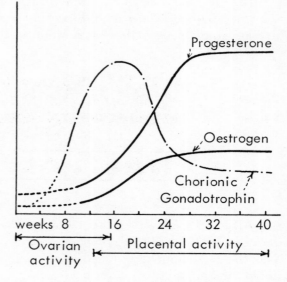

Oestrogens and progesterone are produced mainly by the ovary during the first 12 weeks of pregnancy. During this time chorionic gonadotrophin is secreted by the placenta in large quantities to maintain the corpus luteum. Thereafter the placenta gradually takes over the production of oestrogens and progesterone, the corpus luteum regresses and the secretion of chorionic gonadotrophin is greatly reduced.

Oestrogens and progesterone maintain the growth of the uterus and control its activity during pregnancy. They also are responsible for changes in the maternal body such as growth of the breasts.

Growth hormone-like substances have been isolated from the placenta. The exact function of these is not yet known but they do modify maternal metabolism in such a way as to favour growth of the foetus.

Similarly cortico-steroids are greatly increased in pregnancy and some are produced by the placenta. They also are involved in alterations of maternal metabolism.

A substance resembling posterior pituitary hormone is said to be formed by the placenta but this is still a matter of controversy.

DEVELOPMENT OF MEMBRANES

The membranes are derived from that part of the trophoblast which atrophies as the blastocyst expands – the chorion laeve – plus the amnion.

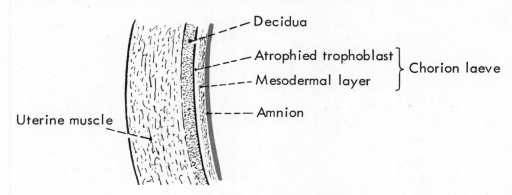

The amnion is easily stripped from the chorion and this helps to distinguish dizygotic (binovular) from monozygotic (monovular) twins.

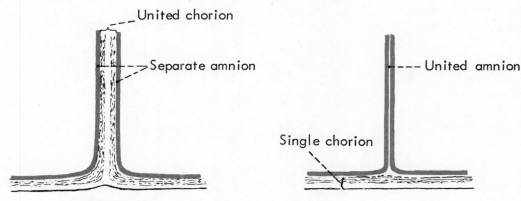

BINOVULAR
(or MONOVULAR DICHORIONIC)

If the membranes are in three distinct layers over the surface in apposition, the twins may be either monovular or binovular.

MONOVULAR

When the membranes in apposition consist only of two layers – the two amnions – the twins are definitely monovular.

CHAPTER 2

MATERNAL PHYSIOLOGY

WEIGHT INCREASE

WEIGHT

There is an increase in weight during pregnancy equivalent to 25 per cent of non-pregnant weight: approximately 28 lb. (12.5 kg) in the average case.

The main increase occurs in the second half of pregnancy. It should not exceed 5 lb. (2.25 kg) per month or 2 lb. (0.9 kg) in any one week and should not be less than $\frac{1}{2}$ lb. (0.22 kg) per week.

The increase is due to growth of the conceptus, enlargement of maternal organs, maternal storage of fat and protein and increase in the maternal blood volume and interstitial fluid.

DISTRIBUTION of WEIGHT INCREASE

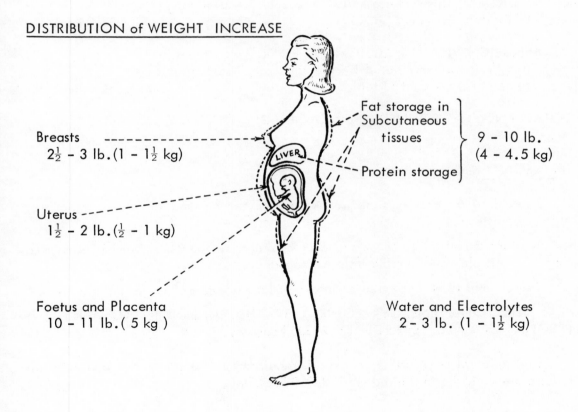

Breasts
$2\frac{1}{2}$ – 3 lb.(1 – $1\frac{1}{2}$ kg)

Fat storage in
Subcutaneous
tissues   9 – 10 lb.
(4 – 4.5 kg)
Protein storage

Uterus
$1\frac{1}{2}$ – 2 lb.($\frac{1}{2}$ – 1 kg)

Foetus and Placenta
10 – 11 lb.(5 kg)

Water and Electrolytes
2 – 3 lb. (1 – $1\frac{1}{2}$ kg)

METABOLISM

The demands for energy derive from:-

A. **BASIC PHYSIOLOGICAL PROCESSES.** Respiration, circulation, digestion, secretion, maintenance of body temperature, growth and repair. These account for 66 per cent of total energy requirements in the non-pregnant female.. 1,440 kcal/day

B. **EVERYDAY ACTIVITIES.** Walking, maintaining posture, speech, other movements - e.g. eating. Equivalent to 17 per cent of total in non-pregnant state .... 360 kcal/day

C. **WORK.** This varies greatly. Probably 7 - 10 per cent of total .... 150 - 200 kcal/day

D. **SPECIFIC DYNAMIC ACTION OF FOOD.** Metabolism appears to be stimulated by the taking of food. In the region of 7 per cent of total .... 144 kcal/day

TOTAL ENERGY REQUIRED IN NON-PREGNANT STATE ... 2,100 kcal/day

IN PREGNANCY

There is a marked increase in "A" due to the demands of foetus, placenta, uterus, breasts etc.

A slight reduction in "B" may occur as pregnancy advances, and it is assumed that "C" will play only a minor role in pregnancy.

There ought to be an increased intake of food and therefore an increase in "D".

THE TOTAL ENERGY REQUIRED BY THE PATIENT IN ADVANCED PREGNANCY WILL BE AROUND 2,500 kcal/day.

During lactation a further increase is required for milk production and the total requirements will be in the region of 3,000 kcal/day.

24

METABOLISM

The total METABOLISM is increased in pregnancy due largely to the foetus.

Oxygen consumption is raised by 20 per cent.

Despite this the rate, expressed as kilocalories per square metre per hour, is only slightly above the non-pregnant level.

To maintain the increased total metabolism there is an increased activity in control mechanisms.

The anterior pituitary probably secretes more thyroid stimulating hormone.

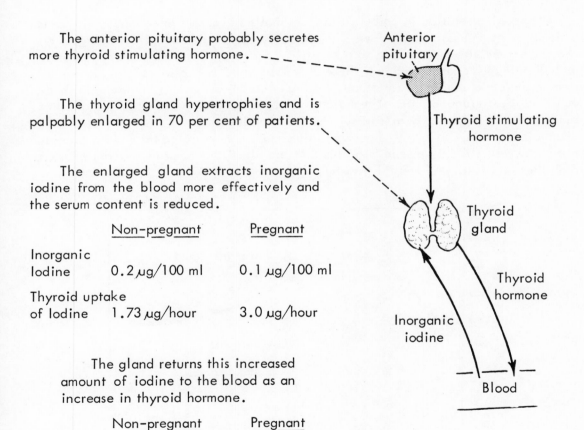

The thyroid gland hypertrophies and is palpably enlarged in 70 per cent of patients.

The enlarged gland extracts inorganic iodine from the blood more effectively and the serum content is reduced.

	Non-pregnant	Pregnant
Inorganic Iodine	0.2 µg/100 ml	0.1 µg/100 ml
Thyroid uptake of Iodine	1.73 µg/hour	3.0 µg/hour

The gland returns this increased amount of iodine to the blood as an increase in thyroid hormone.

	Non-pregnant	Pregnant
Protein bound Iodine	5 µg/100 ml	8 - 10 µg/100 ml

CARBOHYDRATE METABOLISM

In the non-pregnant state ingested glucose is dealt with in four ways. Under the influence of insulin it may be deposited in the liver as glycogen. Some escapes into the general circulation and a proportion of this is metabolised directly by the tissues: some is converted to depot fat and a further portion is stored as muscle glycogen again with the aid of insulin.

The blood sugar is maintained between 80 – 100 mg/100ml. Sugar which passes out in the renal glomerular filtrate is never in excess of the amount which can be reabsorbed by the tubules, and none appears in the urine.

A marked alteration in carbohydrate metabolism occurs in pregnancy. There is a demand on the part of the foetus for an easily convertible source of energy. At the same time there is a need to store energy for future demands such as lactation and the steadily increasing growth of the pregnancy and also to provide a more steady source of energy in the form of a high energy fuel. This the maternal body achieves by storage of fat. The major portion of the diet is carbohydrate and this requires to be redirected to satisfy the above requirements. The first noticeable change occurs in the blood sugar and this can be demonstrated by an oral glucose tolerance test. It can be seen from this that the blood sugar, after a meal, remains high thus facilitating placental transfer.

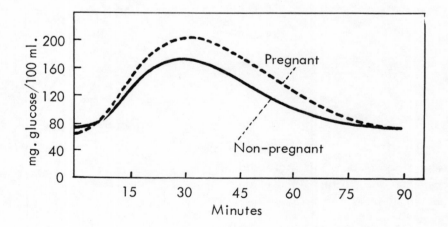

The mechanism governing the changes is not clearly understood but may be as in the following diagram....

CARBOHYDRATE METABOLISM

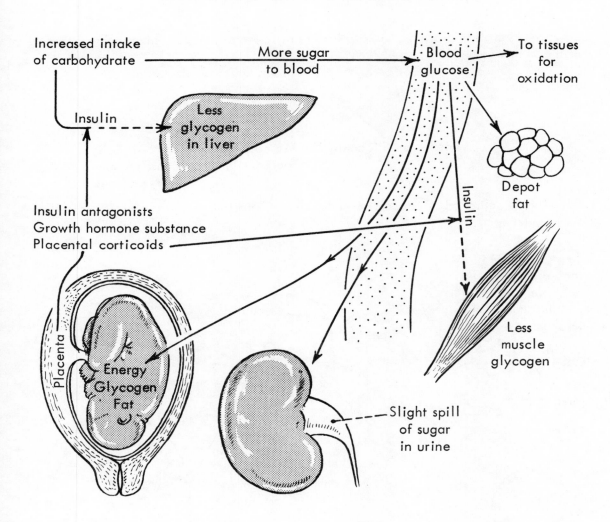

Increased intake of carbohydrate

More sugar to blood

Blood glucose

To tissues for oxidation

Insulin

Less glycogen in liver

Insulin antagonists
Growth hormone substance
Placental corticoids

Depot fat

Insulin

Placenta

Energy
Glycogen
Fat

Less muscle glycogen

Slight spill of sugar in urine

In pregnancy an antagonist to insulin is present. This may be the increased corticoids and growth hormone produced by the placenta. Less glycogen is deposited in the maternal liver and muscles. More sugar circulates for a longer time in the maternal blood. The placenta is able to pass more to the foetus. At the same time rather more passes the glomerulus than can be reabsorbed by the renal tubule and a small amount appears in the urine of most pregnant women.

PROTEIN METABOLISM

The overall picture is one of positive nitrogen balance. This reaches its peak at the 28th week.

By the end of pregnancy 500 grams have been retained.

50%   50%

Foetus and Placenta   Maternal gain (breasts, uterus, increase in blood constituents, N_2 storage)

This is achieved by a complicated series of interlocking mechanisms, not all of them understood.

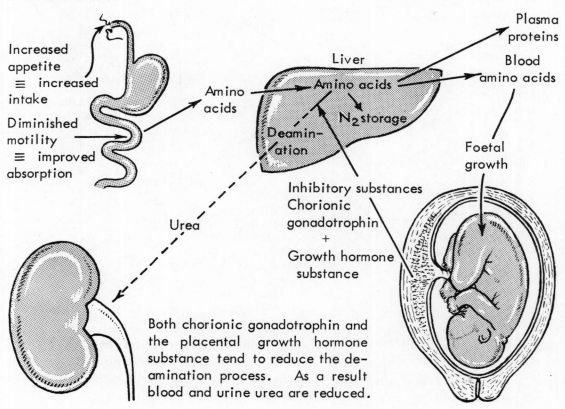

Increased appetite ≡ increased intake

Diminished motility ≡ improved absorption

Amino acids

Urea

Liver

Amino acids

Deamin-ation

N_2 storage

Plasma proteins

Blood amino acids

Foetal growth

Inhibitory substances
Chorionic gonadotrophin
+
Growth hormone substance

Both chorionic gonadotrophin and the placental growth hormone substance tend to reduce the de-amination process. As a result blood and urine urea are reduced.

PROTEIN METABOLISM

The concentration values are altered by haemodilution thus masking the fact that the total amounts are increased in most instances. In the case of urea however the reduction in concentration is greater than can be explained by haemodilution.

	Non-pregnant	Pregnant
Blood amino acid nitrogen	5.0 mg/100 ml.	3.4 – 5.0 mg/100 ml.
Plasma proteins	8.1 g /100 ml.	7.5 g /100 ml.
Albumin/globulin ratio	1.32:1	0.84:1
Blood urea	20 – 40 mg/100 ml.	10 – 12 mg/100 ml.
Non protein nitrogen	32.0 mg/100 ml.	28.0 mg/100 ml.
Uric acid	3.0 mg/100 ml.	3.0 mg/100 ml.
Creatinine	1 – 2 mg/100 ml.	1 – 2 mg/100 ml.

Changes occur in the concentration of several of the plasma proteins, particularly albumin, β-globulin and fibrinogen.

	Non-pregnant (grams)	Pregnant (grams)
Albumin	4.25	3.25
β-globulin	1.0	1.3
Fibrinogen	0.35	0.56

The significance of these changes is unknown.

URINARY NITROGEN	Non-pregnant (grams)	Pregnant (grams)
Total nitrogen/24 hours.	12 – 16	8 – 12
Urea as percentage of total N_2.	80 – 90	70 – 85
Ammonia N_2 as percentage of total.	2.5 – 4.5	3 – 5

FAT METABOLISM

Fat would appear to be the main form of maternal stored energy during pregnancy. By 30 weeks some 4 kg are stored. Little is stored thereafter. Most of this is in the form of depot fat, in the abdominal wall, back and thighs, and perhaps retroperitoneally. Despite the enlargement only some 12 - 20 g are deposited in the breasts.

Blood Fat increases from 3rd month

	Total lipoid	Cholesterol
Non-pregnant	700 mg/100 ml	120 mg/100 ml
Pregnant at term	1,050 mg/100 ml	280 mg/100 ml

The high blood levels and increased deposition are due partly to increased intake and partly to increased conversion of glucose to fat.

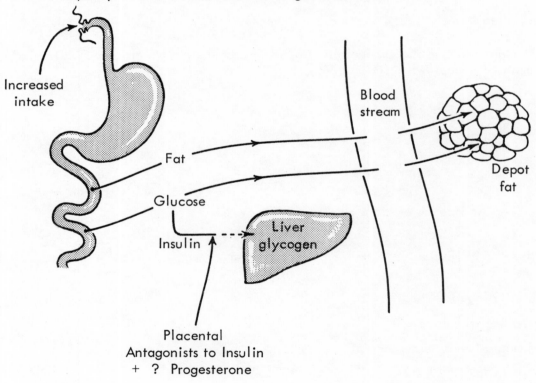

FAT METABOLISM

Three facts have to be related:-

1. The total metabolism and demand for energy is increased in pregnancy.
2. Glycogen stores are diminished and therefore energy obtained directly from carbohydrate will be reduced.
3. Although blood fat is greatly increased only a moderate amount is laid down in fat stores.

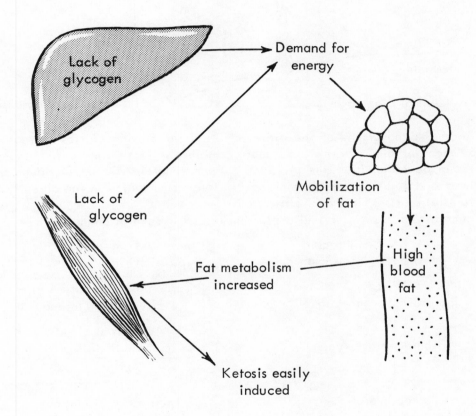

It is well recognised that the pregnant patient easily becomes ketotic whenever any strain, such as labour, is imposed. This is probably directly related to the poor glycogen stores.

RESPIRATORY CHANGES

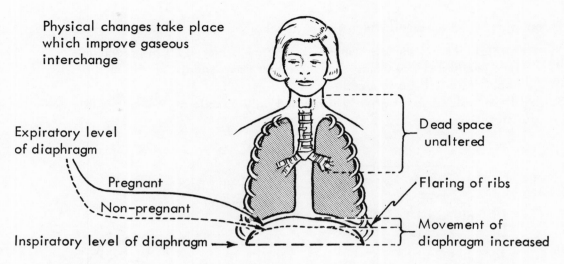

Physical changes take place which improve gaseous interchange

Dead space unaltered

Flaring of ribs

Movement of diaphragm increased

Expiratory level of diaphragm

Pregnant

Non-pregnant

Inspiratory level of diaphragm →

The increased movement of the diaphragm and the flaring of ribs increase the tidal movement of air. Expiration is more complete so that an increased volume of fresh air can be taken in. This increase is approximately 200 ml. The dead space is unaltered and this increase in moving air is accommodated in the alveoli. The minute ventilation rises from 7.25 litres to 10.5 litres.

The increase in inspiration and expiration results in several changes:-

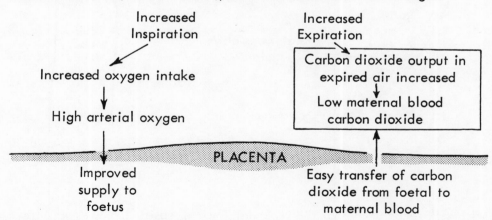

Increased Inspiration

Increased Expiration

Increased oxygen intake

Carbon dioxide output in expired air increased

High arterial oxygen

Low maternal blood carbon dioxide

PLACENTA

Improved supply to foetus

Easy transfer of carbon dioxide from foetal to maternal blood

The diaphragmatic excursion is reduced in late pregnancy and the increased respiratory exchange is maintained by thoracic movement.

RESPIRATORY CHANGES

Foetal plasma carbon dioxide tension exceeds that of maternal plasma by 4–8mm mercury. Therefore it passes easily into the maternal blood. Despite this, due to the pulmonary hyperventilation, the concentration of carbon dioxide in maternal plasma is 6 – 10% less than that of the non-pregnant female.

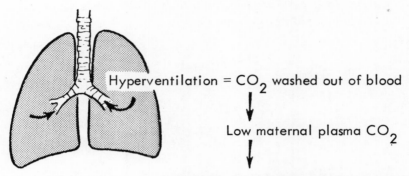

Hyperventilation = CO_2 washed out of blood

↓

Low maternal plasma CO_2

↓

Relatively diminished requirement for circulating cations

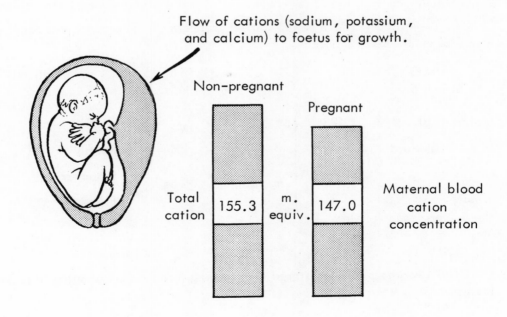

Flow of cations (sodium, potassium, and calcium) to foetus for growth.

Non-pregnant

Pregnant

Total cation   155.3   m. equiv.   147.0   Maternal blood cation concentration

CATION CHANGES

The diminution in maternal circulating cation is only relative, that is, in concentration. The total circulating cation is raised.

SODIUM

850 m-equivalents are retained during pregnancy. This is divided in almost equal proportions between mother and conceptus.

MOTHER		850 m-equiv		CONCEPTUS	
	m-equiv				m-equiv
Maternal blood . . .	145				
Interstitial fluid. . .	155	413 m-equiv	437 m-equiv	Foetus	280
Uterus.	78			Liquor amnii . . .	100
Breasts.	35			Placenta.	57

POTASSIUM

316 m-equivalents are stored during pregnancy. The conceptus receives almost twice as much as the mother.

MOTHER		316 m-equiv		CONCEPTUS	
	m-equiv				m-equiv
Maternal blood . . .	28				
Interstitial fluid . . .	5	117 m-equiv	199 m-equiv	Foetus	154
Uterus	49			Liquor amnii. . .	42
Breasts.	35			Placenta	3

CALCIUM

29.5 m-equivalents are stored late in pregnancy. Almost all of this goes to the foetus.

CARDIOVASCULAR SYSTEM

Marked demands are made on this system, mainly as a result of the growth of the conceptus and the increase in metabolism.

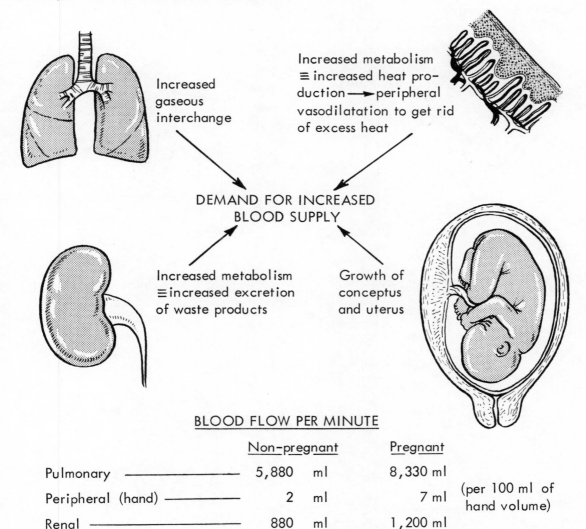

Increased gaseous interchange

Increased metabolism ≡ increased heat production ⟶ peripheral vasodilatation to get rid of excess heat

DEMAND FOR INCREASED BLOOD SUPPLY

Increased metabolism ≡ increased excretion of waste products

Growth of conceptus and uterus

BLOOD FLOW PER MINUTE

	Non-pregnant		Pregnant	
Pulmonary	5,880	ml	8,330	ml
Peripheral (hand)	2	ml	7	ml
Renal	880	ml	1,200	ml
Uterine	51.7	ml	185	ml

(per 100 ml of hand volume)

CARDIOVASCULAR SYSTEM

The demand for an increased blood supply to many parts of the body is met by an increase in blood volume. The mechanism whereby this is achieved is not understood but may be as follows:-

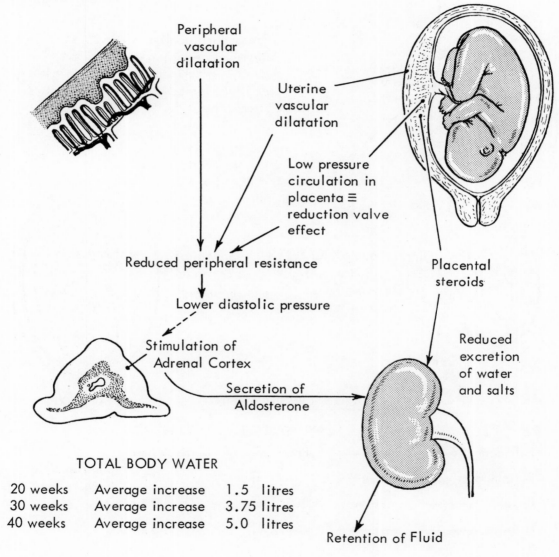

Peripheral vascular dilatation

Uterine vascular dilatation

Low pressure circulation in placenta ≡ reduction valve effect

Reduced peripheral resistance

Lower diastolic pressure

Placental steroids

Stimulation of Adrenal Cortex

Secretion of Aldosterone

Reduced excretion of water and salts

Retention of Fluid

TOTAL BODY WATER

20 weeks	Average increase	1.5	litres
30 weeks	Average increase	3.75	litres
40 weeks	Average increase	5.0	litres

BLOOD VOLUME CHANGES

In non-pregnant individuals water ≡ 72% body weight. Of this 5% is intra-vascular, intracellular fluid makes up 70% and interstitial fluid accounts for the remaining 25%.

In pregnancy, intracellular water appears to be unchanged but both blood and interstitial fluid are increased.

The plasma volume starts to increase early in pregnancy and reaches a peak around the 32nd week. Thereafter it is maintained until towards term when a slight fall occurs. The increase varies from individual to individual but is most marked in multigravid patients.

      Average non-pregnant volume = 2,600 ml.

      Peak volume in primigravida   = 3,850 ml = 41% increase.

      Peak volume in multigravida   = 4,100 ml = 57% increase.

As would be expected this increase in plasma volume entails adjustments and changes in many organs and systems in the body. The most apparent alterations are to be found in the blood itself and in the heart. Some of these changes are relative, others are absolute.

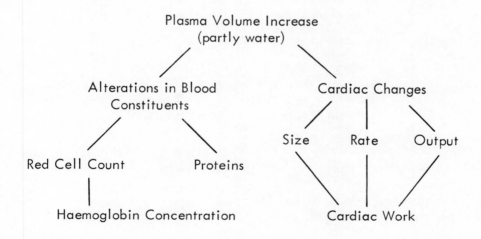

CARDIAC CHANGES

Most changes tend to increase the demands made on the heart and therefore increase the work-load.

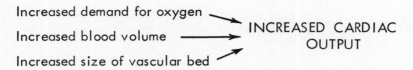

Increased demand for oxygen

Increased blood volume → INCREASED CARDIAC OUTPUT

Increased size of vascular bed

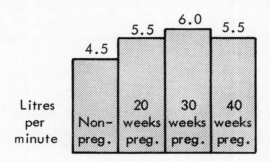

This increase in output is brought about <u>partly</u> by a rise in heart rate

	Heart Rate
Non-pregnant	70/min
20 weeks pregnant	78/min
Late pregnancy	85/min

and <u>partly</u> by an increased stroke volume.

Non-pregnant	64 ml.
20 weeks pregnant	70 ml.
30 weeks pregnant	70 ml.
40 weeks pregnant	64 ml.

The heart is enlarged, partly due to dilatation and partly to hypertrophy. Its volume increases from an average of 670 ml. to 750 ml.

The increase in work-load is modified by changes in the composition of the blood and peripheral vascular dilatation.

CARDIAC CHANGES

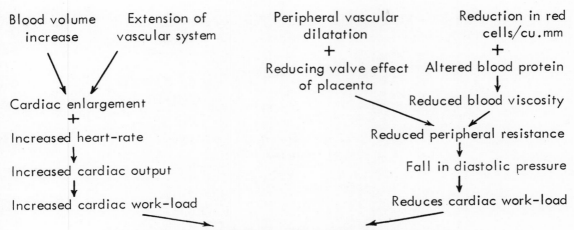

Blood volume increase / Extension of vascular system

↓ ↓

Cardiac enlargement
+
Increased heart-rate
↓
Increased cardiac output
↓
Increased cardiac work-load

Peripheral vascular dilatation
+
Reducing valve effect of placenta

Reduction in red cells/cu.mm
+
Altered blood protein
↓
Reduced blood viscosity

Reduced peripheral resistance
↓
Fall in diastolic pressure
↓
Reduces cardiac work-load

Total Cardiac work-load only moderately increased.

LOCAL VASCULAR CHANGES.   Apart from increased blood supply already mentioned local changes are most apparent in the lower limbs and are due to the pressure exerted by the enlarging uterus on the pelvic veins. Since one third of the total circulating blood is distributed to the lower limbs the increased venous pressure may produce striking effects which can be exaggerated by posture.

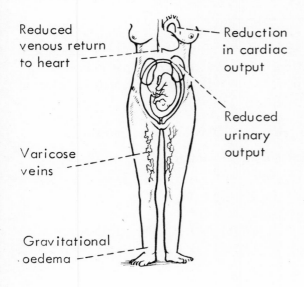

Reduced venous return to heart

Reduction in cardiac output

Reduced urinary output

Varicose veins

Gravitational oedema

These changes are most marked during daytime due to upright posture. They tend to be reversed at night when the patient retires to bed, oedema fluid is resorbed, venous return increases and renal output rises, resulting in nocturnal frequency. If the patient adopts the supine position however, the uterine pressure on the veins increases and there is no reversal of the changes.   In a few cases the supine position has such an influence that the venous return is grossly retarded, hypotension may ensue and the patient may black-out.

BLOOD VALUES

The change in blood values such as haemoglobin content is the result of demands of the growing pregnancy modified by the increase in plasma volume.

Increase in total metabolism

↓

Increase in total oxygen consumption

↓

Demand for increase in total oxygen-carrying capacity of blood

↓

Increase in total red cell volume

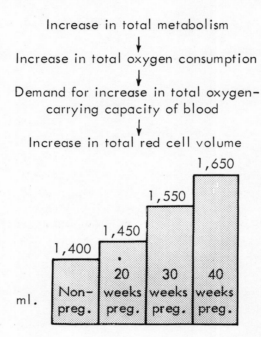

This represents a maximum increase of 18 per cent. The plasma volume increases by 40 – 50 per cent. Thus there is a reduction in the red cell count per cubic millimetre from 4.5 million to around 3.8 million. Towards term as the plasma volume diminishes the red cell count rises slightly.

Similarly the haematocrit falls during pregnancy with a slight rise at term.

	Haematocrit Reading (per cent)
Non-pregnant	40 – 42
20 weeks pregnant	39
30 weeks pregnant	38
40 weeks pregnant	40

BLOOD VALUES

Changes in haemoglobin run parallel with those in red cells. The mean cell haemoglobin concentration in the non-pregnant = 34 per cent, that is each 100 ml. of red cells contain 34 g haemoglobin. This does not alter in pregnancy, therefore, as with the total red cell volume, the total haemoglobin rises throughout pregnancy.

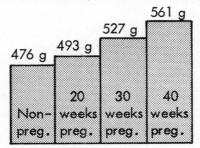

This is a total increase of 85 g, equivalent to 18 per cent.

The increasing plasma volume, however, produces an apparent reduction in haemoglobin. The haemoglobin concentration falls throughout pregnancy until the last four weeks when there may be a slight rise. The fall is apparent by the 12th week and the minimum value is reached at 32 weeks.

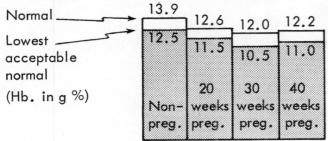

It will be seen from this that no single value can be taken as normal throughout pregnancy. This is important in diagnosing anaemia. At 30 weeks a haemoglobin reading of 10.5 is normal but the same reading at 20 weeks indicates anaemia.

<u>LEUCOCYTES</u>   There is a marked increase in these cells during pregnancy from 7,000 per cu.mm in the non-pregnant to 10,500 per cu.mm in late pregnancy. The increase is due almost entirely to neutrophil polymorphonuclears.

<u>BLOOD PLATELETS</u>   Increase continuously during pregnancy and in the puerperium.

(Counts/cu.mm)   Non-preg. 187,000;   20 weeks preg. 250,000;
30 weeks preg. 275,000;   40 weeks preg. 316,000;   Puerperium 600,000.

This may be related to the need to prevent haemorrhage but the mechanism is obscure.

BLOOD VALUES

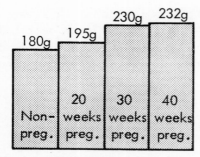

| 180g | 195g | 230g | 232g |
| Non-preg. | 20 weeks preg. | 30 weeks preg. | 40 weeks preg. |

The total plasma proteins increase as pregnancy advances.

| 7.25g | 5.75g | 5.75g | 5.8g |
| Non-preg. | 20 weeks preg. | 30 weeks preg. | 40 weeks preg. |

Due to increase in plasma volume the concentration of protein diminishes.

(Proteins are usually estimated in serum, fibrinogen being considered separately.)

The changes in protein are much more complex, involving the individual protein fractions. Albumin concentration falls steeply and the fall is proportionately greater than that of total protein. Total globulin shows a considerable increase in concentration, due mainly to increases in α and β globulins. As a result the albumin/globulin ratio falls from the non-pregnant value of 1.32 to 0.84 in late pregnancy. The reason for these changes is not known. Globulins act as transport mechanisms for many substances in the blood such as hormones and iron. Cortisol, oestrogens, progesterone, aldosterone and other steroids are greatly increased in pregnancy, so also is the transport of iron. This may account for some of the protein changes.

FIBRINOGEN

This protein shows a steady rise in concentration throughout pregnancy. From a non-pregnant level of 0.26 g per 100 ml. to 0.4 g per 100 ml., equivalent to more than 100 per cent increase in total circulating fibrinogen.

Together with the increase in platelets this could, in one sense, be regarded as a protection against haemorrhage.

One of the results of the increase in fibrinogen and globulins is an increased tendency to clumping of red cells. As a consequence the erythrocyte sedimentation rate in pregnancy is greatly increased, and this estimation is of little or no value in the diagnosis of disease.

GASTRO-INTESTINAL TRACT

Changes in the gastro-intestinal tract appear to be of minor degree but may have a marked cumulative effect in some cases. The main change is one of decreased motility which may be due to the effect of increased circulating steroid.

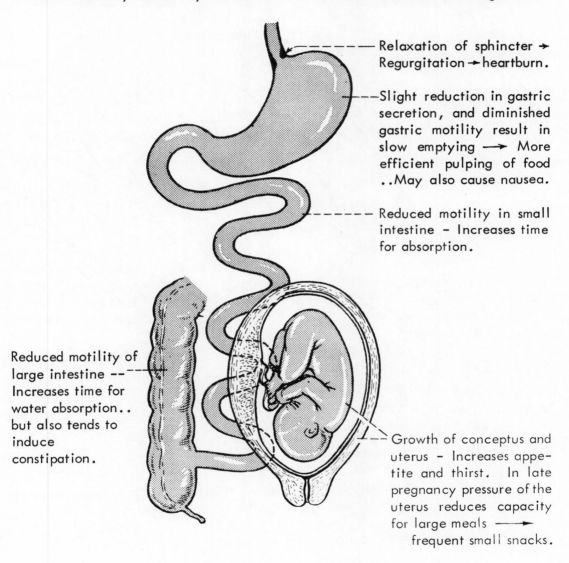

Relaxation of sphincter → Regurgitation → heartburn.

Slight reduction in gastric secretion, and diminished gastric motility result in slow emptying → More efficient pulping of food ..May also cause nausea.

Reduced motility in small intestine – Increases time for absorption.

Reduced motility of large intestine – Increases time for water absorption.. but also tends to induce constipation.

Growth of conceptus and uterus – Increases appetite and thirst. In late pregnancy pressure of the uterus reduces capacity for large meals → frequent small snacks.

RENAL SYSTEM

Frequency of micturition is a common symptom in early pregnancy and again at term. This is due to changes in pelvic anatomy and is a 'normal' feature of pregnancy.

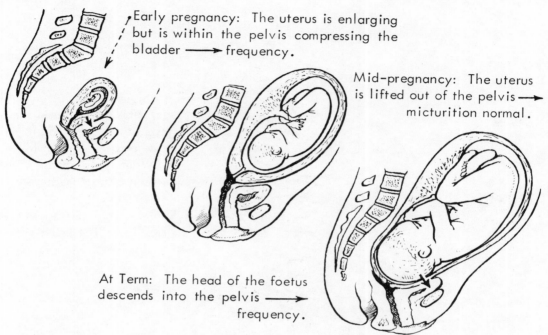

Early pregnancy: The uterus is enlarging but is within the pelvis compressing the bladder ⟶ frequency.

Mid-pregnancy: The uterus is lifted out of the pelvis ⟶ micturition normal.

At Term: The head of the foetus descends into the pelvis ⟶ frequency.

Other anatomical changes occur which may be due to the influence of hormones, possibly progesterone. There is a general loss of tone in smooth muscle. This affects the bladder and ureters.

The ureters are said to dilate greatly and again urine may stagnate.

Relaxation of bladder may result in incomplete emptying and collection of residual urine.

Both of these tend to favour the onset of urinary infection.

RENAL SYSTEM

Urinary output on a normal fluid intake tends to be slightly diminished. This seems paradoxical in view of the increased flow of blood to the kidneys.

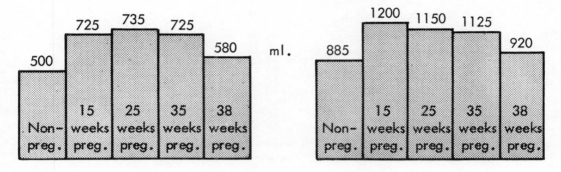

Renal plasma flow per minute is greatly increased.

Total renal blood flow runs almost parallel with plasma flow but with increasing haemodilution the red cell volume/100 ml. decreases and this alters the figures.

As a result the amount of fluid filtered off the plasma through the renal glomeruli is similarly increased and 100 extra litres of fluid pass into the renal tubules each day. Despite this the urinary output is diminished. Obviously there must be an increased tubular reabsorption. It is estimated that extracellular water is increased by 6 to 7 litres during pregnancy. Along with this water sodium and other electrolytes are reabsorbed by the tubules to maintain body osmolarity. Under test the pregnant patient only excretes 80 per cent of the total found in the urine of non-pregnant subjects.

The mechanism whereby this is achieved is not yet known, but it is thought that the increased amounts of aldosterone, progesterone and oestrogen are responsible.

Owing to the lag type of blood sugar curve following ingestion of carbohydrate, and the production of lactose, glycosuria of mild degree occurs in 35 - 50 per cent of all pregnant women. It is a normal feature, but in some cases it may make the diagnosis of diabetes mellitus difficult.

ENDOCRINE SYSTEM

Knowledge of endocrine changes during pregnancy is scant but the following is a summary of such knowledge regarding steroid substances and their supposed activity.

PROGESTERONE is produced by the corpus luteum in the first few weeks of pregnancy. Thereafter it is derived from the placenta. Output reaches a maximum of at least 250 mg per day. <u>Possible actions:-</u>

1. Reduces smooth muscle tone. Stomach motility diminishes—may induce nausea. Colonic activity reduced — delayed emptying — increased water reabsorption — constipation. Reduced uterine tone — diminished uterine activity. Reduced bladder and ureteric tone — stasis of urine.
2. Reduces vascular tone — diastolic pressure reduced. Venous dilatation.
3. Raises temperature.   4. Increases fat storage.
5. Induces over-breathing — alveolar and arterial carbon dioxide tension reduced.
6. Induces development of breasts.

OESTROGENS.   In early pregnancy the source is the ovary. Later oestrone and oestradiol are probably produced by the placenta and are increased a hundredfold. Oestriol, however, is a product resulting from the interaction of the placenta and the foetal adrenals and is increased one thousandfold. The output of oestrogens reaches a maximum of at least 30 – 40 mg per day. Oestriol accounts for 85 per cent of this total. <u>Possible actions:-</u>

1. Induce growth of uterus and control its function.
2. Responsible, together with progesterone, for the development of the breasts.
3. Alter the chemical constitution of connective tissue, making it more pliable — stretching of cervix possible, joint capsules relax, pelvic joints mobile.
4. Cause water retention.   5. May reduce sodium excretion.

CORTISOL. The maternal adrenals are the sole source in early pregnancy but later considerable quantities are thought to be produced by the placenta. Some 25 mg are produced each day. Much of this is protein bound and therefore may not be generally active. <u>Possible actions:-</u>

1. Increases blood sugar.   2. Modifies antibody activity.

ALDOSTERONE is almost certainly wholly derived from the maternal adrenals. The amounts produced during pregnancy are much increased. It is probably related to the retention of sodium and water.

CHAPTER 3

OBSTETRICAL ANATOMY

VULVA

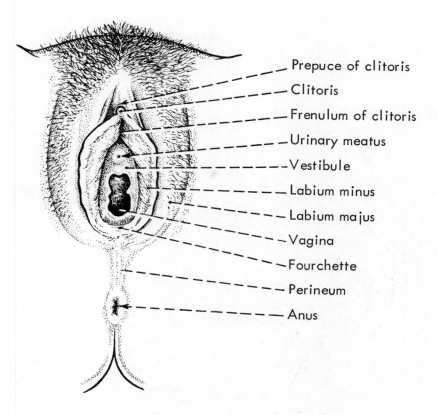

Prepuce of clitoris
Clitoris
Frenulum of clitoris
Urinary meatus
Vestibule
Labium minus
Labium majus
Vagina
Fourchette
Perineum
Anus

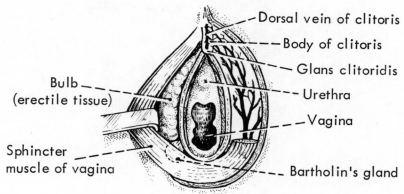

Dorsal vein of clitoris
Body of clitoris
Glans clitoridis
Urethra
Vagina
Bartholin's gland

Bulb
(erectile tissue)

Sphincter
muscle of vagina

PELVIC ORGANS

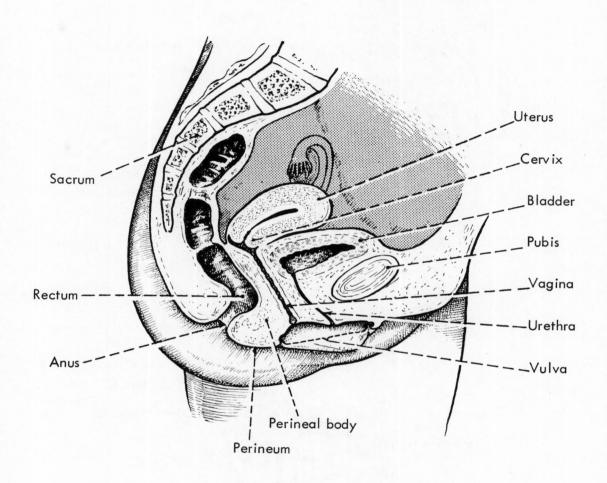

Uterus

Cervix

Bladder

Pubis

Vagina

Urethra

Vulva

Sacrum

Rectum

Anus

Perineal body

Perineum

PERINEUM

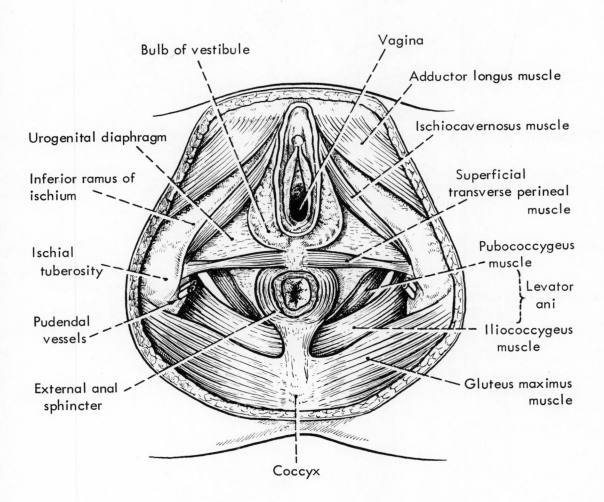

Bulb of vestibule

Vagina

Adductor longus muscle

Urogenital diaphragm

Ischiocavernosus muscle

Inferior ramus of
ischium

Superficial
transverse perineal
muscle

Ischial
tuberosity

Pubococcygeus
muscle

Levator
ani

Pudendal
vessels

Iliococcygeus
muscle

External anal
sphincter

Gluteus maximus
muscle

Coccyx

PELVIC FLOOR

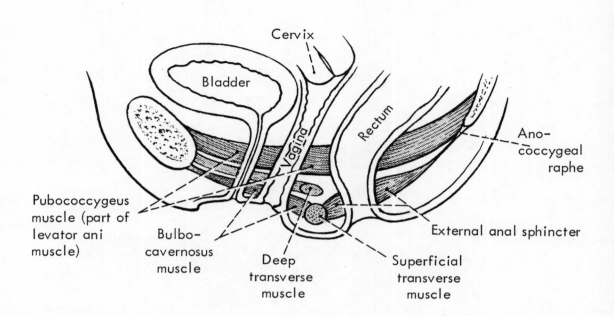

Cervix

Bladder

Rectum

Ano-
coccygeal
raphe

Pubococcygeus
muscle (part of
levator ani
muscle)

Bulbo-
cavernosus
muscle

Deep
transverse
muscle

Superficial
transverse
muscle

External anal sphincter

SOFT TISSUES OF THE OBSTETRIC
PELVIS (Schematic)

A muscular basin with an
opening below at the front.
The muscular tissues are
supported by and enclosed
in the pelvic bones.

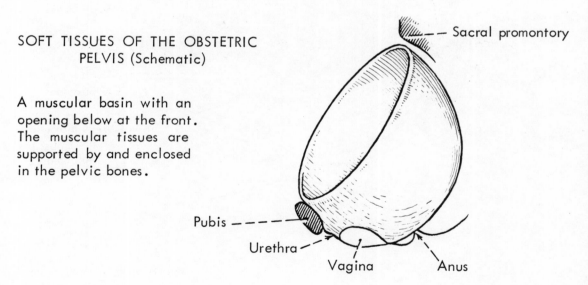

Sacral promontory

Pubis

Urethra

Vagina

Anus

PELVIC FLOOR

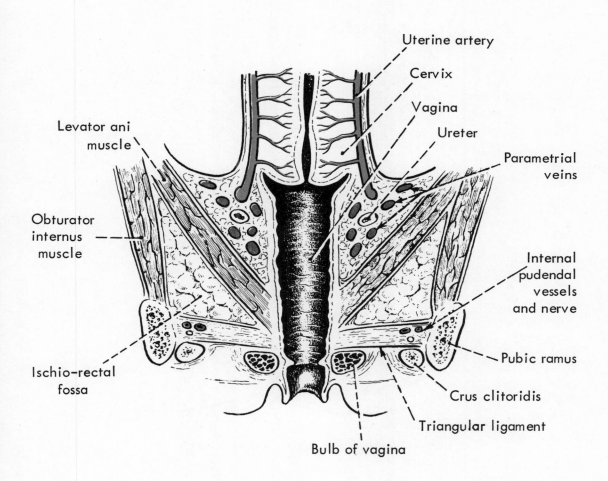

Uterine artery

Cervix

Vagina

Ureter

Parametrial veins

Levator ani muscle

Obturator internus muscle

Internal pudendal vessels and nerve

Ischio-rectal fossa

Pubic ramus

Crus clitoridis

Triangular ligament

Bulb of vagina

ISCHIORECTAL FOSSA

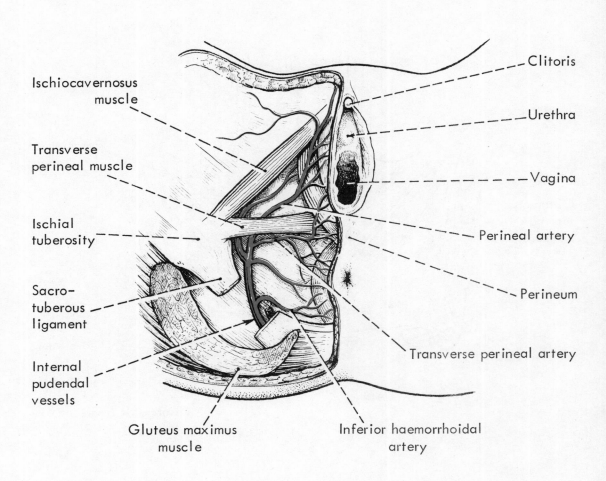

Ischiocavernosus muscle

Transverse perineal muscle

Ischial tuberosity

Sacro-tuberous ligament

Internal pudendal vessels

Gluteus maximus muscle

Clitoris

Urethra

Vagina

Perineal artery

Perineum

Transverse perineal artery

Inferior haemorrhoidal artery

ISCHIORECTAL FOSSA

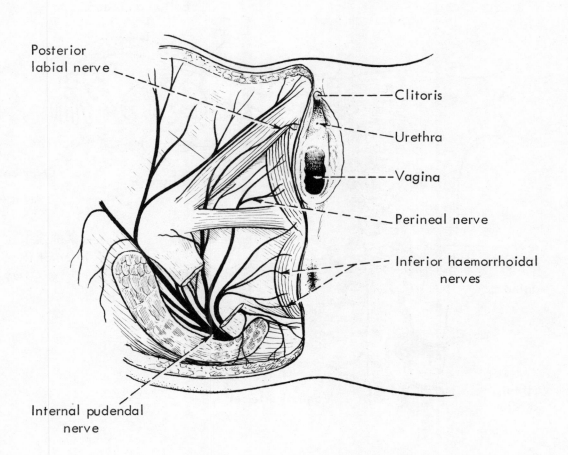

Posterior labial nerve

Clitoris

Urethra

Vagina

Perineal nerve

Inferior haemorrhoidal nerves

Internal pudendal nerve

PELVIC BLOOD SUPPLY

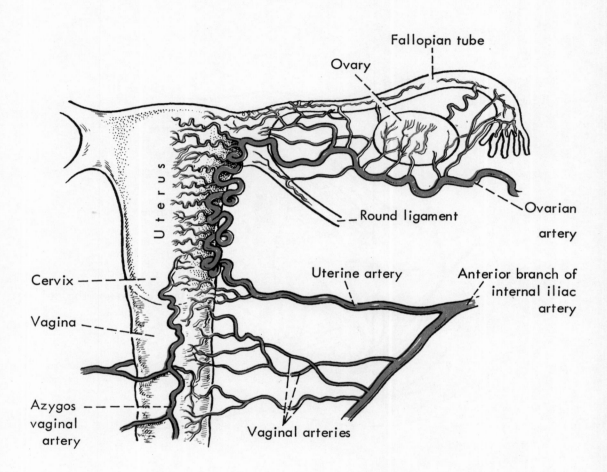

Note coiling of vessels to allow stretching as uterus grows in pregnancy.

PELVIC SYMPATHETIC NERVES

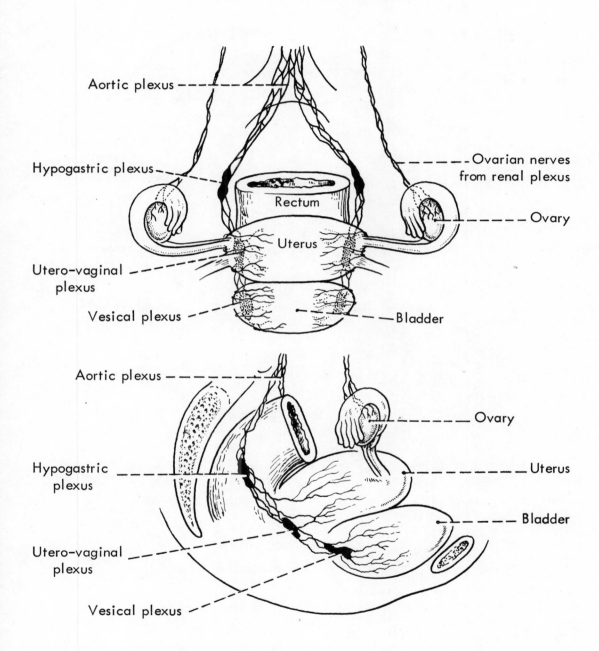

Aortic plexus

Hypogastric plexus

Utero-vaginal plexus

Vesical plexus

Rectum

Uterus

Ovarian nerves from renal plexus

Ovary

Bladder

Aortic plexus

Hypogastric plexus

Utero-vaginal plexus

Vesical plexus

Ovary

Uterus

Bladder

57

SUPPORTS OF UTERUS

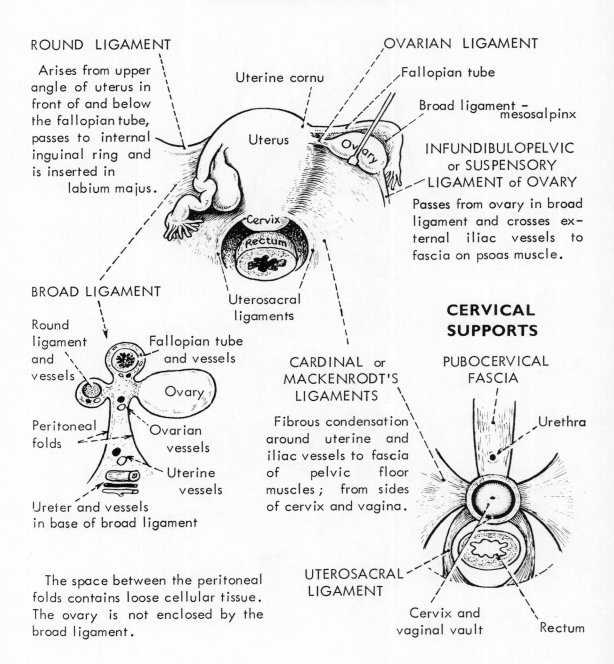

ROUND LIGAMENT

Arises from upper angle of uterus in front of and below the fallopian tube, passes to internal inguinal ring and is inserted in labium majus.

Uterine cornu

Uterus

Cervix

Rectum

OVARIAN LIGAMENT

Fallopian tube

Broad ligament – mesosalpinx

Ovary

INFUNDIBULOPELVIC or **SUSPENSORY LIGAMENT of OVARY**

Passes from ovary in broad ligament and crosses external iliac vessels to fascia on psoas muscle.

Uterosacral ligaments

BROAD LIGAMENT

Round ligament and vessels

Fallopian tube and vessels

Ovary

Peritoneal folds

Ovarian vessels

Uterine vessels

Ureter and vessels in base of broad ligament

CARDINAL or MACKENRODT'S LIGAMENTS

Fibrous condensation around uterine and iliac vessels to fascia of pelvic floor muscles; from sides of cervix and vagina.

CERVICAL SUPPORTS

PUBOCERVICAL FASCIA

Urethra

UTEROSACRAL LIGAMENT

Cervix and vaginal vault

Rectum

The space between the peritoneal folds contains loose cellular tissue. The ovary is not enclosed by the broad ligament.

58

UTERINE MUSCULATURE

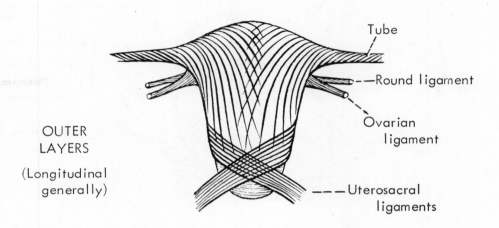

Tube

Round ligament

Ovarian ligament

Uterosacral ligaments

OUTER LAYERS

(Longitudinal generally)

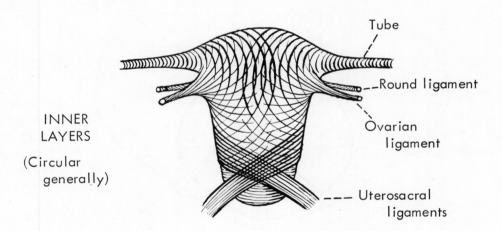

Tube

Round ligament

Ovarian ligament

Uterosacral ligaments

INNER LAYERS

(Circular generally)

BONY PELVIS—BRIM

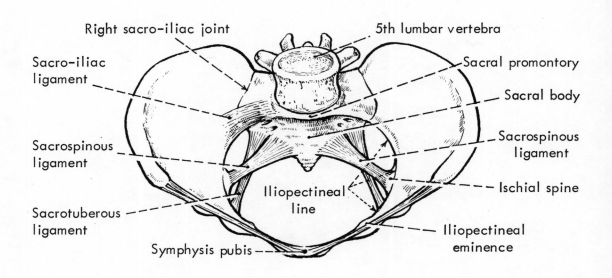

Right sacro-iliac joint

5th lumbar vertebra

Sacro-iliac ligament

Sacral promontory

Sacral body

Sacrospinous ligament

Sacrospinous ligament

Iliopectineal line

Ischial spine

Sacrotuberous ligament

Iliopectineal eminence

Symphysis pubis

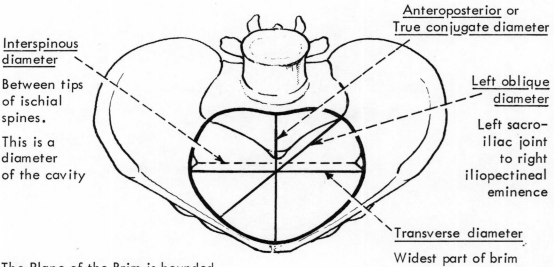

Interspinous diameter

Between tips of ischial spines.

This is a diameter of the cavity

Anteroposterior or True conjugate diameter

Left oblique diameter

Left sacro-iliac joint to right iliopectineal eminence

Transverse diameter

Widest part of brim

The Plane of the Brim is bounded
   Anteriorly by the Pubis,
   Laterally by the Iliopectineal lines,
   Posteriorly by the Alae and Promontory of the Sacrum.

BONY PELVIS—SAGITTAL VIEW

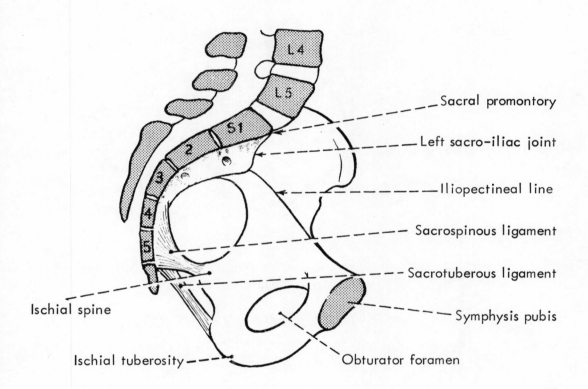

Sacral promontory

Left sacro-iliac joint

Iliopectineal line

Sacrospinous ligament

Sacrotuberous ligament

Symphysis pubis

Ischial spine

Obturator foramen

Ischial tuberosity

BONY PELVIS—CAVITY

The Pelvic Cavity is bounded
    Above by the Plane of the Brim,
    Below by the Plane of the Outlet,
    Posteriorly by the Sacrum,
    Laterally by Sacrosciatic ligaments
        and Ischial bones and
    Anteriorly by Obturator Foraminae,
        Ascending Rami of Ischia
        and Pubis

Note that pelvic outlet plane
is in two parts angled to each
other.

Plane of Mid cavity or Plane of Greatest Pelvic Diameters

Mid pubis to junction of second and third sacral vetebrae.

Plane of Least Pelvic Diameters

Symphysis pubis through ischial spines to end of sacrum.

True Conjugate of Brim

From sacral promontory to upper and inner border of symphysis pubis.

Diagonal Conjugate Diameter of Brim

From sacral promontory to under border of symphysis pubis.

Antero-Posterior Diameter of Outlet

Under body of symphysis pubis to end of sacrum or coccyx if fused.

Inclination of pelvic brim 50° – 60°
(Usually 55°)

BONY PELVIS—OUTLET

The Plane of the Outlet is bounded
   Anteriorly by Pubic Arch
   Laterally by Great Sacrosciatic Ligaments
     and Ischial Tuberosities
   Posteriorly by Tip of Coccyx if fused
     or to End of Sacrum

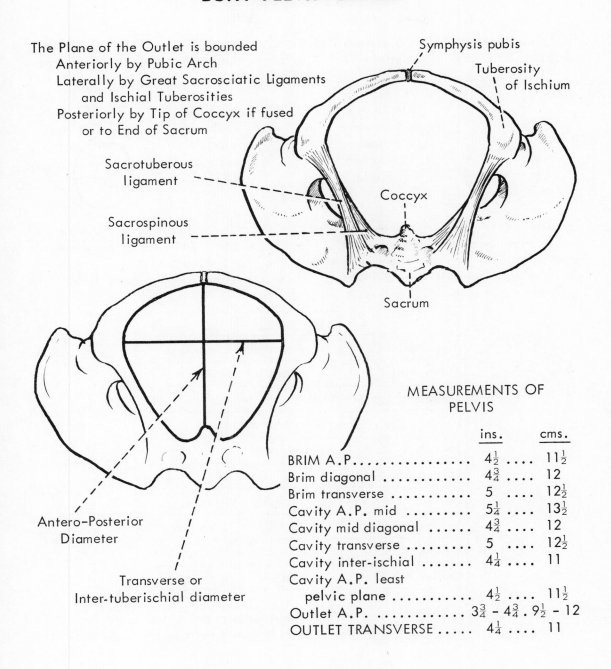

MEASUREMENTS OF
PELVIS

	ins.	cms.
BRIM A.P.	$4\frac{1}{2}$	$11\frac{1}{2}$
Brim diagonal	$4\frac{3}{4}$	12
Brim transverse	5	$12\frac{1}{2}$
Cavity A.P. mid	$5\frac{1}{4}$	$13\frac{1}{2}$
Cavity mid diagonal	$4\frac{3}{4}$	12
Cavity transverse	5	$12\frac{1}{2}$
Cavity inter-ischial	$4\frac{1}{4}$	11
Cavity A.P. least pelvic plane	$4\frac{1}{2}$	$11\frac{1}{2}$
Outlet A.P.	$3\frac{3}{4} - 4\frac{3}{4}$	$9\frac{1}{2} - 12$
OUTLET TRANSVERSE	$4\frac{1}{4}$	11

PELVIC TYPES

Four types of pelvis are described — Gynaecoid (50%), Anthropoid (25%), Android (20%) and Platypelloid (5%).   In many cases the pelvis is of mixed type.

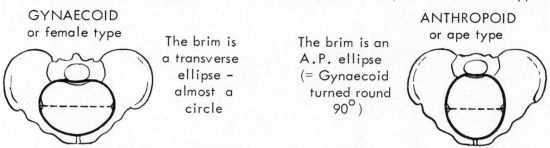

GYNAECOID
or female type

The brim is a transverse ellipse — almost a circle

The brim is an A.P. ellipse (= Gynaecoid turned round 90°)

ANTHROPOID
or ape type

The transverse diameter (widest part of brim) and the available transverse diameter (at mid-point of antero-posterior diameter of brim) coincide in the gynaecoid and anthropoid pelves. The hind pelvis is the area behind the transverse diameter and the fore pelvis the area in front. These areas are roughly equal in both the gynaecoid and anthropoid pelves.

	Gynaecoid	Anthropoid
Sacral angle	Approximately 100°	
Sacral line	Parallel to pubis	
Sacrosciatic notch	Shallow, wide	Shallow, wider
Ischial spines	Not prominent	
Sacrum	Broad, shallow, concave	
Cavity side walls	Parallel	
Pubis	Light, shallow	
Sub-pubic angle	At least 85°	More than 80°
Bituberous diam.	Wide	Narrower
Outlet A.P. diam.	Long	Longer

Gynaecoid

Anthropoid

The delivery of the foetal head through these types of pelvis has equal mechanical problems at all levels, i.e. if it is easy at brim it should be easy in cavity and outlet.

PELVIC TYPES

ANDROID
or male type

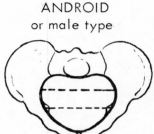

Brim is roughly triangular. Trans.diameter near sacrum. 'Available trans.' diameter is shortened.

Brim is kidney shaped. Transverse and 'available transverse' diameters coincide.

PLATYPELLOID
or flat type

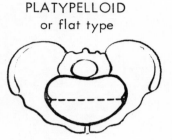

The area of the hind pelvis is reduced and shallow. Area of the fore pelvis is reduced and narrowed at front.

The hind pelvis is shallow and the area reduced. Fore pelvis is shallow and the area reduced.

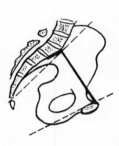

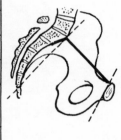

	Android	Platypelloid
Sacral angle	90° or less	more than 90°
Sacral line	convergent	divergent
Sacrosciatic notch	narrowed	wide, shallow
Ischial spines	prominent, heavy	prominent
Sacrum	flattened, narrow, long	broad, short, concave
Cavity side walls	converge	diverge
Pubis	heavy, deep	shallow
Sub-pubic angle	narrowed	more than 85°
Bituberous diam.	reduced	increased
Outlet A.P.diam.	narrow	longer

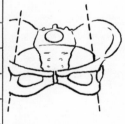

The delivery of a foetal head through this pelvis gives increasing problems the further it descends.

The delivery of a foetal head through this pelvis meets problems at the brim but thereafter the difficulties decrease with descent.

FOETAL SKULL

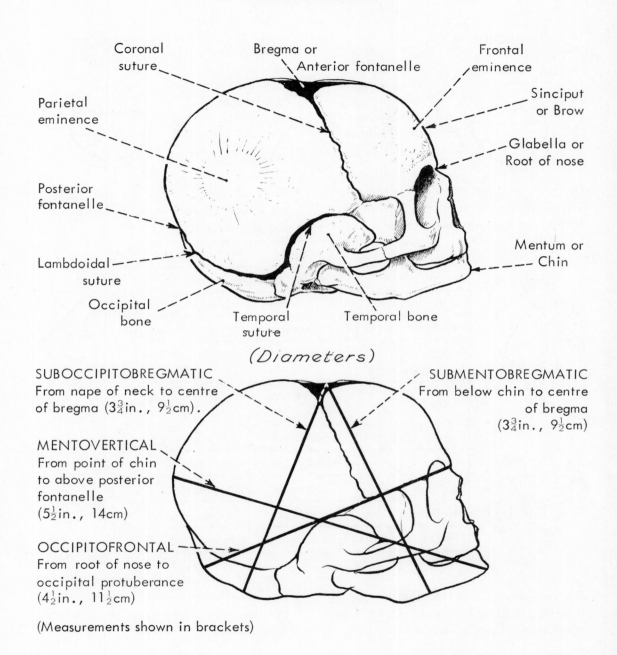

Coronal suture

Bregma or Anterior fontanelle

Frontal eminence

Parietal eminence

Sinciput or Brow

Posterior fontanelle

Glabella or Root of nose

Lambdoidal suture

Mentum or Chin

Occipital bone

Temporal suture

Temporal bone

(Diameters)

SUBOCCIPITOBREGMATIC
From nape of neck to centre
of bregma ($3\frac{3}{4}$in., $9\frac{1}{2}$cm).

SUBMENTOBREGMATIC
From below chin to centre
of bregma
($3\frac{3}{4}$in., $9\frac{1}{2}$cm)

MENTOVERTICAL
From point of chin
to above posterior
fontanelle
($5\frac{1}{2}$in., 14cm)

OCCIPITOFRONTAL
From root of nose to
occipital protuberance
($4\frac{1}{2}$in., $11\frac{1}{2}$cm)

(Measurements shown in brackets)

FOETAL SKULL

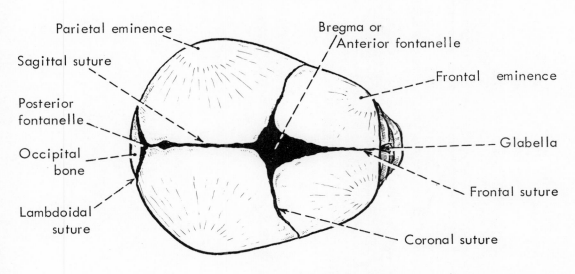

Parietal eminence

Sagittal suture

Posterior fontanelle

Occipital bone

Lambdoidal suture

Bregma or Anterior fontanelle

Frontal eminence

Glabella

Frontal suture

Coronal suture

(Diameters)

BIPARIETAL ($3\frac{3}{4}$ in., $9\frac{1}{2}$ cm)
Between two parietal eminences

BITEMPORAL ($3\frac{1}{4}$ in., $8\frac{1}{2}$ cm)
Greatest distance between two halves of coronal suture

(Circumferences)

SUBOCCIPITOBREGMATIC
    x BIPARIETAL (11 in., 28 cm)
These are engaging diameters of well flexed vertex presentation.

OCCIPITOFRONTAL
    x BIPARIETAL (13 in., 33 cm)
These are engaging diameters of deflexed vertex presentation and found in Occipito-posterior positions.

(The vertex is the area bounded by the anterior and posterior fontan-elles and the parietal eminences.)

MENTOVERTICAL x BIPARIETAL (14 in., $35\frac{1}{2}$ cm)
This is the largest circumference of the head and is found in Brow presentation.

67

CHAPTER 4

DIAGNOSIS OF PREGNANCY

SYMPTOMS AND SIGNS OF PREGNANCY

(The more useful symptoms and signs are shown in full line).

WEEKS

0 4 8 12 16 20 24 28 32 36 40

Pregnancy Test
Amenorrhoea
Morning Sickness
Breast Changes
Bladder Symptoms
Cervical Changes
Palpable Uterine Changes
Vaginal and Vulval Changes
Hegar's Sign
Uterus Palpable Abdominally
Ultrasound
Ballottement
X-ray Signs
Quickening (Multipara)
Abdominal Enlargement
Quickening (Primigravida)
Palpable Uterine Contractions
Palpable Foetal Movement
Foetal Heart Audible
Palpable Foetal Parts

LABORATORY DIAGNOSIS OF PREGNANCY

All pregnancy tests depend on the fact that, 14 days after fertilization, the chorion of the embedded blastocyst secretes Chorionic Gonadotrophin in increasing quantities. A peak is reached in 10 – 12 weeks, and the hormone is excreted in the mother's urine.

There are two kinds of test:-   BIOLOGICAL and IMMUNOLOGICAL

BIOLOGICAL tests make use of the power of human chorionic gonadotrophin to stimulate the gonads of certain animals.

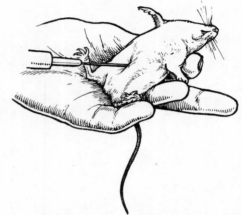

In the ASCHHEIM-ZONDEK test the urine is injected into a mouse which is killed after 5 days. A positive reaction is the presence of corpora lutea and hae-morrhagic follicles in the mouse ovary. In the FRIEDMAN test the rabbit is used and a result can be obtained in 2 days.

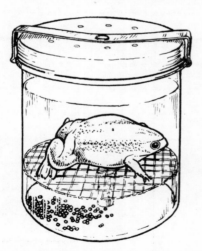

In the HOGBEN test a positive urine injected into the female Xenopus toad will cause it to ovulate within 12 – 14 hours. The ova pass through the grating and can be seen at the bottom of the jar.

If a male toad is used a positive urine will produce spermatozoa in cloacal fluid (withdrawn by pipette) in 2 hours.

All these tests are expensive and troublesome, involving the breeding of animals and, in the case of toads, requiring special environmental conditions and priming to keep the gonads in a suitable state.

IMMUNOLOGICAL TESTS FOR PREGNANCY

Human chorionic gonadotrophin (HCG) is a protein and will induce antibody formation in other animals. The antiserum can be used to detect the presence of the hormone in the urine but it is necessary to make the reaction visible.

1. Standard HCG is adsorbed on to particles or cells in suspension.
2. To this are added antiserum (immune body – IB) and some of the patient's urine.
3. If the urine contains HCG it will neutralise the antiserum, leaving none to react with the HCG on the particles, and the suspension will remain unchanged. This is a Positive result.

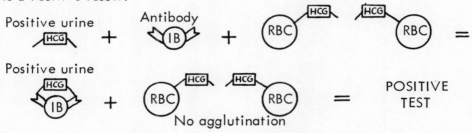

4. If there is no HCG in the patient's urine, the antiserum will be free to react with the hormone on the particles which will flocculate – a Negative result.

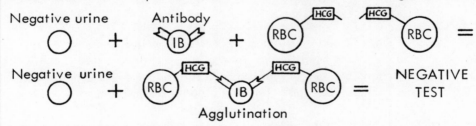

The particles used are either Latex ('Gravindex') or tanned red cells ('Prognosticon'; 'Prepuerin' tests).

During the first 40 days the HCG levels are low and the tests are unreliable. Negative tests should be repeated 41 days from the last menstrual period. From the 110th day onwards the test will usually remain positive.

Fallacies occur in both biological and immunological methods which are not, in themselves, pregnancy tests but merely indicate the presence or absence of large quantities of gonadotrophin. Both false negatives and positives are met with, and tests should not replace clinical diagnosis.

SYMPTOMS AND SIGNS

4 weeks AMENORRHOEA

Causes such as ovarian-pituitary imbalance, emotional upset, local infection, must be considered. Ovulation may have occurred earlier or later in the cycle than normal. Women do not always recall such dates with precision.

4 weeks MORNING SICKNESS

The majority of women suffer some gastric upset in the early months, from nausea and anorexia to repeated vomiting, especially in the morning. The cause is unknown, but probably the increased amount of circulating oestrogen has a temporary effect on liver metabolism. It also decreases gastric motility.

6 weeks BLADDER SYMPTOMS

Increased frequency of micturition in the 2nd and 3rd months is due to a combination of increased vascularity, and pressure from the enlarging uterus. Near term, frequency may again appear, due by then to lack of room for the bladder to expand.

SIGNS OF PREGNANCY DUE TO INCREASED VASCULARITY

(These are of less importance since the development of quick, sensitive laboratory tests for pregnancy.)

Cervical softening.. 6 weeks
Increased pulsation in lateral fornices (Osiander's Sign).............. 8 weeks
Darkening of vaginal mucous membrane (Jacquemier's Sign)........... 8 weeks
Vulval varicosities (Kluge's Sign) .... 10 weeks

SYMPTOMS AND SIGNS

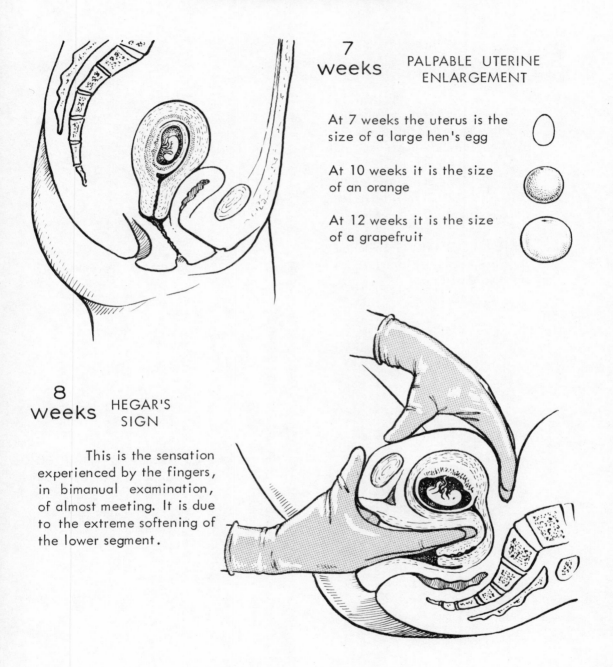

7 weeks   PALPABLE UTERINE ENLARGEMENT

At 7 weeks the uterus is the size of a large hen's egg

At 10 weeks it is the size of an orange

At 12 weeks it is the size of a grapefruit

8 weeks   HEGAR'S SIGN

This is the sensation experienced by the fingers, in bimanual examination, of almost meeting. It is due to the extreme softening of the lower segment.

75

SYMPTOMS AND SIGNS

6-8 weeks

The earliest symptoms and signs – increased vascularity and sensation of heaviness, almost of pain – appear at 6 weeks. By 8 weeks the nipple and surrounding area – the PRIMARY AREOLA – have become more pigmented.

MONTGOMERY'S TUBERCLES – abortive accessory lactiferous ducts are also prominent

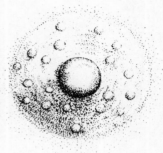

The breast at 8 weeks

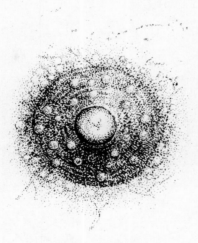

The breast at 16 weeks

16 weeks

By 16 weeks a clear fluid (colostrum) is secreted and may be expressed. By 20 weeks the secondary areola – a mottled effect due to further pigmentation – has become prominent.

SYMPTOMS AND SIGNS

14 weeks — INTERNAL BALLOTTEMENT

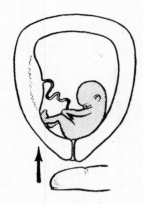 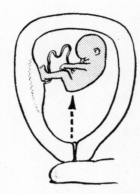 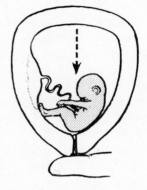

Tap upwards and hold finger against cervix.

The foetus is knocked upwards.

The foetus sinks and a gentle tap is felt on the finger.

24 weeks — EXTERNAL BALLOTTEMENT

One hand taps the abdomen and sends the foetus across the uterine cavity.

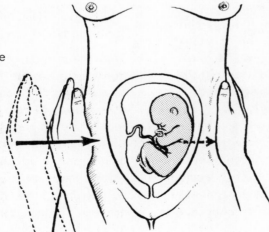

The other hand lying on the uterus perceives the impulse.

16 weeks

ABDOMINAL ENLARGEMENT

The uterus becomes abdominal by 12 weeks and increase in abdominal size is apparent by 16 weeks.

The reduction in fundal height which occurs between 38 and 40 weeks is called "lightening", and is due to the descent of the foetus as the lower segment and cervix prepare for labour. It often does not occur in women who have had a previous pregnancy
(multiparae).

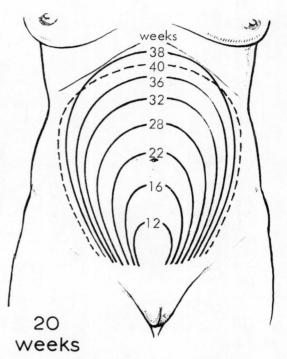

16-18 weeks

QUICKENING ("FEELING LIFE")

The sensation of foetal movement transmitted as far as the parietal peritoneum which has somatic innervation. It is a very faint sensation to begin with and is perceived more readily by the multipara. It is not a completely reliable sign; the mother may be unwilling to admit its absence even to herself; and hysterical women undergoing imaginary pregnancy ('pseudocyesis') can easily convince themselves of its presence.

20 weeks

PALPABLE UTERINE CONTRACTIONS (Braxton Hicks' sign)

The uterus undergoes irregular painless contractions from the 9th to 10th week onward, which become palpable by the 20th week, at first on bimanual examination, later per abdomen. They have no rhythm, but become more frequent as pregnancy advances, and in the last weeks may interfere with abdominal palpation. The distinction between Braxton Hicks contractions and early labour is not always clear.

24 weeks — AUSCULTATION OF THE FOETAL HEART

The foetal heart is heard with a foetal stethoscope pressed on the abdomen over the back of the foetus. Sounds are most clearly heard over the left foetal scapula; so the point of maximum intensity will vary with the position of the foetus.

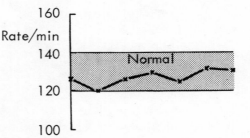

The rate varies between 120 and 140/minute and the rhythm should be regular.

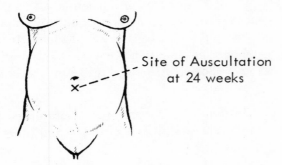

Site of Auscultation at 24 weeks

Sounds to be distinguished from foetal heart :—

1. The maternal pulse, transmitted by aorta.
2. The uterine souffle, a blowing sound caused by the pulsation of blood through enlarged uterine arteries.

---

20 weeks — PALPABLE FOETAL MOVEMENTS

This sensation is felt at first as a faint flutter. Movements are stronger in the later months, and may be perceived as a definite impulse on the examiner's ear when the foetal stethoscope is being used.

26 weeks — PALPABLE FOETAL PARTS

The outlines of the foetus, the head and limbs, begin to be palpable at this time. A fibromyoma is the only tumour that may falsely suggest foetal parts: but diagnosis of pregnancy cannot be made on this sign alone.

PIGMENTATION IN PREGNANCY

This probably represents an excess of precursors of adrenal hormones
(cf. Addison's Disease).

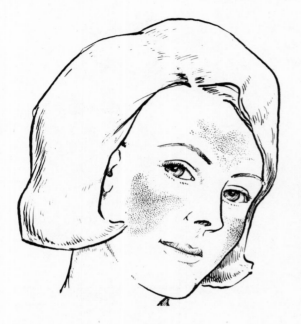

Areas already pigmented become more so (nipples, external genitalia and anal region). Some fresh pigmentation appears on the face (chloasma) and on the abdomen (linea nigra) and striae gravidarum.

('Chloasma' is from a Greek word meaning the greenish tint of a growing shoot or bud.)

Striae gravidarum are depressed streaks on the skin of the fat areas (abdomen, breasts and thighs). After delivery they regress and persist as striae albicantes. They are due to stretching, but may also be associated with increased secretion of ACTH.

CHAPTER 5

ANTENATAL CARE

ANTENATAL CARE

Its PURPOSE

1. To MAINTAIN the mother in the best possible state of health, so that she may give birth to a healthy child.

2. To RECOGNISE abnormalities and complications at an early stage.

3. To EDUCATE the mother in the duties of mother-hood, and dispel the ignorance and fears of pregnancy and labour.

Its BRANCHES

Diagnosis of pregnancy

Medical Care and Obstetrical Care

General Hygiene

Physiotherapy

Mothercraft

RESPONSIBILITY for maternity services in Great Britain is shared by the General Practitioner, the Public Health Maternity Department and the Hospital. The patient first applies to her Doctor at an early stage in her pregnancy.

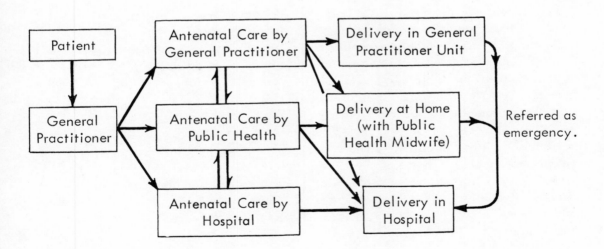

THE FIRST VISIT

A full general history is taken, with the object of recording any condition or abnormality which may affect the present pregnancy.

SOCIAL HISTORY: Age, date of birth, religion, husband's occupation, next-of-kin, are all essential. The social background provides a rough measure of the patient's family income, her standard of education and nutrition, the quality of her home conditions.

MENSTRUAL HISTORY.

How certain is the patient of the date of her Last Menstrual Period (L.M.P.)? Are her periods normally regular?

The maturity of the pregnancy is calculated from the date of the L.M.P. The patient may be wrong, she may have forgotten, she may be deliberately misleading. The average pregnancy lasts 40 ± 1 weeks. To calculate the Estimated Date of Delivery (E.D.D.) from the L.M.P. this formula is used:-
L.M.P. – 3 months + 1 year + 7 days = E.D.D.
(Go back 3 months from L.M.P. and add a year and a week) Thus:-
L.M.P. 9.7.1968
Go back 3 months 9.4.1968
Add 1 year 9.4.1969
Add 7 days . . . .16.4.1969 = E.D.D.

MEDICAL HISTORY

In Particular:-

Cardiac function
Previous Rheumatic Fever?
Any Congenital Condition?

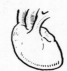

Respiratory function
Any Tuberculosis, Asthma, Chronic Bronchitis?

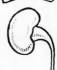

Renal function
Any Pyelonephritis?
Any Congenital Condition?
Any Hypertension?

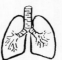

SURGICAL HISTORY

In Particular:-

Previous Blood Transfusion?
(This question leads to any history of trauma.)

Previous Operations on Genital Tract?
(A previous amputation of cervix might cause difficulty in labour.)

Previous Abdominal Operations?
(Adhesions may interfere with the position of the uterus. There may have been a previous Caesarean section.)

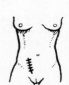

THE OBSTETRIC HISTORY

The patient shown in this example of a fairly typical obstetric history is known as a Para 4 + 1 (i.e. 4 babies and one abortion) or as Gravida 5 + 1 (bearing her 5th child).

No.	Year	Place	Maturity	Length of Labour	Delivery	Baby Wt.	Sex	Result	Complications
1	2/2 1958	Royal Maternity	40	24 hr.	Spon-taneous	8lb 13oz	M	alive	None
2	Nov 1958	Royal Infirmary	3 month abortion			—	D+C	—	2 pints blood
3	7/12 1959	At Home	40	12 hr	Spon-taneous	8lb 8oz	M	alive	none
4	8/6/62	At Home	32	6 hr	Spon-taneous	very small	F	D	Died at birth — prematurity
5	5/5/65	Royal Maternity	41	6 hr	Spon-taneous	8lb 1oz	M	alive	Post-partum haemorrhage / Blood transfusion

Also required is information about the patient's married state, duration of marriage and whether her pregnancies have been deliberately spaced.

All this information is essential and must be available. The object is to discover any previous abnormalities that may recur in or influence the present pregnancy.

MARRIED STATE etc. This gives some idea of the fertility of the patient and the ease or otherwise with which she conceives.

DATES AND PLACES. These help the patient towards clear and accurate recall.

LENGTH OF LABOUR AND TYPE OF DELIVERY. These are the most objective assessments of performance in labour, and are an indication of what may be looked for this time.

DETAILS OF BABY. Incidents such as still births must obviously be recorded. Birth weights are the best indication of pelvic capacity.

COMPLICATIONS. Haemorrhage after normal delivery may occur again, and the attendants must be forewarned. Patients are often terrified of a repetition of some complication and must receive reassurance.

THE FIRST EXAMINATION

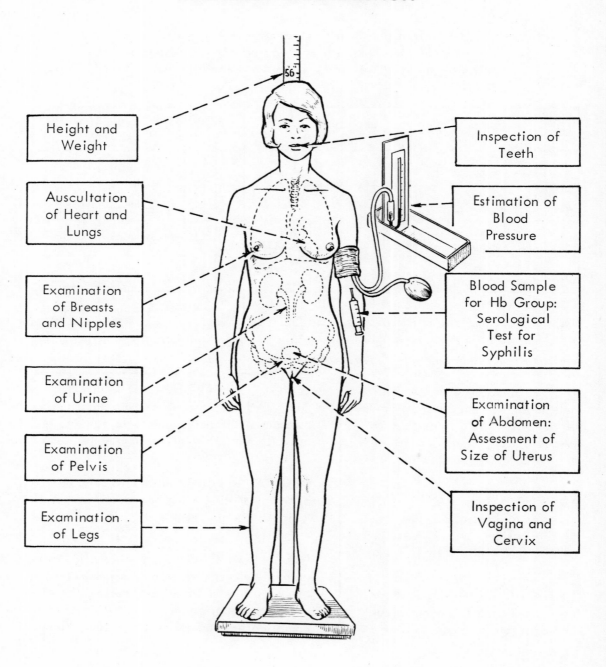

Height and Weight

Auscultation of Heart and Lungs

Examination of Breasts and Nipples

Examination of Urine

Examination of Pelvis

Examination of Legs

Inspection of Teeth

Estimation of Blood Pressure

Blood Sample for Hb Group: Serological Test for Syphilis

Examination of Abdomen: Assessment of Size of Uterus

Inspection of Vagina and Cervix

THE BLOOD IN ANTENATAL CARE

In obstetrical practice, the ever present risk is HAEMORRHAGE. Blood transfusion may be required at very short notice.

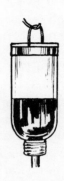

THE ABO and Rh BLOOD GROUP MUST BE KNOWN.

If the mother is Rh–negative the baby, if Rh-positive, may be affected by Haemolytic Disease of the Newborn, and require emergency treatment.

THE MOTHER'S Rh FACTOR MUST BE KNOWN.

Venereal disease may infect the foetus during pregnancy and parturition, causing serious harm and perhaps even death.

SEROLOGICAL TESTS FOR SYPHILIS MUST BE CARRIED OUT.

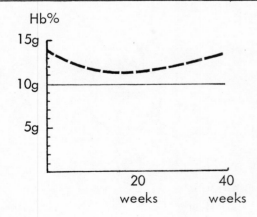

Anaemia is common in women because of the menstrual loss. The pregnant woman must satisfy the demands of the foetus.

THE HAEMOGLOBIN LEVEL MUST BE CHECKED AT LEAST AT MONTHLY INTERVALS.

VAGINAL EXAMINATION

Usually two examinations are made, an early one to detect abnormal uterine position, and ovarian tumours: and a late one near term to assess pelvic capacity. If the patient is tense and frightened, vaginal examination will be useless.

FIRST EXAMINATION: The patient lies in the dorsal position, and first one then two lubricated fingers are gently inserted, pressing against the perineum rather than the vestibule. The size, shape and position of the uterus can be felt between the two hands, and the fornices palpated. Afterwards the cervix is examined with a speculum and any complaint of discharge is dealt with.

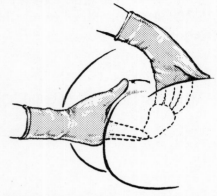

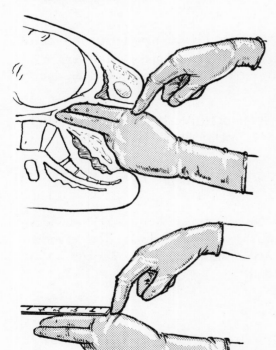

SECOND EXAMINATION: Usually at the 36th week. The diagonal conjugate is measured, and some idea of the size and shape of the pelvic cavity obtained by palpating the side walls and sacrum.

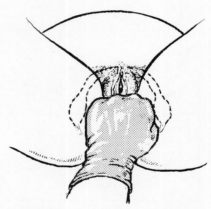

The inter-tuberischial diameter is measured with the fist and the pubic arch is palpated.

88

POSITION OF THE FOETUS

PRESENTATION   is the part of the foetus overlying the external os, e.g. vertex, breech, shoulder.

ATTITUDE   is the "posture" of the foetus, e.g. flexion, deflexion, extension.

DENOMINATOR   is an arbitrary part of the presenting part, e.g. occiput in vertex presentation, sacrum in breech presentation.

The pelvis is divided into eight segments for the purposes of description and location of the presenting part.

The denominator is in one of these segments and takes its position from it. For example, the occiput is the denominator of the vertex presentation and if the occiput is close to the left iliopectineal eminence the position is described as the left occipito-anterior or L.O.A.

ATTITUDES

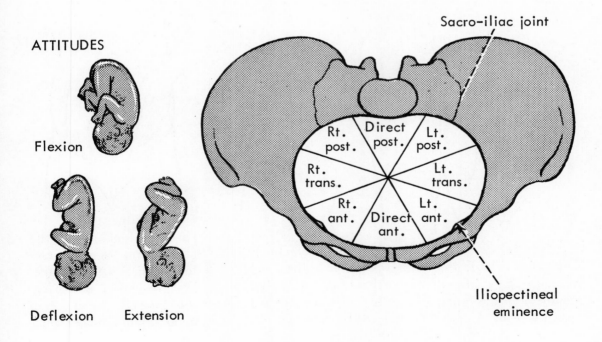

Flexion

Deflexion   Extension

Sacro-iliac joint

Rt. post.   Direct post.   Lt. post.

Rt. trans.   Lt. trans.

Rt. ant.   Direct ant.   Lt. ant.

Iliopectineal eminence

ABDOMINAL PALPATION

This examination must be made systematically.

Remember that the following tissue layers may interpose between your fingers and the foetal head.

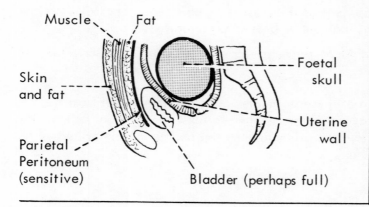

Muscle   Fat

Skin and fat

Parietal Peritoneum (sensitive)

Bladder (perhaps full)

Foetal skull

Uterine wall

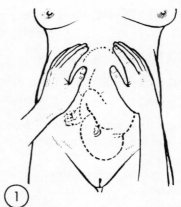

① The fundus is palpated and the breech identified.

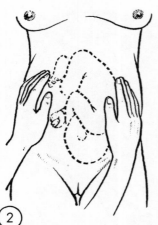

② The hands palpate the contours of the uterus, identifying the back and the limbs.

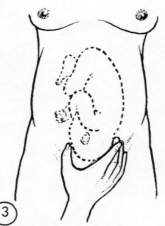

③ The lower pole is palpated. The head should be identified and if not engaged will be mobile.

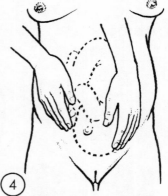

④ The examiner faces the patient's feet and gently pushes two fingers into the pelvis. This is the best method of palpating the foetal head and determining engagement.

ABDOMINAL PALPATION

The Examiner must ask himself, and answer, SIX questions.

① Is the FUNDAL HEIGHT consistent with the estimation of maturity made from the date of the L.M.P? See p. 84. (The date might be wrong: there might be twins: the foetus might be dead etc.)

---

② Is the LIE Longitudinal?

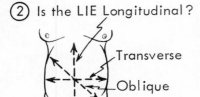

Transverse

Oblique

The Lie is the position of the long axis of the foetus relative to the mother. Only a longitudinal lie is normal.

---

④ Is the CEPHALIC PRESENTATION a VERTEX? This depends on the ATTITUDE of the foetus i.e. the relationship of its different parts to each other. The normal attitude is FULL FLEXION.

In full flexion, every foetal joint is flexed.

Sometimes the head may be extended.

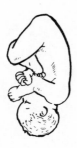

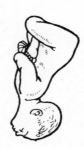

This gives a vertex presentation, the only normal presentation.

This gives a face presentation, which is highly abnormal.

③ Is the PRESENTATION Breech?

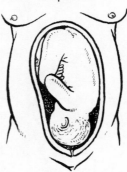

or Cephalic?

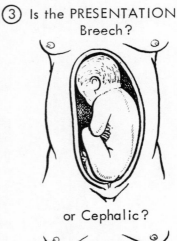

The presenting part is that part of the foetus which occupies the lower pole of the uterus. Only a cephalic presentation is normal.

ABDOMINAL PALPATION

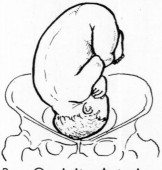

R.   Occipito-Transverse
(R.O.T.)   25%

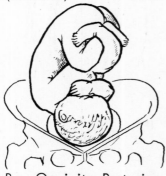

R.   Occipito-Anterior
(R.O.A.)   10%

R.   Occipito-Posterior
(R.O.P.)   10%

⑤ What is the POSITION
    of the VERTEX ?

The position is the relationship of the presenting part to
the mother's pelvis. It is
conveniently expressed by
referring to the position of
one area of the presenting
part known as the
          DENOMINATOR.
The denominator of the
vertex is the OCCIPUT; and
there are eight recognised
positions. (Direct anterior
or posterior positions, not
shown here, rarely occur).

The percentages given here
refer to the position at the
pelvic brim, and transverse
and anterior are regarded as
normal.

Position is important in
obstetrics because if the
foetus takes up a posterior
position in the pelvis (i.e.
if the occiput rotates towards
the sacrum and the foetus
faces forwards) the labour is
likely to be long and
difficult. There may be some
analogy with the experience
of trying to put a right foot
into a left shoe.

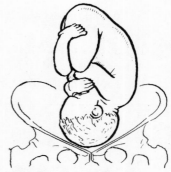

Left Occipito-Transverse
40%   (L.O.T.)

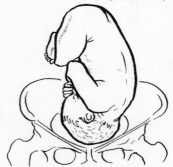

Left Occipito-Anterior
12%   (L.O.A.)

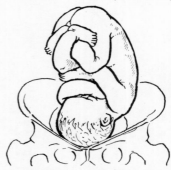

Left Occipito-Posterior
3%   (L.O.P.)

ABDOMINAL PALPATION

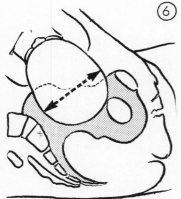

(6) Is the VERTEX ENGAGED?

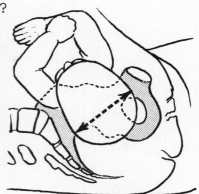

Engagement means the descent of the biparietal plane through the pelvic brim. Note that if the vertex is at the level of the ischial spines the head must be engaged, unless there is large caput formation.

Engagement often occurs in primigravidae in the last two weeks of pregnancy, but with multiparae it is usually a phenomenon of labour. The determination of engagement is important, because if it has occurred, disproportion between the foetal head and pelvic brim (and probably the whole pelvis) can be ruled out and vaginal delivery will be feasible.

In the antenatal clinic engagement is usually determined by abdominal palpation.

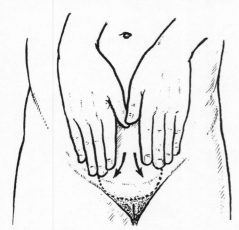

The fingers diverge when the head is engaged.

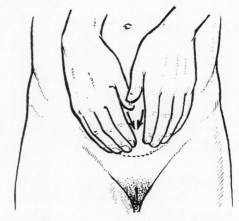

The fingers meet round the presenting part when the head is not engaged.

SUBSEQUENT VISITS

Visits are made 4-weekly to 26 weeks, then fortnightly to 36 weeks and then weekly to term.

Wk	BP	Urine	Wt lb.	Oedema	Fundal Height	Foetus	FH	Remarks
16	116/80	trace acetone	142	nil	16	—	-	Still some nausea
20	120/78	clear	146	nil	20	—	-	Feels life
24	118/80	clear	149	nil	24	—	✓	Well
26	125/80	trace sugar	151	nil	26	Foetal parts felt	✓	Well
28	120/78	clear	152	nil	28	Foetal parts felt	✓	Slight Backache
30	120/80	clear	154	nil	30	Breech	✓	Well
32	126/82	trace sugar	156	nil	32	Vertex	✓	Constipated
34	130/84	clear	158	ring tight	34	Vertex free	✓	Well
36	126/82	clear	160	ring tight	36	Vertex LOA free	✓	Well
37	130/84	clear	161	ring tight	37	"	✓	Feels a lot of movement
38	130/80	clear	162	trace	38	"	✓	Can't sleep Rx soneryl 100 mg.
39	126/78	clear	163	trace	near term	Vertex engaging	✓	Well
40	130/80	clear	163	trace	near term	Vertex LOA engaged	✓	Feels 'pressure'

(Findings not strictly normal are underlined.)

Blood pressure: Normal is 120/80 or less. Abnormal is over 140/90. Readings should be taken on a rested patient.

Urine: Traces of acetone or sugar are not significant, but there should be no albumin.

Oedema: The first 10% of retained fluid does not show as oedema ('occult oedema'). The fingers may swell, causing the ring to feel tight. There should be no pitting oedema.

Weight: The normal increase is about 1 lb a week, from the 13th week onwards.

Fundal Height: This should correspond to the maturity estimated from the date of the L.M.P. (in the first column).

Foetal Heart: If this is difficult to hear, foetal movements should be felt for, and the patient asked about feeling life.

Remarks: This column must include among other things a note of all drugs prescribed.

DIET IN PREGNANCY

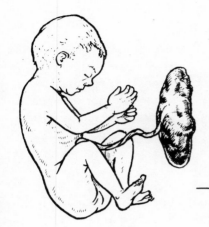

The body of a 7½lb.(3.4 kg) baby at birth contains:-

400g	Protein	25g	Ca	The Placenta	
220g	Fat	16g	P	contains	
80g	CHO	0.4g	Fe	55g Protein	

Two-thirds of this development takes place in the last 3 months.

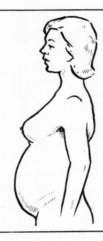

The mother also lays down new protein in the uterus and breasts (perhaps up to 500g) and at term her basal metabolism has increased by 25% or about 350 kcal/DAY. If she is breast-feeding, the baby will at one month require 7.0g Protein, 0.2g Ca and 300 kcal DAILY

The pregnant and lactating woman needs above all else a substantial increase in dietary protein, mostly of animal origin, and especially in the third trimester.

Estimated DAILY requirements for Diet in Pregnancy:-

Protein	100g	410 kcal	P	1.9g
Fat	100g	920 kcal	Ca	1.5g
CHO	300g	1230 kcal	Fe	15mg
			Vit.A	6,000 I.U.
		2560 kcal	B complex	25 mg
			Vit.C	100mg
			Vit.D	600 I.U.

Phosphorus requirements are always met when a good protein diet is taken.
The object should be to provide a good mixed diet, palatable to the mother, with additional fat-soluble vitamins(A,D), ascorbic acid and iron.

Cow's milk is the only naturally balanced food containing nearly 20g of first-class protein per pint, minerals, all the vitamins, and fat.

GENERAL HEALTH

EXERCISE

Most mothers get enough exercise looking after their own homes and families. In hot weather gentle pursuits such as sea bathing do no harm.

CLEANLINESS

Regular and frequent washing especially of the genito-anal region is desirable. There is inevitably an increase in sweating and discharge in pregnancy.

COITUS

Coitus during pregnancy is normal in the human species and its frequency should depend on the mother's inclination. A previous history of abortion might be an indication for avoiding coitus during the first three months.

SMOKING

Women who are heavy smokers should be advised to cut down the number of cigarettes they smoke each day. Nicotine in excess does cause vasoconstriction and may therefore affect placental function.

CLOTHING

Clothing must be loose and comfortable, and tight girdles and suspender belts should not be worn. Fashionable shoes are permissable if safe and comfortable.

BOWELS

Constipation is almost the rule in pregnancy and a bowel motion every second day is a reasonable compromise. Otherwise laxatives should be taken. Attention to diet may help.

TEETH

The teeth require the same care as in the non-pregnant state. If the mother is healthy there is no objection to the use of local analgesia or nitrous oxide for dental treatment.

WORK

Industrial work of a strenuous type should not be undertaken in the third trimester. The mother should be able to rest as she chooses.

CARE OF THE BREASTS

The nipple and areola should be kept clean with soap and water to avoid the formation of crusts of colostrum. Such crusts, if present, may be removed with a little ether.

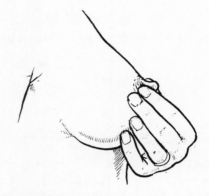

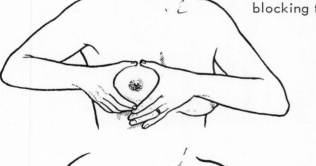

The nipple and areola should be soft and protractable.

During the last two months of pregnancy, the breasts should be massaged to 'milk' the colostrum and prevent it from blocking the ducts.

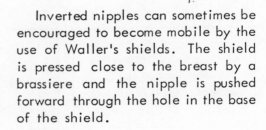

Inverted nipples can sometimes be encouraged to become mobile by the use of Waller's shields. The shield is pressed close to the breast by a brassiere and the nipple is pushed forward through the hole in the base of the shield.

MENTAL PREPARATION

Many of the physical complications which
arise in labour have psychological origins.

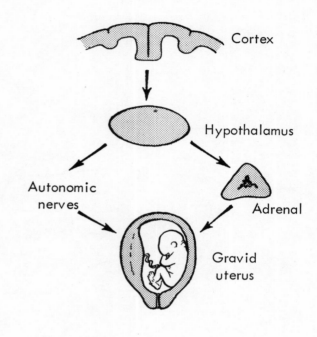

Cortex

Hypothalamus

Autonomic
nerves

Adrenal

Gravid
uterus

Fear of the unknown acts
through the cortex and hypothalamus on the sympathetic
system. Tension is produced,
neither the patient nor her
uterus can properly relax,
and exhaustion follows.

Fear of labour, fear of the
unknown is universal, and the
most effective antidote is a
doctor-patient relationship
which allows the mother to
repose an absolute trust and
confidence in her attendants.
Close personal involvement of the doctor is not always possible in the circumstances
of present-day obstetric practice, but antenatal instruction has been systematised.

To help the mother avoid psychological tension she is given:-

Lectures on pregnancy and labour to DISPEL IGNORANCE.	Lectures on the care of the baby when it comes; the mother is READY.	Instruction on means of inducing actual MUSCULAR RELAXATION.

EXERCISE AND RELAXATION

The patient is instructed in simple EXERCISES to be done every day.

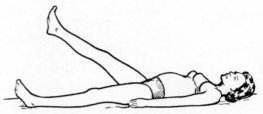

Legs raised alternately. Strengthens abdominal muscles and improves their tone.

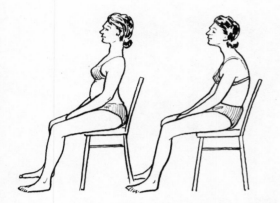

Knee bending strengthens back muscles and keeps leg and hip joints supple.

The back is alternately arched and curved. Strengthens back and abdominal muscles.

A position of RELAXATION is assumed and by deep, regular breathing and conscious relaxation of different groups of muscles the patient, with practice, learns to reach a state almost of somnolence at will. She will make use of this between contractions when in labour.

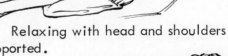

Relaxing with head and shoulders supported.

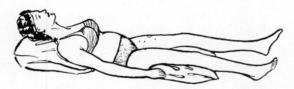

Relaxing with thighs supported.

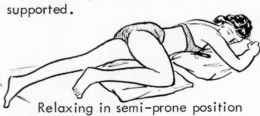

Relaxing in semi-prone position with two pillows.

MINOR COMPLAINTS

HEARTBURN

Probably due to oesophageal reflux of gastric acid. The enlarging uterus encourages some degree of hiatus hernia as pregnancy advances. Sleeping in a semi-recumbent position helps, so do alkalies, especially when containing a local anaesthetic which acts directly on the painful mucosa.

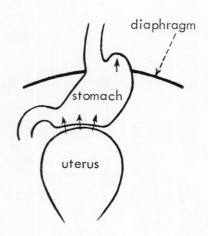

LEG CRAMPS
BACHACHE
SCIATIC PAIN
FEMORAL NERVE PAIN

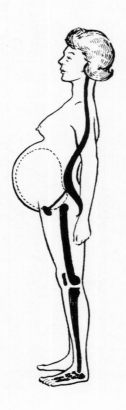

None of these complaints can be easily explained, but they probably have some connection with the postural changes of pregnancy – the "Pride of pregnancy". Alterations in the centre of gravity cause a characteristic lordosis; and this along with the softening of ligaments caused by the steroid hormones may produce pressure on nerve roots (leading to nerve pain and cramps) and muscle spasm (leading to bachache). Treatment is directed mainly towards resting the muscles and preventing undue flexion of the vertebral joints by getting the patient to sleep with boards under her mattress.

MINOR COMPLAINTS

SUBJECTIVE COMPLAINTS

Fatigue, somnolence, headache, 'blackouts'. These are most marked in the early months and their cause is uncertain. Insomnia is best treated by mild soporifics.

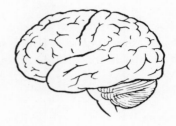

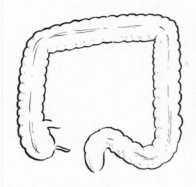

CONSTIPATION

Due in part to oestrogenic effect on smooth muscle, in part to obstruction by the foetal head. Attention to diet is the first step, but the patient is miserable if a bowel motion is not achieved every second or third day and laxatives are often required.

MORNING SICKNESS

The cause is not known, but is probably due to the effect of steroids on the liver and to reduced gastric motility. It is aggravated by cooking and by fatigue. The treatment of mild cases includes rest, light carbohydrate diet in the morning (biscuits and milk) and a variety of drugs including antihistamines (for their anti-emetic and sedative effects) and antispasmodics such as belladonna derivatives. These are all given empirically.

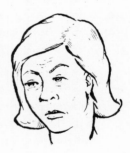

PRESSURE in the PELVIS

This gradually obstructs venous return and leads to haemorrhoids, varicose veins of legs, and varicosities of vulva and abdominal wall. Treatment must of course be symptomatic. The haemorrhoids can be helped by suppositories and only in rare cases is haemorrhoidectomy required. The legs can be clothed in special thigh stockings.

VAGINAL DISCHARGE

The normal vaginal discharge increases in pregnancy because of the greater vascularity of the vagina. The desquamation from the surface and the transudation through the walls is increased. The acidity is reduced and the pH is raised.

Normal

The normal discharge is milky in character but the quantity is not enough to cause irritation or to require a pad.

The increased moisture of the vulva and perineum during pregnancy allow abnormal organisms to spread into the vagina. Many of these bacteria originate in the bowel and tend to cause foetor.

The treatment is by ordinary hygiene, loose absorbent clothing, and talcum powder.

Yeasts

Glycosuria in pregnancy creates favourable conditions for yeasts such as monilia to flourish. The yeasts cause a marked reddening of the mucosa with small white flakes and plaques adhering to the wall and a smegma-like discharge. Local hygiene will help and there are a number of local treatments which are effective e.g. nystatin (nystan), amphotericin B (fungilin), noxytiolin (gynaflex) and gentian violet and its derivatives.

Trichomonads

Trichomonal vaginitis has a greenish-yellow discharge, sometimes with tiny vacuoles in it and a vague malodour. There may also be blood staining. Treatment is by local hygiene and vaginal medication e.g. hydrargaphen (penotrane), nifurantil (magmilor).

There is an oral treatment by metronidazole (flagyl) but this is inadvisable in the first half of pregnancy.

The husband should be treated too as intercourse may cause reinfection.

Gonorrhoea

Gonorrhoea must be kept in mind as a cause of purulent discharge.

PELVIC JOINT PAINS

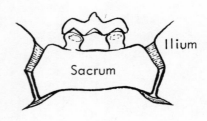

The Pelvic Joints and Ligaments are relaxed during pregnancy. This may give slight mechanical advantage as the pelvis is not so rigid as in the non-pregnant state, but it also impairs the natural locking mechanism of the sacrum to rotation of the ilium. The weight bearing strain is then heavy on the ligaments, causing sacro-iliac strain usually affecting one side more than the other.

Treatment in severe cases is to relieve the weight-bearing by confining the patient to lying flat on a bed with fracture boards. In extreme cases a plaster shell may be needed.

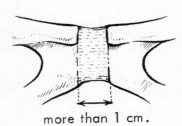

more than 1 cm.

The Symphysis Pubis may separate in late pregnancy and cause pain both at the pubis and the sacro-iliac joints on walking. The symphysis is painful to touch and sometimes a finger can be placed between the two edges of the symphysis. Flexion of one thigh will show that there is undue mobility and independence of the two pubic bones. On X-ray examination a gap of more than 1 cm is regarded as diagnostic.

Treatment is by rest in bed but severe cases may require to be nursed with a sling round the hips. Bandaging or strapping round the pelvic girdle may give relief.

Engagement of the head acts as an internal splint and may relieve symptoms so that the major period of discomfort is in the puerperium.

Subluxation of the symphyseal joint has the advantage of giving an increase in pelvic size and thus an easier labour.

Coccydynia

This condition is sometimes a cause of discomfort in the antenatal period as the ischial ligaments drag on a tender coccyx, but more commonly the discomfort is in the puerperium due to the excessive displacement of the coccyx and rupture of the ligaments in labour or to the mobilising of a coccyx which had been fused.

Treatment is by rest, and time will heal, but in severe cases peri-articular steroid injections will relieve pain.

NERVE PAINS

Sciatica

This is described as a traumatic neuritis of the puerperium (page 314) but it may occur during the pregnancy as a pain in the area supplied by the sciatic nerve. Altered posture may be a cause, compressing the nerve in the foramen between L5 and S1. The foetal head may press on the nerve at the pelvic brim or in the cavity.

Treatment is difficult though the patient may find her own way of relieving her discomfort. The following movements often help:-
1. Lying supine on a flat hard surface (e.g. floor) and stretching.
2. Sitting on a hard chair and leaning forward.
3. Standing on one leg and flexing the other thigh.
4. Lying on one side.

Carpal Tunnel Syndrome

This is due to compression of the median nerve by oedema of the surrounding tissues in the carpal tunnel at the wrist. There is tingling and numbness in the hands and fingers especially noted on waking. Pain however may be referred to the elbow or shoulder and may cause confusion with brachial plexus pain.

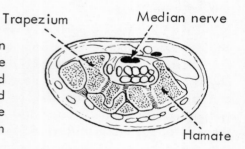

Treatment: Diuretics and low salt intake may help. Finger flexions may also help especially if the hand and arm are held up above the head. If these treatments are inadequate the hand is immobilised by supporting bandages or a splint maintaining the hand in a neutral position. If all else fails then the transverse carpal ligament is divided. The condition usually disappears spontaneously in the puerperium but care of the baby may cause relapse.

Brachial Plexus Pain

This is due to excessive shoulder droop with traction on the cords of the brachial plexus in the neck or to pressure on the plexus and vessels of the arm between the first rib and clavicle. Oedema probably plays a part.

The patient complains of tingling and numbness affecting the radial and median nerve areas.

Treatment: Diuretics and resting the arm in a sling may relieve, though elevation of the arm above the head is also helpful.

NERVE PAINS

Meralgia Paraesthetica

This condition is due to compression of the lateral cutaneous nerve of the thigh at the lateral end of the inguinal ligament or as it penetrates the dense fascia lata.

There is paraesthesia of the lateral side of the thigh sometimes with a burning quality. The symptoms are made worse by standing and walking. The distension of pregnancy is probably a contributory factor and also the oedema of the tissues. The symptoms disappear spontaneously after delivery.

Intercostal Neuralgia

This may not be a nerve pain but be due to muscle spasm. The pain is intermittent in character. It is found in late pregnancy and sometimes is of 'girdle' type, usually unilateral.

The pain is often caused by sitting in a relaxed position and is relieved by posture. A straight backed chair, a lumbar cushion and lateral flexion of the trunk away from the affected side will all relieve the pain.

Facial Nerve (Bell's) Palsy

Caused probably by oedema, this occurs rarely in the last trimester of pregnancy or the early puerperium and is usually temporary, clearing up spontaneously 3 or 4 weeks after confinement.

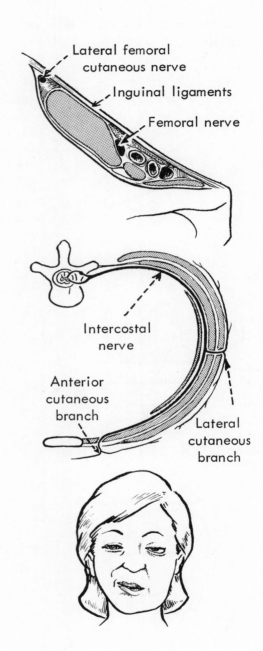

Lateral femoral cutaneous nerve

Inguinal ligaments

Femoral nerve

Intercostal nerve

Anterior cutaneous branch

Lateral cutaneous branch

X-RAY PELVIMETRY

Radiological study of the pelvis is usually reserved for cases of doubt because of the risk of radiation to maternal and foetal gonads. (3 views commonly taken)

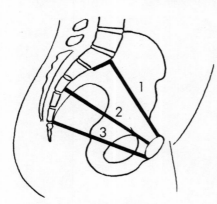

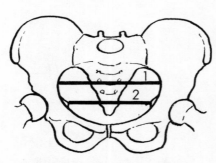

ERECT LATERAL VIEW

The ERECT LATERAL VIEW shows:-
1. Obstetric conjugate diameter, sacral angle and the angle of inclination of the brim.
2. Antero-posterior diameter of mid-pelvic cavity.
3. Antero-posterior diameter of outlet.

It also shows shape of sacrosciatic notch, length and curvature of sacrum and shape of ischial spines. The thickness and depth of the symphysis pubis can be estimated and the presenting part and its relationship to the brim assessed.

The ANTERO-POSTERIOR VIEW shows:-
1. Transverse diameter of inlet.
2. Interspinous diameter.

The general shape and symmetry of the pelvic brim can be assessed and the breadth and shape of the sacrum observed.

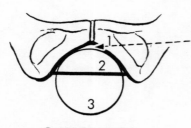

ANTERO-POSTERIOR VIEW

OUTLET VIEW

The OUTLET VIEW shows:-
1. Shape of subpubic arch. The angle may be measured by the lines joining the lower border of the symphysis pubis to the ischial tuberosities.
2. Inter-tuberischial diameter. This is measured 1 cm. above the tuberosities.
3. Assessment of subpubic capacity. A circle 9.3 cm. in diameter is applied to the subpubic area and the distance between the symphysis and the circumference is measured. This measurement is the "waste space of Morris" and should not exceed 1 cm.

The foetal head in labour, well flexed and moulded, should approximate to 9.3 cm. ($3\frac{3}{4}$ins).

X-RAY PELVIMETRY

There is another view sometimes taken with the patient reclining at an angle of 60° to bring the pelvic brim into the horizontal. This gives an excellent view of the brim shape but means a high dosage of X-ray for the foetal gonads in vertex presentation (nearly twice as much as for the three other views). It is not commonly employed.

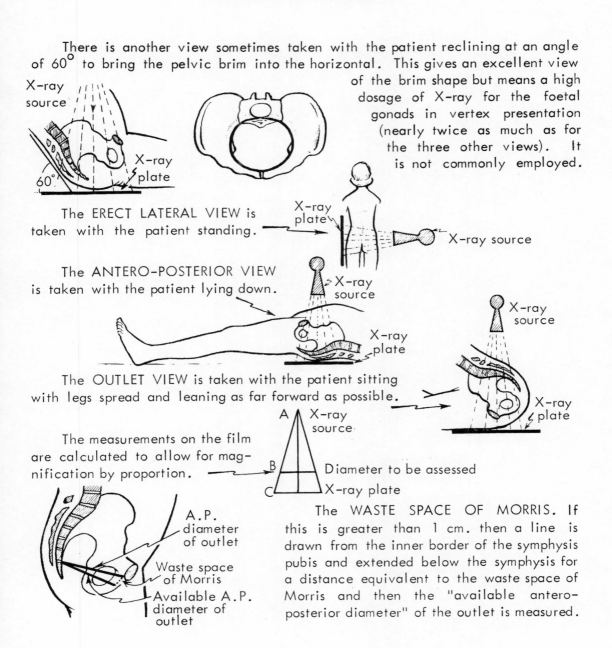

The ERECT LATERAL VIEW is taken with the patient standing.

The ANTERO-POSTERIOR VIEW is taken with the patient lying down.

The OUTLET VIEW is taken with the patient sitting with legs spread and leaning as far forward as possible.

The measurements on the film are calculated to allow for magnification by proportion.

A — X-ray source
B — Diameter to be assessed
C — X-ray plate

A.P. diameter of outlet

Waste space of Morris

Available A.P. diameter of outlet

The WASTE SPACE OF MORRIS. If this is greater than 1 cm. then a line is drawn from the inner border of the symphysis pubis and extended below the symphysis for a distance equivalent to the waste space of Morris and then the "available antero-posterior diameter" of the outlet is measured.

CHAPTER 6

SYSTEMIC DISEASES IN PREGNANCY

CARDIAC DISEASE

In normal non-pregnant subjects approximately 5,000 ml of blood are pumped through the lungs every minute by the right ventricle. To balance this the same amount must be put out by the left ventricle.

During pregnancy the blood volume increases progressively to reach a peak around 28 to 32 weeks. The output of the ventricles is raised to 6,000 ml per minute and the rate of flow through the valves and vessels from right to left must increase considerably.

Mitral stenosis is the usual lesion associated with cardiac failure in pregnancy. It obstructs the flow from right to left. The rate of flow through an orifice is roughly inversely proportional to the radius raised to the 4th power. If the radius of the mitral is reduced by one half the rate of flow is cut to one sixteenth and the cardiac output will be reduced greatly. In overcoming this two changes take place:-

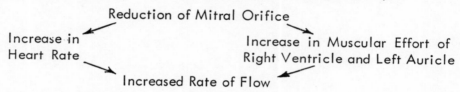

Reduction of Mitral Orifice

Increase in Heart Rate

Increase in Muscular Effort of Right Ventricle and Left Auricle

Increased Rate of Flow

While these changes may maintain a normal circulation they reduce the cardiac reserve and the following further changes will tend to occur if there is additional strain.

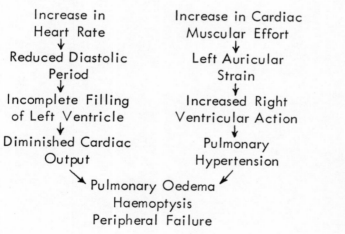

Increase in Heart Rate
↓
Reduced Diastolic Period
↓
Incomplete Filling of Left Ventricle
↓
Diminished Cardiac Output

Increase in Cardiac Muscular Effort
↓
Left Auricular Strain
↓
Increased Right Ventricular Action
↓
Pulmonary Hypertension

Pulmonary Oedema
Haemoptysis
Peripheral Failure

The balance is precarious and in effect depends on myocardinal efficiency and the degree of tachycardia influencing the diastole.

CARDIAC DISEASE

It must be remembered that the patient suffering from mitral stenosis enters pregnancy with a cardiac reserve which is already reduced even if there are no signs of failure.

Cardiac failure may come on gradually in pregnancy as the demand for a rise in cardiac output accompanies the increasing blood volume. Acute failure in the form of pulmonary oedema may occur early in pregnancy when the blood volume begins to increase or when it is approaching its maximum. Most commonly however acute failure is precipitated by some other incidental change. Usually it is some circumstance which causes tachycardia in excess of 110 per minute thus reducing the diastolic period, the filling of the left ventricle and the cardiac output. This in turn leads to obstruction of the pulmonary blood flow and to oedema of the lungs.

Common aggravating factors are:-

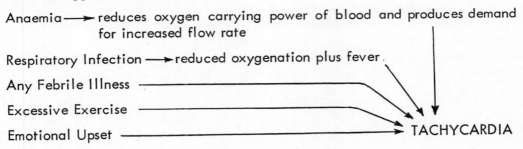

Anaemia⟶ reduces oxygen carrying power of blood and produces demand for increased flow rate

Respiratory Infection ⟶reduced oxygenation plus fever

Any Febrile Illness

Excessive Exercise

Emotional Upset ⟶ TACHYCARDIA

Acute failure may also occur immediately after the third stage of delivery due to the sudden increase in the circulating volume, which may exceed the capacity of the mitral valve to pass blood.

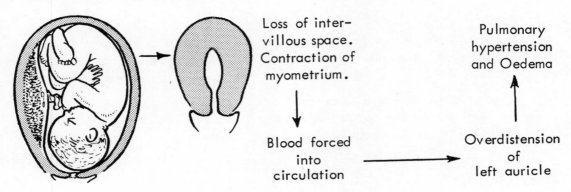

Loss of intervillous space. Contraction of myometrium.

↓

Blood forced into circulation ⟶ Overdistension of left auricle

↑

Pulmonary hypertension and Oedema

CARDIAC DISEASE

Diagnosis

The diagnosis of mitral stenosis is not difficult and in many cases the patient is already known to have the lesion.

Owing to slight changes in timing a third sound may be heard at the apex even when the heart is normal.

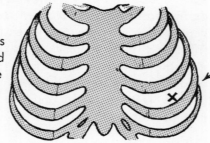

The apex beat is commonly altered in position in pregnancy.

4th interspace and further to the left than in non-pregnant.

Also misleading is the absence of signs of congestive cardiac failure. The failure is almost always a forward failure associated with diminished left ventricular output. Cyanosis, turgid neck veins, enlarged tender liver and cardiac oedema are rarely observed. When congestive cardiac failure does occur its onset is gradual and it responds to the usual treatment (bed rest, digitalis, cardophyllin).

The common symptoms of cardiac failure in pregnancy are dyspnoea, limitation of activity, fatigue, palpitations, and sometimes pain of an anginal type.

Management

The anatomical lesion is not so important as the functional grading.

This is carried out at the first visit and the patient placed in one of the following grades.

Grade 1
Patient has no symptoms and no limitation of physical activity.

Grade 2
Patient is comfortable at rest. Ordinary physical activity causes fatigue, palpitations and dyspnoea.

Grade 3
The patient is comfortable at rest. Any activity causes palpitations, dyspnoea and possibly anginal pain.

Grade 4
Even when resting the patient is dyspnoeic.

The condition of the patient must be assessed at regular intervals throughout pregnancy.

CARDIAC DISEASE

Forty per cent of patients with mitral stenosis enter pregnancy with no symptoms but almost all deteriorate one grade as pregnancy progresses.

Grades 1 and 2

Attend to teeth, gums. Bacterial endocarditis is a constant danger.

Weigh patient regularly. Try to prevent excessive blood volume change. Restrict salt intake. Prevent excessive weight gain. Give high protein low carbohydrate diet.

See frequently. In all cases advise daily rest.

All febrile illnesses are dangerous. Sulphonamides may be given as a prophylactic.

Anaemia is common and produces deterioration of at least one grade. Treat vigorously with intramuscular iron if necessary.

Hospitalise for week or two at 28 weeks. Reassess at this time and every 2 weeks thereafter.

Hospitalise once more for at least 2 or 3 weeks. Premature labour is common and the immediate puerperium is dangerous.

General ante-natal care is important. Forewarning of obstetric difficulties is essential. Malpositions should be corrected.

If early signs of failure develop:-
1. Complete bed rest.
2. Give sedatives liberally.
3. Digoxin may be given with care. Be guided by pulse rate.
4. Restrict fluid intake and give diuretics.
5. No disturbance of the pregnancy can be contemplated until all symptoms have disappeared.

Grade 3 patients should be in hospital throughout pregnancy.

Grade 4 patients should not only be in hospital but must be totally confined to bed.

CARDIAC DISEASE

As indicated acute pulmonary oedema may occur at any time. It is of sudden onset. The main feature is intense dyspnoea with bronchospasm.

Treatment is required urgently and has five objectives.

1. Relieve anxiety. Give morphine gr $\frac{1}{4}$ (15 mg) intravenously.
2. Increase oxygenation. Give oxygen by mask until oxygen tent available.
3. Reduce blood volume. Remove 500 - 600 ml of blood by rapid venesection.
4. Control tachycardia. Give digoxin but watch pulse rate. If slowed too much, the output of the right ventricle may exceed capacity of mitral valve.
5. Relieve bronchospasm. Give intravenous aminophylline 250 mg.

Throughout the treatment the patient must be propped up. When immediate danger is over diuretics may be given.

The cause of the acute failure must be treated if still present and precautions taken to avoid further episodes.

Termination of Pregnancy

There is almost no place for this in the treatment of cardiac patients. After 12 weeks when the blood volume begins to increase the risks are greater than those of continuing the pregnancy. The stress of operation, the anaesthetic and the danger of infection are all important factors.

Equally, at the other end of pregnancy there is little indication for inducing labour. Again the possibility of infection is a real danger.

LABOUR

Penicillin 0.5 mega-units should be given twice daily throughout labour. Usually labour is easy. There is no place for trial of labour. Elective Caesarian section is not a method of choice but must be carried out if obstetric problems exist which will make delivery difficult.

First Stage

Anxiety will cause tachycardia and breathlessness. Give liberal sedation. Morphia gr $\frac{1}{4}$ (15 mg) is recommended.

CARDIAC DISEASE

Patients in grades 3 and 4 should remain propped up. If symptoms of failure appear give continuous oxygen and carry out venesection. Give digoxin if pulse rate exceeds 110 or respirations 24 per minute. Cardiac failure in the first stage is not in itself a reason for Caesarean section. Interference should be avoided at all costs and the patient nursed through to the second stage when delivery becomes possible. If for some reason delivery is considered imperative the obstetrician has a choice of three methods.

1. Delivery using traction with a small ventouse cup.
2. Caesarean section.
3. Incision of cervix under local anaesthesia and extraction of foetus by forceps or ventouse.

Gas and oxygen should not be given as oxygen saturation of blood will be reduced and tachycardia induced. Trilene or halothane are used as general anaesthetics.

Second Stage

Curtail effort on the part of the patient, bearing down should be avoided. Normal uterine contractions are sufficient to cause descent of the head. To speed delivery episiotomy is carried out under pudendal block.

Forceps or ventouse should only be used if delivery has not occurred 20 minutes after full dilatation.

Third Stage

There should be no hurry at this point. Time must be allowed for circulatory adjustment. Oxytocics such as ergometrine are not advisable as a routine treatment. Venesection of one pint may be useful at this juncture.

Suturing of the episiotomy may be carried out under local anaesthesia.

As soon as delivery is complete the patient should be propped up. Give morphia and oxygen. No attempt should be made to stop blood loss unless it become excessive.

PUERPERIUM

The first 12 hours when circulatory changes are taking place, are critical. Blood which would otherwise be filling the chorio-decidual space and supplying the uterus is now added to the general circulation and the right ventricle may be overloaded.

The patient should have a minimum of 14 days rest or until all signs of incipient failure have disappeared. Breast feeding is not advisable.

CARDIAC DISEASE

Caesarean Section

This should by avoided if possible. The strain of operation and anaesthetic exceeds that of vaginal delivery. It should only be considered if there is a marked delay or other obstetric problems e.g. placenta praevia.

Prognosis

Maternal: Cardiac disease is responsible for 10% of all maternal deaths in the United Kingdom.

Mortality Rate in Cardiac Cases

Overall	2.5%
Grades 1 and 2	less than 0.5%
Grade 3	5.0%
Grade 4	22.0%

If auricular fibrillation occurs 70% of cases go in to failure and the mortality rate soars to 41%. After the age of 35 the risk is doubled in all grades.

Foetus: The prognosis is related to maternal cardiac failure.

Still birth rate	3% (corrected to 1%)
Neonatal death rate	2%

Premature labour is common:	Overall incidence	16%
	In cardiac failure	43%

Subsequent Pregnancies

Patients in grades 1 and 2 should be advised to allow 2 years to elapse before contemplating another pregnancy.

Another pregnancy should not be contemplated by patients in grades 3 and 4 and sterilisation should be considered.

Valvotomy during Pregnancy

Opinion varies regarding the advisability of valvotomy during pregnancy but a considerable number of successes have been reported.

There seems little danger in performing the operation in suitable cases during the first half of pregnancy.

ANAEMIA

Pregnancy makes considerable nutritional demands on the mother. It is not surprising therefore that anaemia is a common complication.

The main nutritional factors involved are Iron, Folic acid and other Vitamins of the B group, and Protein.

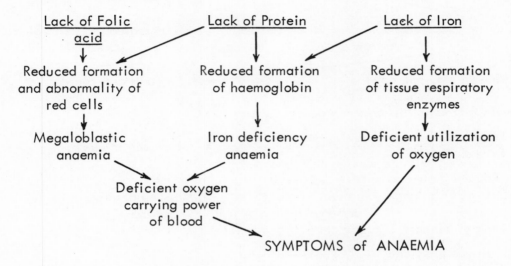

Although there are two distinct anaemic conditions each apparently due to deficiency of a single factor (iron deficiency anaemia and megaloblastic anaemia due to folic acid deficiency) it should be remembered that a single deficiency is almost an impossibility.

The deficiency of any substance may be due to:-

1. Diminished intake.
2. Abnormal absorption.
3. Reduced storage.
4. Abnormal utilization.
5. Abnormal demand.

The aetiology of anaemia must be considered in relation to these principles.

IRON DEFICIENCY ANAEMIA

During pregnancy there is an increased demand for iron amounting to approximately 1,230 mg. There is however a saving of 220 mg. due to 9 months amenorrhoea. The total amount of extra iron required will be 1,010 mg.

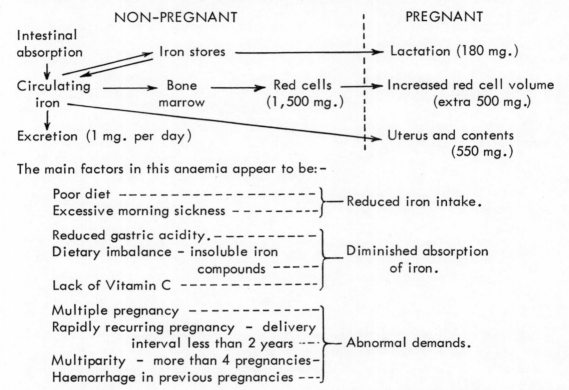

The main factors in this anaemia appear to be:-

Poor diet ------------------------- ⎫
Excessive morning sickness --------- ⎬— Reduced iron intake.

Reduced gastric acidity. ----------- ⎫
Dietary imbalance - insoluble iron
                      compounds ----- ⎬— Diminished absorption
                                              of iron.
Lack of Vitamin C ----------------- ⎭

Multiple pregnancy ------------- ⎫
Rapidly recurring pregnancy - delivery
               interval less than 2 years --- ⎬— Abnormal demands.
Multiparity - more than 4 pregnancies-
Haemorrhage in previous pregnancies ---⎭

<u>SYMPTOMS</u>:- The majority of patients make no complaint even if the anaemia is moderately severe. Subjective feelings are accepted as part of the 'burden of pregnancy'.

Equally, due to the peripheral vasodilatation of pregnancy (heat loss mechanism) pallor is not a feature of anaemia of pregnancy. IT IS THEREFORE IMPERATIVE THAT THE HAEMOGLOBIN VALUE SHOULD BE ASCERTAINED IN EVERY PREGNANT PATIENT.

Close questioning may reveal the same symptoms as in non-pregnant anaemic subjects.

IRON DEFICIENCY ANAEMIA

BLOOD CHANGES

The progressive haemodilution in pregnancy makes it impossible to set a single point on the haemoglobin scale which will divide anaemic from non-anaemic subjects. In healthy non-pregnant individuals the haemoglobin reading is usually 12.6 g per 100 ml. or over. This value declines during pregnancy.

At term the value may be as low as 10.8 g per 100 ml. This is a decline of almost 2 g per 100 ml. The lowest acceptable normal in pregnancy probably ought to be 10.5 g but this applies only to late pregnancy. A patient with this reading in early pregnancy will be anaemic at a later stage.

A rough prediction may be made as follows:-
Haemoglobin reading at 12 weeks minus 2 g (or 14 per cent on Haldane scale)
= Haemoglobin reading at term.

Ideally the aim is to have the patient's haemoglobin value at 11 g or over per 100 ml. at term. This would mean a value of 13 g per 100 ml. in early pregnancy. In practice a reading of 12.5 g per 100 ml. in early pregnancy is considered reasonably satisfactory. Below this figure anaemia is present. At mid-pregnancy the lowest normal reading is 11.5 g per 100 ml., and at term 10.5 g.

MORPHOLOGY

Except in the severest grades anisocytosis (alteration in size) is unusual. Poikilocytosis (change in shape) is rarely seen and the cells appear uniformly coloured.

TREATMENT

This will vary with the severity of anaemia and the duration of pregnancy.

EARLY PREGNANCY

Oral iron is the treatment of choice. Ferrous sulphate tablets, 200 mg. 3 times per day, are given. This will produce a haemoglobin increase of 1g/100 ml./month. This is a satisfactory rate of response provided the anaemia is not of gross degree e.g. 6 g or less per 100 ml. Lack of response is generally due to failure to take the treatment. This may be due to sickness caused by the iron. Organic salts of iron - gluconate, succinate or fumarate, - may be tried. If there is no response and the patient is known to have taken the tablets a more complete haematological investigation should be undertaken.

IRON DEFICIENCY ANAEMIA

LATE PREGNANCY

After 30 weeks and in all cases of very severe anaemia the response to oral iron is too slow and parenteral iron will be required. This may be given in two ways:-

A. <u>Repeated intramuscular injections</u>. 250 mg of iron will raise haemoglobin by 1 g per 100 ml. Injections are given every other day. A response of almost 1 g Hb per 100 ml. occurs within a week.

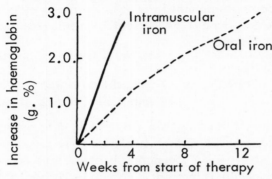
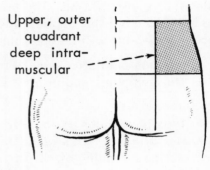

B. <u>Total dose infusion</u>. By this method the total iron deficiency is corrected by a single intravenous infusion of iron-dextran in 1,000 ml. saline given slowly over several hours.

The deficiency in haemoglobin in g x 250 = mg of iron which must be given. To allow for depleted iron stores, blood loss at delivery and foetal demands this figure must be increased by 50 per cent.

Example:
> Haemoglobin reading of patient = 8 g per 100 ml.
> Haemoglobin reading desired   = 12 g per 100 ml.
> Haemoglobin deficit   = 4 g per 100 ml.
> Iron required for maternal haemoglobin = 4 x 250 = 1,000 mg
> Iron required for storage, foetus and delivery = 500 mg
> Total dose for infusion = 1,500 mg

Anaphylactoid reactions may occur. This method must never be used in patients with a history of allergy.

An oral antihistamine tablet is given 30 minutes before infusion. Iron solution is given at the rate of 10 drops per minute for 30 minutes. If there is no reaction the rate may then be increased to 45 drops per minute.

IRON DEFICIENCY ANAEMIA

SEVERE ANAEMIA NEAR TIME OF DELIVERY

Up to the 35th week parenteral iron may be given. Beyond this time, in view of the usual uncertainty in dates and the possibility of premature labour, a transfusion of packed red cells may be given. This is an emergency treatment and should only be used if the patient's haemoglobin is below 9 g per 100 ml. It must be realised that while the haemoglobin and therefore the oxygen carrying power of the blood will be increased the respiratory enzymes (iron containing) of the tissues will be unaffected. The tissues are unhealthy, particularly the myocardium. The transfusion must be given very slowly and preferably in two or more stages to avoid cardiac failure. One pint of blood raises the haemoglobin value by approximately 0.7 g per 100 ml.

The main reason for blood transfusion in this condition is not primarily correction of anaemia but that any further loss of blood at delivery will be dangerous and may be fatal.

REFRACTORY ANAEMIAS

In most cases seemingly refractory anaemia is due to failure to take the prescribed treatment. If however the anaemia truly fails to respond to treatment remember that nutritional deficiencies are rarely single. Folic acid deficiency should be suspected and looked for. If the haemoglobin still fails to rise further investigation is required to eliminate the possibility of a rarer blood disease.

To Summarise:

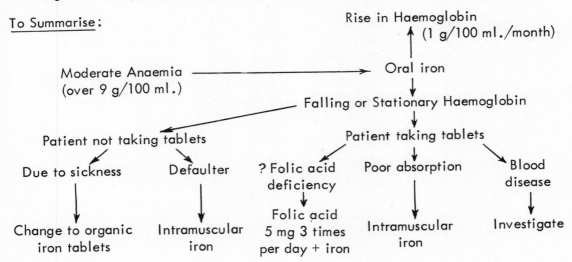

FOLIC ACID DEFICIENCY

Folic Acid is necessary for the formation of nucleic acids and therefore nuclei. Its absence leads to reduction of cell proliferation. Where the deficiency is partial those tissues, such as bone marrow, which are constantly proliferating, show the main effects.

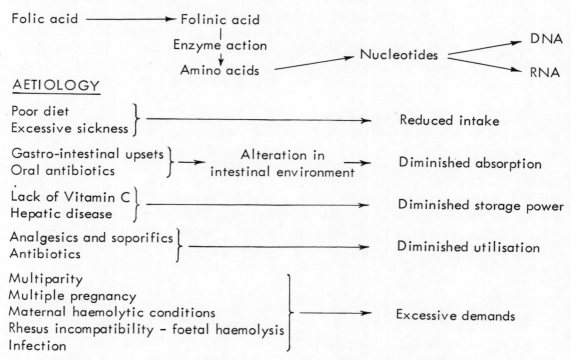

AETIOLOGY

Poor diet
Excessive sickness } ⟶ Reduced intake

Gastro-intestinal upsets
Oral antibiotics } ⟶ Alteration in intestinal environment ⟶ Diminished absorption

Lack of Vitamin C
Hepatic disease } ⟶ Diminished storage power

Analgesics and soporifics
Antibiotics } ⟶ Diminished utilisation

Multiparity
Multiple pregnancy
Maternal haemolytic conditions
Rhesus incompatibility – foetal haemolysis
Infection } ⟶ Excessive demands

The main factors are poor intake coupled with the excessive demands of pregnancy.

CLINICAL FINDINGS

These depend on the severity of the deficiency. In the early stages the patient may have no symptoms and no apparent signs apart from a moderately low haemoglobin value. The diagnosis is frequently made when, despite continued iron therapy, the haemoglobin value first increases and then remains static. The deficiency in these cases is a double one and may be visualised as follows:-

FOLIC ACID DEFICIENCY

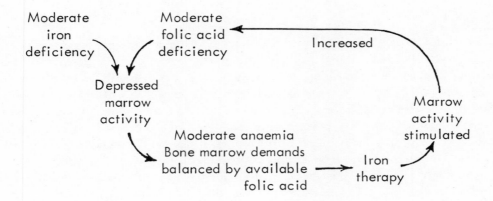

In its severe form this deficiency is characterised by a megaloblastic anaemia. Cases are most often seen among patients with haemoglobin values below 8 g per 100 ml. Almost invariably these patients have symptoms of anaemia – breathlessness, giddiness, palpitations, swelling of feet and ankles. Signs of nutritional deficiency may be present – glossitis, oral fissures, and irregularities of the nails. The spleen is commonly enlarged and in very severe cases there may be vomiting, diarrhoea and pyrexia and even a purpuric rash.

LABORATORY DIAGNOSIS

In almost all cases the diagnosis can be made by examination of the peripheral blood, and apart from the low haemoglobin value most of the changes are seen in a blood film. These consist of:-

a.   Macrocytosis.
b.   Poikilocytosis in very severe cases.
c.   Giant multi-segmented polymorphs.
d.   Slight shift to left in white cells.
e.   Low platelet count.
f.   Low white cell count.
g.   Megaloblasts are present in severe cases but may only be found after centrifuging the blood and examining a film made from the buffy coat.

In mild cases only the first three changes may be seen. Frequently the macrocytes are poorly coloured due to concomitant iron deficiency. Very occasionally it may be necessary to examine the bone marrow when megoblasts will be found.

FOLIC ACID DEFICIENCY

TREATMENT

Folic acid is specific for this condition and the dosage is 15 – 20 mg per day orally. In severe cases it may at first be given parenterally. Response is rapid but folic acid must be maintained until pregnancy is over. It should be discontinued early in the puerperium, whenever normal blood levels are attained. In patients who have had little or no antenatal care this anaemia may appear in the puerperium. Anaemia is almost certainly present antenatally. The apparent sudden onset is due to the added strain of loss of blood at delivery. Treatment is as before but the folic acid must be stopped as soon as possible and certainly within three months of delivery. Such a case is best dealt with under hospital laboratory control in order to avoid aggravating a possible developing Addisonian pernicious anaemia.

In all cases of folic acid deficiency, antenatal or puerperal, iron should also be given.

POTENTIAL ANAEMIAS AND PROPHYLAXIS

Many patients seen in early pregnancy will have border-line haemoglobin values. Oral iron supplements can be given after the stage of sickness has passed. Alternatively, all antenatal patients, whatever their haemoglobin values, may be given iron supplements. It has been suggested that folic acid supplements should also be given to 'normal' pregnant patients. Approximately 200 – 300 μg may be given daily and there are a number of preparations combining both folic acid and iron. Even so, the patient's haemoglobin must be checked at regular intervals. Biological problems are rarely completely solved by this kind of simplification.

Finally, pills and potions are only supplements and never a substitute for a good mixed diet.

Other anaemias which may be encountered are:-

1. Acquired haemolytic anaemia. This may manifest itself in pregnancy. The treatment is the same as for the non-pregnant case.

2. Drug induced haemolytic anaemias. This is usually encountered in Eastern Mediterranean and negro populations and may be related to glucose-6-phosphate dehydrogenase deficiency of the red cells. Drugs such as anti-malarials, sulphonamides, nitrofurans, phenacetin and other analgesics can cause its manifestation.

3. Thalassaemia minor.

All of these haemolytic conditions tend to induce a folic acid deficiency.

PUERPERAL ANAEMIA

This is a common condition arising as a result of incidents at the time of delivery or lack of antenatal care. Frequently both factors are involved in the same patient, and the anaemia is often megaloblastic.

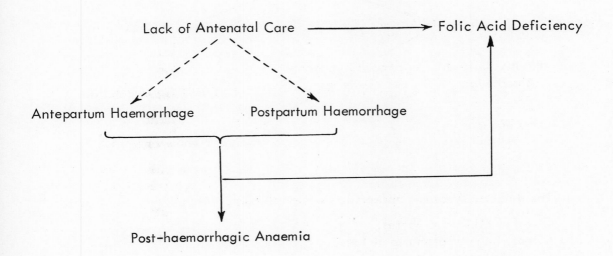

COMPLICATIONS DUE TO ANAEMIA

Anaemia increases the incidence of a number of complications in pregnancy. The main effects are as follows.

Premature labour ——————————— 2 – 3 times overall incidence

Infection – urinary or genital tract ——— twice as common

Antepartum haemorrhage
Postpartum haemorrhage } ——————— said to be more common but this is doubtful.

DIABETES

Metabolic changes induced by pregnancy make it difficult to control diabetes during gestation. In a sense pregnancy tends to be diabetogenic.

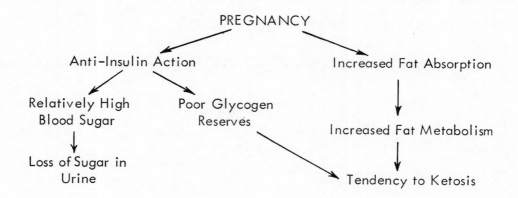

The diabetic syndrome appears to develop through three phases.

1. Overt or clinical diabetes.
2. Latent, non-symptomatic diabetes.
3. Pre-diabetes.

All three are influenced by the diabetogenic effect of pregnancy.

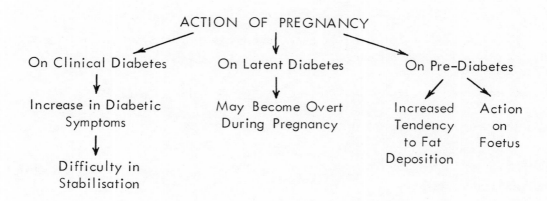

DIABETES

Clinical Diabetes

Almost all cases of this type are already diagnosed and being treated before attending the ante-natal clinic. The problem of those cases arising during pregnancy or discovered at ante-natal visits is considered under latent diabetes.

While pregnancy tends to influence the diabetic condition, diabetes also has considerable effect on the pregnancy and both aspects have to be considered in management of the patient.

Effect of Pregnancy on Diabetes

1. The carbohydrate tolerance is reduced, especially in the last trimester.

2. Insulin requirements increase and fluctuate during the same period.

3. Glycosuria occurs in greater degree and may be misleading as a measure of the diabetic state.

4. Acidosis is more easily induced. In combating this state with insulin, hypoglycaemia may occur.

5. Diabetic lesions such as retinopathy tend to worsen.

Effect of Diabetes on Pregnancy

1. The fertility rate in untreated diabetes is low (25 - 30%). With good treatment it becomes normal.
2. Hydramnios is always present and severe in 25%. It is thought to be related to sugar excreted in the foetal urine.
3. The incidence of pre-eclampsia (20%) is high.
4. Malpresentations and premature labour are common, possibly related to hydramnios.
5. Dystocia is frequent due to the increase in foetal size. Inertia may be a problem.
6. Infection is an ever present danger.
7. Congenital abnormalities are said to be more frequent.

Management

This will obviously depend on the severity of the diabetic condition. Mild or 'chemical' diabetes may be controlled by diet alone. Severe diabetes is frequently difficult to control.

DIABETES

Moderate to Severe Diabetes

Early pregnancy

No change from pre-
pregnant treatment

30 weeks   Admit to hospital.
Estimate fasting blood sugar daily.
Adjust diet – 30 cal per kg (include 150 g of carbohydrate).
Use soluble insulin to control any fluctuations in blood
   sugar.
Watch patient's weight. If evidence of fluid retention –
   chlorothiazide 1 – 2 g daily.
Base treatment on blood sugar not urinary sugar.
Watch out for monilial infection.

36 weeks   X-ray patient –
   Check for skeletal deformity in foetus; estimate maturity.
   Beware of wrong assessment of maturity. Babies are longer
   than normal if diabetic control is poor.

Interruption of
Pregnancy.

Intra-uterine death is more common after 36 weeks and pregnancy is usually interrupted in the 37th week, but the optimum time depends on several factors:-

1. The presence of pre-eclampsia.
2. The degree of hydramnios.
3. The severity of the diabetic condition.
4. The patient's age.
5. The patient's obstetric history.

Elective Caesarean Section

This is usually carried out in:-

1. all severely diabetic patients.
2. elderly patients.
3. any case where difficulty in labour or delivery is anticipated.

DIABETES

Surgical Induction

This is employed in the following cases:-

1. Multipara with a history of previous satisfactory spontaneous vaginal deliveries.
2. Primigravida with no obstetric abnormalities.
3. Where there is congenital deformity incompatible with life.

Induction of labour is carried out in late afternoon. After an evening meal plus insulin the patient is stabilised and no further insulin is required till the following morning. Delivery is usually achieved by 8.00 a.m. in two thirds of the patients. If labour is not well established in 12 hours Caesarean section is carried out. Trial of labour has no place in the management of the pregnant diabetic patient.

Labour

Prolonged labour will cause ketosis due to poor carbohydrate intake, dehydration and possibly vomiting. Prevent by giving intravenous glucose drip – 10 g glucose per hour. If the condition threatens to become unstable give 40 g glucose plus 20 units insulin immediately. Where means are available the acid-base balance should be monitored on an Astrup apparatus and base deficit corrected.

Prolonged labour should be avoided if possible by performing Caesarean section. Prophylactic antibiotics may be given where labour is long.

Puerperium

There is a sharp fall in insulin requirements and the dose must be readjusted. The danger of infection remains a problem.

Baby

If the diabetes is well controlled the baby is usually normal but it is often oedematous and lethargic. If control has been poor the baby is commonly very large. The stomach is frequently full of liquor due to the inevitable hydramnios. In addition respiratory efforts are poor and it is prone to atelectasis.

1. Aspirate pharynx, larynx, trachea and stomach.
2. Provide intermittent positive pressure oxygen therapy if necessary.
3. Repeat aspirations every few hours for 48 hours.
4. Give no feeds for 48 hours.

DIABETES

Foetal Prognosis

Perinatal mortality is high even with good control. The reasons are not completely understood. Some of the factors involved in prognosis are:-

A. Control of Diabetes
   1. Controllability
      The younger the diabetic mother the more severe her diabetes and the more difficult it is to control.
   2. Degree of Control
      Poor control ⟶ blood sugar greater than 200 mg per 100 ml 3 hours after a meal. The mortality rate is at least 37%
      Good control ⟶ blood sugar less than 150 mg per 100 ml 3 hours after a meal. Mortality rate is reduced to 7.6%.

These figures depend on the presence of complications. Even with good control the overall mortality rate is 13%.

With good control: 50% of deaths occur in utero.
                    25% occur during labour.
                    25% are neonatal.
Most of the neonatal deaths take place within 48 hours.

B. Obstetric Complications
   1. Hypertension, either of essential nature or due to pre-eclampsia. The perinatal loss may reach 45%. Avoid pre-eclampsia by good control of diabetes and prevention of excessive weight gain.
   2. Hydramnios. This increases mortality by causing malpresentation. Asphyxia may result from inhalation of fluid. The severity of the hydramnios is directly related to the efficiency of diabetic control.

C. Premature Delivery
   Spontaneous due to hydramnios and baby size in poorly controlled cases or artificial interruption of pregnancy. The usual dangers of prematurity arise and expert paediatric care is essential.

D. Congenital Abnormalities
   These are said to be commoner in poorly controlled cases.

E. Neonatal Infection.

DIABETES

Latent Diabetes

In this condition the patient is on the verge of clinical diabetes and the diabetogenic influence of pregnancy may tip the scales and induce the chemical diabetes or even clinical diabetes.

The diagnosis may be difficult. Certain patients may be suspected to be especially at risk:-

1. Patients with a family history of diabetes.
2. Patients with a history of unexplained stillbirths.
3. Patients with a history of unexplained premature labours.
4. Patients who have produced babies over 10 lb birth weight or whose successive babies show a marked increase in birth weight.
5. Patients who are obese and show an excessive weight gain during pregnancy.
6. Patients with hydramnios.
7. Older patients.
8. Patients with signs of pre-eclampsia.

Test urine of all ante-natal patients for glucose

Clinistix
or Testape

Positive :
possible diabetic

Negative

Test urine for
Ketones

Member of pop-
ulation at risk

No suspicious
factors – normal

Positive

Negative

Test at intervals and
watch size of pregnancy

Almost
certainly
diabetes

Fasting blood
sugar

High

Abnormal

Glucose
tolerance
test

Member of popu-
lation at risk

Provocative
cortisone test

No suspicious factors. Probably normal.
Repeat fasting blood sugar at intervals
and watch size of pregnancy.

DIABETES

Glucose Tolerance Tests

The oral tests are usually satisfactory in diagnosing actual diabetes. Glucose itself is nauseating but it may be given as Ferguzade or Lucozade (250 ml contain 50 g glucose). Difficulty may be experienced due to delay in absorption giving a very flat curve.

Intravenous glucose tolerance tests eliminate the difficulty of intestinal absorption but in mild 'latent' cases interpretation of all tests is not easy since normal pregnant patients may have a lag curve.

Provocative cortisone or prednisone tests may be helpful.

The dangers and prognosis of latent diabetes are the same as those in mild clinical diabetes and the management is identical.

Pre-Diabetes

This is a condition which antedates clinical diabetes by some years. While the signs, symptoms and more obvious biochemical changes are absent, there is an alteration in physiology during pregnancy such that the woman produces large and successively larger babies and she herself tends to become obese. Thirty-three per cent of woman bearing babies weighing more than 10 lb subsequently develop diabetes. The average lapse of time is said to be 24 years.

The diagnosis is frequently retrospective but the population at risk is the same as listed under latent diabetes and the condition should be anticipated as far as possible. Biochemical tests should not be carried out before the 7th month but even so they are rarely helpful.

The foetal loss in pre-diabetes is approximately 23%, partly due to complications at birth because of the baby's size, but also because the baby tends to be oedematous, lethargic and apnoeic. Frequently it has a Cushing-like appearance. The liver, spleen and heart are enlarged, and at postmorten hyperplasia and increase in number of the pancreatic islets is found. Male babies frequently show increase in the number of the testicular interstitial cells.

If the condition is suspected the patient should be admitted to hospital at 32 weeks. The fasting blood sugar should be measured frequently. The diet should be the same as that prescribed in clinical diabetes.

URINARY TRACT INFECTION

Pregnant women are especially liable to this condition, especially if there has been a previous episode of infection. The main predisposing causes are stasis of urine, and an increased susceptibility to ascending infection.

Stasis

Progesterone normally produces atony of the muscle of the renal pelvis and ureters, and in the days when pyelography was frequently done in pregnancy, it was usual to observe some dilatation and kinking of the ureters. As a result the rate of flow of urine is reduced and bacterial growth encouraged.

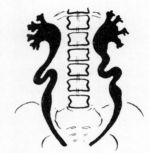

Pyelogram in acute pyelonephritis

Increased Susceptibility to Ascending Infection.

There is a much higher incidence of urinary infection among women compared with men, presumably because of the ease with which bacteria can gain access to the bladder through the short female urethra. During pregnancy there is a great increase in the moistness and in the bacterial population of the vestibule and vagina (cf. the increase in symptoms of urinary infection and Bartholin's gland infection brought about by excessive sexual intercourse).

Sites of Infection

When the urine is infected there is always the likelihood that the renal parenchyma is involved. In pregnancy it must be assumed that this is so and that the disease is a pyelonephritis and not just a pyelitis or cystitis.

Organisms

By far the commonest is E.coli. Other organisms sometimes found include B. proteus, Strept. faecalis and sometimes Pseudomonas aeruginosa.

Other Associations

Urinary infection is related to the standard of personal hygiene maintained by the individual; and there is therefore a social gradient. It is also thought to be related to asymptomatic bacteriuria which may proceed to acute pyelonephritis if untreated.

URINARY TRACT INFECTION

A Mid-Stream Specimen of Urine

Because of the risks of catheter infection, urine for diagnosis is now collected from voided mid-stream specimens. Various attempts are made to reduce the inevitable contamination, all of them troublesome and somewhat objectionable to the patient at an outpatient clinic. Present practice ranges between no vulval toilet at all, and scrupulous cleansing with antiseptic, followed by plugging the vagina with a tampon, before asking the patient to pass urine. Too heavy a contamination as is likely in pregnancy, makes interpretation of culture and bacterial counts difficult, and too much antisepsis will destroy significant organisms during micturition. The bacteriologist must be aware of the exact technique used; and if the specimen is not to be cultured within an hour it is essential to refrigerate it at 4° C until the laboratory can receive it.

Bacterial Counts in Urine

A count of over 100,000 bacteria per ml. means that bacteria are actively multiplying in the bladder and that the urine is infected. A normal clean specimen of urine should not contain more than 10,000. Full quantitative counts (culturing a urine diluted to such an extent that each colony is assumed to come from one bacterium) takes time and trouble, and various semi-quantitative methods are in use, all involving a degree of error. When combined with the error inherent in the MSSU, it will be realised that very often more than one specimen may need to be cultured before diagnosis is definite. When doubt persists, urine may be collected by suprapubic aspiration of the full bladder, which avoids all contamination.

Asymptomatic Bacteriuria

About 5% of women attending an antenatal clinic have an infected urine (according to the bacterial count) without symptoms of infection. If untreated, about one quarter of these will develop acute pyelonephritis during that pregnancy; and it is possible that these patients are exposed to a greater than average risk of developing chronic renal disease in later years. The screening of all antenatal patients for bacteriuria has been suggested, but at present no simple and accurate test exists, and the proposal is still a subject of controversy. At present the obstetrician must decide whether the benefit received by the patient justifies the effort and expense of collecting and culturing urine from each patient (often several times) and treating a condition which may not be significant.

URINARY TRACT INFECTION

Clinical Features: These are variable and often vague.

1. Dysuria. The patient says that the urine 'felt hot' or that it was 'like passing needles'.
2. Fever. Temperature may be raised to 102° F (43.7° C) and pulse rate is also elevated.
3. Loin Pain. This sign is diagnostic. Tenderness may be elicited over one or both kidneys.
4. Abdominal Pain. This is usually referred to the lower quadrants and is presumably related to the inflammatory process in the ureters and bladder.
5. There may be nausea and vomiting.
6. A positive urine culture may be obtained.

Laboratory Investigations
A mid-stream specimen of urine must be collected and swabs from the throat and vagina should be sent at the same time.

Differential Diagnosis
Both patient and doctor often mistake the condition for the onset of premature labour. Loin tenderness should be diagnostic. Appendicitis is much less common, and the urine should be normal. Concealed accidental haemorrhage may in the early stages cause confusion, but there is no pyrexia, and again the urine should be sterile although protein will be present.

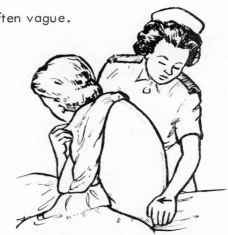

To elicit loin tenderness, first palpate the spine gently to accustom the patient to the touch, then tap gently with the thenar eminence over the loin. If positive, the patient gives an unmistakeable wince.

Treatment
The patient is put to bed, given mild analgesics and encouraged to drink. A 'holding antibiotic' such as sulphadimidine or nitrofurantoin should be given until the sensitivity is reported. Antibiotic treatment is maintained for 10 days and the urine should be sterile on completion.

Very rarely an acute hydronephrosis may develop and this must be dealt with by drainage for 24 hours through a ureteric catheter. In such cases an X-ray pyelogram is justified to prove the obstruction before proceeding to pass a ureteric catheter.

URINARY TRACT INFECTION

Prognosis

The infection is quite likely to recur later on in the pregnancy and especially during the puerperium, (see page 329) and a full renal tract investigation should be carried out once the pregnancy is over. Congenital abnormalities of the renal tract are not uncommon.

Chronic Renal Disease

This is a serious complication in pregnancy. There is argument as to whether the pregnancy has a permanently damaging effect on diseased kidneys; but there is no doubt about the effect of renal disease on pregnancy. Hypertension, if not already present, nearly always occurs and placental function is affected. The foetal prognosis is poor; and if renal impairment is severe the added stress of pregnancy may be fatal for the mother. If the patient has severe nephritis it is best to advise termination.

In less severe cases, and when termination is refused, renal function must be observed closely in addition to the usual intensive antenatal supervision, and treatment modified to suit the circumstances. If possible a physician specialising in renal disease should be asked to share the management, and if renal function is deteriorating, the pregnancy should be terminated by section as soon as the foetus is judged large enough to survive.

Renal Function Tests

These tests are less reliable in pregnancy because of the physiological retention of fluid and the alteration in metabolite levels due partly to the haemodilution and partly to the negative nitrogen balance of pregnancy.

Specific Gravity

A concentration and dilution test should show a range between 1.025 and 1.003. In severe impairment the S.G. tends to remain static at about 1.010.

Blood Urea Level

The normal pregnancy level is between 10 and 20 mg%. Forty per cent of urea is reabsorbed by the tubules, and a blood level over 50 mg% suggests a serious fall in glomerular filtration rate.

Clearance Tests

Creatinine clearance is clinically the most useful. The non-pregnant rate of about 170 litres/24 hr shows a 40% increase by 12 - 14 weeks, gradually returning to normal by term. The rate should not fall below the non-pregnant figure. A steady deterioration in function tests is particularly sinister if accompanied by the presence of casts and red cells in the urine.

JAUNDICE

Jaundice is an uncommon complication of pregnancy. The incidence is 1 in 1,500 pregnancies.

Aetiology

A. Pregnancy jaundice
1. Acute fatty liver.
2. Cholestatic jaundice.
3. Complicating pre-eclampsia and eclampsia.

B. Intercurrent jaundice
1. Viral hepatitis.
2. Obstructive jaundice due to gall-stones.

C. Iatrogenic jaundice
1. Hepatotoxic drugs.
2. Drugs interfering with conjugation of bilirubin.
3. Drugs causing haemolytic conditions.

The most common causes of jaundice in pregnancy are:-

Viral hepatitis: 41%
Cholestatic jaundice: 21%
Obstructive jaundice: less than 6%

Viral Hepatitis

In epidemics the incidence is the same in pregnant and non-pregnant adult females but sporadic cases are more likely to occur in mothers. This is due to the fact that hepatitis is most common in children and this exposes mothers to infection.

The disease runs the same course as in the non-pregnant and the prognosis is good provided the patient is well nourished. Folic acid deficiency is likely to develop due to the inability of the infected liver to store the vitamin. There is no indication for termination. In early pregnancy abortion may result and premature birth is said to be common if the condition occurs later.

Recurrent Cholestatic Jaundice of Pregnancy

This is a mild jaundice of unknown aetiology occurring in the last trimester. Jaundice may be absent and pruritis the only feature. The urine is usually dark and the stools pale. It recurs with each pregnancy.

This jaundice may be related to the high blood steroid level in pregnancy. A recurrent jaundice occurs in some patients given oral contraceptives and these drugs would not be prescribed for any patient who has suffered from cholestatic jaundice in pregnancy.

JAUNDICE

Acute Fatty Liver of Pregnancy (Acute Yellow Atrophy of Pregnancy)

This is a fatal disease occurring in the last trimester of pregnancy characterised by a liver in which the cells are filled by small vacuoles of lipid surrounding a central nucleus.

The patient has severe nausea and vomiting, abdominal pain, haematemesis and becomes jaundiced. Headaches are severe and convulsions may occur. She becomes stuporose, lapses into coma; and death commonly takes place several days after delivery. The course is the same as in fulminating viral hepatitis. Acute pyelonephritis is frequently present and the patient is undernourished. Azotaemia, hyperuricaemia and acidosis occur.

In recent times this condition has followed the administration of large doses of tetracycline. This acts as an inhibitor of cell metabolism, interfering with acetate metabolism, oxidative phosphorylation and preventing the incorporation of glutamate into protein.

Treatment is largely symptomatic. Vitamins such as B_{12} and folic acid plus lipotrophic substances like choline may be given but their efficiency is doubtful. The prognosis is extremely poor. The mother usually dies and the foetus is stillborn.

Avoid tetracyclines in late pregnancy.

Pre-Eclampsia-Eclampsia

In this condition the serum transaminase and alkaline phosphatase are commonly raised but jaundice is infrequent. When it does occur it is of haemolytic type and is usually a terminal event. It is related to haemorrhage in the liver.

Gall-Stones

These are associated with obesity and parity but not necessarily with multiparity. Jaundice due to gall-stones is uncommon in pregnancy. The management is the same as in the non-pregnant patient.

JAUNDICE

Drugs and Jaundice

Tetracycline has already been mentioned in relation to fatty liver.

Chlorpromazine, phenothiazine, diabenase and anabolic steroids can cause a mild cholestatic jaundice.

Jaundice due to repeated administrations of halothane is extremely rare but can be fatal.

Sulphonamides tend to displace bilirubin from its sites of conjugation and novobiocin inhibits conjugation of bilirubin in the liver. They should therefore be avoided in the newborn since they may lead to jaundice and kernicterus.

Glucose 6-phosphate dehydrogenase deficiency occurs in Mediterranean races. Phenacetin given to a mother bearing a child with such a deficiency may precipitate jaundice in the baby. Isoniazid and P.A.S. can cause a severe jaundice resembling viral jaundice. Serum transaminase rises before jaundice appears.

	Serum Bilirubin	Serum Transaminase	Alkaline Phosphatase
Viral Hepatitis	Increased	Very high	Slightly increased
Recurrent Cholestatic Jaundice	Increase of conjugated bilirubin	Normal. Occasionally high	Increased
Acute Fatty Liver	Increased	Moderate increase	Moderate increase
Gall-Stones	Increase of conjugated bilirubin	Normal	Increased

Jaundice can be a terminal event in severe hyperemesis but this is a rare occurrence. Milder jaundice may be caused by haemolytic blood diseases e.g. acholuric jaundice, sickle-cell anaemia, haemoglobinopathies.

HYPERTHYROIDISM

This causes impaired fertility so pregnancy is uncommon but anti-thyroid treatment improves the chance of conception.

Thyrotoxicosis may declare in pregnancy.

Diagnosis

The usual symptoms are present.

Tachycardia sleeping and waking, sweating, anxiety, muscular tremor, absence of weight gain or even loss of weight without apparent cause.

The Basal Metabolic Rate (B.M.R.) is unhelpful as it normally rises in pregnancy by about 20%.

The thyroid gland normally enlarges in pregnancy.

The serum cholesterol level rises in normal pregnancy.

The protein-bound iodine (P.B.I.) level also rises in pregnancy but 6 - 9 ug% can be considered euthyroid.

Anaemia, glycosuria, albuminuria and pyrexia are found in thyrotoxicosis.

There is a risk of abortion, intra-uterine death and premature labour.

Treatment

Rest in bed plus sedation e.g. barbiturates or tranquillisers

Radioactive isotope treatment in pregnancy is dangerous as the isotopes cross the placenta and will injure the foetal thyroid causing foetal goitre or cretinism.

Anti-thyroid drugs (e.g. carbimazole) also cross the placenta but are more controllable and should be regulated to give an euthyroid or slightly thyrotoxic state though there is still risk of foetal goitre or cretinism.

Potassium perchlorate may be used for a short time initially though it is suspected of causing agranulocytosis in prolonged dosage.

Partial thyroidectomy is sometimes practised but fine judgement is required to avoid hypothyroidism after pregnancy.

With adequate control the pregnancy should be normal.

HYPERTHYROIDISM

The baby should be examined carefully after birth.

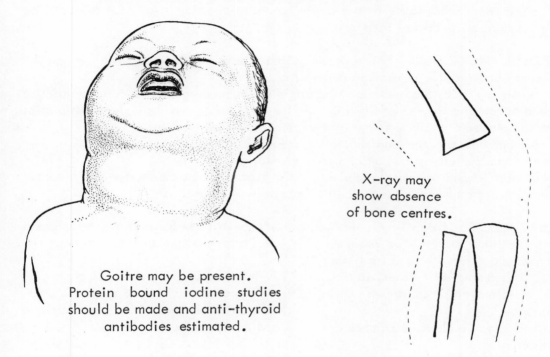

Goitre may be present.
Protein bound iodine studies
should be made and anti-thyroid
antibodies estimated.

X-ray may
show absence
of bone centres.

The baby should not be breast fed as the anti-thyroid drugs are excreted in the milk.

HYPOTHYROIDISM

Hypothyroidism causes reduced fertility but under treatment with thyroid subsitutes fertility may be restored.

Thyroxine may be needed throughout pregnancy in varying dosage because of the altering demands as pregnancy advances. In some cases the thyroid gland hypertrophies and increases its function so that the thyroid substitution therapy can be reduced or stopped.

RESPIRATORY DISEASES

PNEUMONIA. Lobar pneumonia is rare but has a high foetal mortality so early exhibition of suitable antibiotics is important.

Viral pneumonia leads to premature labour or abortion. Antibiotics should be given to control secondary invaders.

CHRONIC BRONCHITIS. This saps the patient's stamina, increases the load on the heart and reduces pulmonary reserve.

Treatment is by bed rest at intervals during the pregnancy and by antibiotics depending on the degree of severity of the handicap. Broad spectrum antibiotics cross the placenta and may lodge in the foetal skeleton.

Anaemia is common and should be treated vigorously. Physiotherapy is important to help clear sputum and improve breathing.

During labour oxygen may be required. Labour should be shortened if need be by the use of local anaesthesia and the forceps or ventouse.

TUBERCULOSIS. Pregnancy does not affect the progress or prognosis.

Treatment is with specific therapy (e.g. para-amino salicylates, isoniazid and streptomycin) continued during pregnancy.

There is a tendency for anaemia to develop.

Physiotherapy is important.

Labour is treated as in bronchitis if there is much incapacity.

The baby should be given B.C.G. and kept apart from the mother for 6 weeks (see page 338) or the baby is given isoniazid resistant B.C.G. and the mother can nurse the baby.

Patients who have had treatment for tuberculosis need careful observation as the increased metabolism of pregnancy may reactivate the focus of infection.

BRONCHIECTASIS. The problems and treatment are similar to bronchitis.

ASTHMA. The effect of pregnancy is very variable. In most cases the condition is unaffected but some improve while others become worse.

Treatment is with epinephrine hydrochloride 0.5 ml of 1:1000 solution intramuscularly or 0.03 g of ephedrine sulphate orally. Aminophylline 500 mg intravenously may also be useful. Many patients use isoprenaline (medihaler) for the spasms and this is usually adequate.

Corticoids and A.C.T.H. are undesirable because of risk of crossing the placenta and interfering with foetal adrenal activity, but may be required if the patient fails to respond to treatment with bronchodilator drugs.

VENEREAL DISEASES

SYPHILIS

The foetus can be infected in utero with resulting abortion or stillbirth, and the liveborn baby may be congenitally syphilitic. The syphilitic placenta is a large pale organ very like the placenta in hydrops foetalis, and showing the microscopic changes of endarteritis and fibrosis.

Serological Tests. Blood for the Wasserman complement-fixation and the Kahn flocculation tests should be taken at the first antenatal visit and again at 36 weeks, in case the disease was latent at the time of the first test. If positive they should be repeated, as false positives are common with the Kahn test. More specific tests such as the Reiter or treponemal antigen tests must be performed before a definite diagnosis is made.

Clinical Signs are rarely seen antenatally. The primary chancre is usually on the labia and the inguinal glands enlarged. Signs of secondary syphilis include condylamata lata, mucous patches, and a generalised rash.

Treatment. 0.9 mega-units of procaine penicillin G given daily for a fortnight will protect the foetus and cure it if already infected. Both mother and child will require follow-up examination after delivery.

GONORRHOEA

Symptoms in the female are so slight that they are often unnoticed. The patient may then develop a salpingitis especially in the puerperium, with resultant sterility.

The infection is transmitted to the baby during labour, and gonococcal ophthalmia appears about the 4th day. It is a serious condition which will lead to blindness if not treated.

Diagnosis. Smears must be taken from the urethral meatus or the cervix, and the presence of intra-cellular Gram negative diplococci is highly suggestive. Material for culture must be sent off in transport medium.

Treatment. A two-day course of penicillin or streptomycin or tetracycline is sufficient. When infection is or has been present, a smear for culture should be taken from the baby's eyes at birth and prophylactic antibiotic treatment given.

The patient's sexual partner or partners must also be investigated, and referral to a venereological clinic is the best way of doing this. The obstetrician's immediate responsibility is to ensure that the woman is adequately treated and that the foetus is protected.

ACUTE ABDOMINAL CONDITIONS IN PREGNANCY

BOWEL OBSTRUCTION

Usually caused by adhesion bands altering in position with the rising uterus, but volvulus is sometimes found. Colic, distension, vomiting, diminished or absent bowel sounds are signs that laparotomy is required.

APPENDICITIS

The point of maximum tenderness is higher in pregnancy, and the high steroid levels will reduce the usual response to inflammation. There is usually sickness; and if doubt persists after a period of observation, laparotomy should be carried out. If pus is present, wound drainage should be continued for at least a week. Acute pyelonephritis may present much the same clinical picture, but loin tenderness and urine findings help in diagnosis.

URINARY CALCULUS

This causes acute pain radiating to the groin and haematuria is present. Treatment is conservative unless hydronephrosis develops and ureteric drainage is required.

DEGENERATING FIBROIDS

Necrobiosis causes pain, vomiting, tenderness and pyrexia, and diagnosis is difficult. The condition should settle with rest and sedation, and operation is only likely to be indicated when there is torsion of the pedicle of a fibroid.

PERFORATION OF ACUTE PEPTIC ULCER

This is very rare in pregnancy because of the high steroid level. The clinical appearances in the early months are unmistakeably of perforation, but are less clear in the 3rd trimester. There is little rigidity, but shock is marked and air may be palpated or shown by X-ray, under the diaphragm.

OVARIAN CYST

Torsion of the pedicle causes acute pain, tenderness, vomiting and often pyrexia. Under anaesthesia a mass separate from the uterus may be distinguished, and laparotomy must be performed.

Laparotomy for these conditions often brings on labour or abortion, although removal of an untwisted ovarian cyst is usually safe enough. Section is not advisable in the presence of intra-abdominal infection.

CHAPTER 7

DISEASES OF PREGNANCY

RHESUS INCOMPATIBILITY

In each individual Rhesus genes are carried on two chromosomes either of which may be handed on to the succeeding generation. There are six main Rhesus genes, three carried on each chromosome. Of the six, three are dominant C, D and E and three, their alleles, c, d, e are recessive. Each chromosome has a C locus, a D locus and an E locus which may be occupied by a dominant or recessive gene of the particular type. The genesis of Rhesus incompatibility in pregnancy is best considered by tracing the genes through successive generations.

From this it will be seen that the mother has the same series of Rhesus genes on both chromosomes – she is homozygous at all loci. Note also that all of the genes are of recessive type.

The most important gene in Rhesus incompatibility is the dominant D gene. Persons possessing this gene are commonly termed Rhesus positive. When it is absent from both chromosomes and its place is occupied by the recessive d allele, the individual is termed Rhesus negative.

In the above diagram the mother is Rhesus negative. Consider now the next generation.

The child has received a chromosome with recessive genes from its homozygous Rhesus negative mother and another with two dominant genes (C and D) from its homozygous Rhesus positive father. The latter chromosome is the one which causes the trouble. It is foreign to the mother and should the foetal cells escape into the maternal circulation they will stimulate the formation of antibodies by the mother.

RHESUS INCOMPATIBILITY

This is the basis of Rhesus iso-immunisation. Theoretically if the child possesses a Rhesus gene not present in the mother's chromosomes the mother may form an antibody to that gene. In practice the capacity of the various Rhesus genes to stimulate antibody formation varies. D is the strongest antigen and d is the weakest. More than 95% of cases of Rhesus incompatibility are due to the dominant D.

Two other factors play a part in the immunisation. The genetic make-up of the father is most important. Examine the following diagrams representing two families.

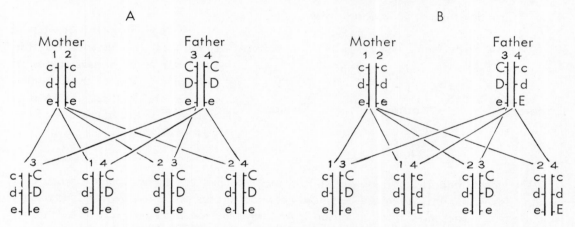

In family A where both mother and father are homozygous the Rhesus genetic make-up of their off-spring will always be the same c⊢C d⊢D e⊢e. If, as is likely, the mother forms antibodies, every child will be affected and the outcome of each succeeding pregnancy will tend to be more hazardous than the previous.

In family B the outcome of a pregnancy will depend on which chromosome is handed on by the father. If chromosome 3, C⊢ D⊢ e⊢ is transmitted to the foetus then antibody formation will result. On the other hand chromosome 4, ⊢c ⊢d ⊢E, is unlikely to stimulate antibody formation. In circumstances such as these, the disease may only affect every other child in the family.

RHESUS INCOMPATIBILITY

The other factor which determines whether the process of immunisation is initiated in the mother or not, is the ABO blood group of the mother and foetus. The immunisation of the mother is brought about by the escape of foetal red cells into the maternal circulation. If the foetal cells are ABO compatible with those of the mother they will persist in her circulation and will stimulate antibody formation. If they are ABO incompatible they will be destroyed rapidly and no immunisation will occur.

The circumstances might be as follows.

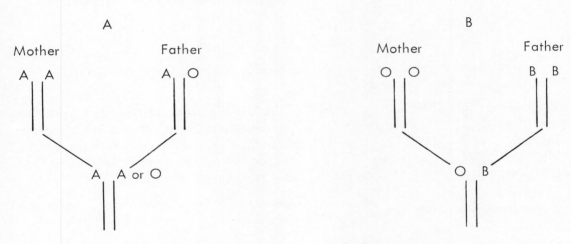

In family A the foetal blood is compatible with the maternal, and foetal cells will continue to live after escape into the maternal circulation. If the mother is Rhesus negative and the foetus Rhesus positive antibodies will form. The foetal cells in example B are incompatible with the maternal blood and will be rapidly destroyed on entry into the maternal circulation. No antibodies are likely to form even if there is Rhesus incompatibility.

Before Rhesus immunisation is likely to occur the red cells of the foetus must have a blood group either the same as the mother or group O, and must possess a Rhesus gene usually dominant D not found in the mother.

RHESUS INCOMPATIBILITY

STATISTICS

The possible combinations of genes on one chromosome in descending order of frequency are:-

CDe	R_1
cde	r
cDE	R_2
cDe	R_o
cdE	r"
Cde	r'
CDE	R_2
CdE	R_y

The commonest genotypes i.e. the mixture of genes on two chromosomes in descending order of frequency are:-

CDe/cde	R_1r	30 – 32%
CDe/CDe	R_1R_1	17 – 18%
cde/cde	rr	13.5%
CDe/cDE	R_1R_2	10 – 12%
cDE/cde	R_2r	10 – 11%

Other combinations are rare.

83% of the U.K. population are Rhesus positive i.e. possess at least one dominant D gene.

17% of the U.K. population are Rhesus negative i.e. do not possess a dominant D gene, but have two recessive d genes.

It follows that 17% of the female population are Rhesus negative.

Probable Genotype of Males marrying Rhesus Negative Females

Rhesus negative males	17%
Rhesus positive males	83%

The latter are made up as follows:-

Homozygous Rhesus positive males	35%
Heterozygous Rhesus positive males	48%

RHESUS INCOMPATIBILITY

ANTENATAL DIAGNOSIS

Every effort must be made to detect the patient likely to bear an affected baby – the Rhesus negative woman.

Routine laboratory testing of the blood of every pregnant woman is essential.

Antibodies may appear at any time during a pregnancy. The following regime may be followed.

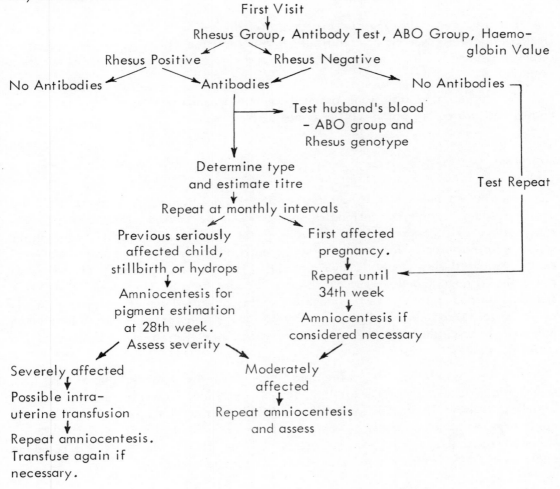

151

RHESUS INCOMPATIBILITY

SALINE ANTIBODY

This is the first antibody to appear in the maternal blood and it agglutinates Rhesus positive cells suspended in saline. It is a large molecule and does not usually cross the placenta.

ALBUMIN ANTIBODY

In most cases this type appears soon after the saline antibody and may replace it altogether. It will only agglutinate Rhesus positive cells suspended in plasma, serum or albumin. It is a small molecule and crosses the placenta easily to affect the baby.

The detection of this type of antibody may be improved by making use of test Rhesus positive cells treated with enzymes such as papain.

COOMBS IMMUNE ANTI-GLOBULIN TEST (I.A.G.T.)

The test depends on the fact that antibodies are globulins. If these globulins are injected into animals antibodies to them will be formed. These antibodies in turn can be used to detect the presence of the original antibodies. In the above tests agglutination may fail to take place even if antibody is present in the maternal serum. Nevertheless the antibody, a globulin, will have attached itself to the test red cells. If now animal serum containing antibodies to globulin, so-called Coombs reagent, is added to the test mixture the antiglobulin will react with the antibody attached to the red cells and cause agglutination. Being very sensitive this test can be used to provide a better measure of the concentration of antibodies in the maternal serum than ordinary agglutination tests.

This test is also applied to the cord blood of babies suspected of suffering from erythroblastosis. Although maternal albumin antibody crosses the placenta and attaches itself to foetal red cells these cells are not agglutinated. It is obviously necessary to make a diagnosis as quickly as possible. Immune anti-globulin (Coombs reagent) added to a suspension of the foetal red cells will produce agglutination if maternal Rhesus antibody is attached to these cells.

RHESUS INCOMPATIBILITY

FOETUS

Advanced disease in foetal life occurs in the minority of cases and usually only after several pregnancies have been affected. The disease may result in intra-uterine death, stillbirth or a live born child showing hydrops foetalis. Frequently the diagnosis of hydrops foetalis can be made ante-natally by X-ray examination.

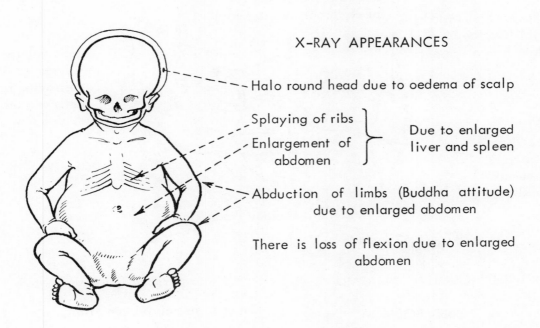

X-RAY APPEARANCES

Halo round head due to oedema of scalp

Splaying of ribs ⎫
Enlargement of   ⎬ Due to enlarged
abdomen   ⎭ liver and spleen

Abduction of limbs (Buddha attitude) due to enlarged abdomen

There is loss of flexion due to enlarged abdomen

Incidence of Stillbirth in Rhesus Incompatible Pregnancies

Over-all risk	15 per cent
In first affected pregnancies	8 per cent
If previous infant severely affected	50 per cent
If previous stillbirth	70 per cent

RHESUS INCOMPATIBILITY

INFANT

The basis of the disease is a haemolytic anaemia brought about by the action of the maternal anti-Rhesus albumin antibody.

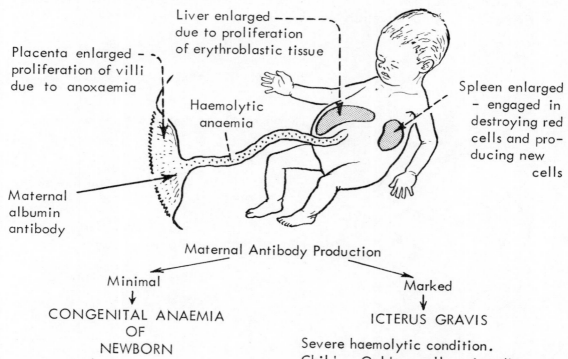

Liver enlarged due to proliferation of erythroblastic tissue

Placenta enlarged - proliferation of villi due to anoxaemia

Haemolytic anaemia

Spleen enlarged - engaged in destroying red cells and producing new cells

Maternal albumin antibody

Maternal Antibody Production

Minimal

Marked

CONGENITAL ANAEMIA OF NEWBORN

A mild haemolytic condition.
Child : Pale.
Liver : Slightly enlarged.
Spleen : Slightly enlarged.
Blood : Mild anaemia. Hb 13 - 15 g per 100 ml.
         Few reticulocytes.
         Bilirubin scarcely increased. Less than 2 mg per 100 ml.
Urine : Negative test for bile.

ICTERUS GRAVIS

Severe haemolytic condition.
Child : Golden yellow jaundice appears within minutes of birth.
Liver : Greatly enlarged.
Spleen : Much enlarged.
Blood : Rapidly increasing anaemia. Numerous reticulocytes, erythroblasts, normoblasts, and early white cells. Indirect and direct bilirubin increased and rising.
Urine : Positive test for bile.

RHESUS INCOMPATIBILITY

PROGNOSIS

An assessment of prognosis in the antenatal period is based on the history of the patient and several laboratory tests.

Obstetric History

First child unaffected in 90% of marriages of Rhesus negative female with Rhesus positive male. Following birth of an affected baby each subsequently affected child is likely to have a more severe form of erythroblastosis.

Maternal History

Any history of a previous blood transfusion in a Rhesus negative woman is to be regarded as ominous. A Rhesus incompatible transfusion causes marked sensitisation. If the patient subsequently has a Rhesus incompatible pregnancy, even if it is her first, antibodies will appear early and in high concentration.

ANTENATAL PERIOD

Antibody Titre

The titre of albumin antibody is of considerable value in the first affected pregnancy. A concentration of 1 in 32 is the danger line. Above this serious disease is likely.

Paternal Genotype

Homozygous "D". The chance of producing an affected second child is 1 in 12. Each succeeding pregnancy will be affected.

Heterozygous "D". The chance of producing an affected second child is 1 in 15. Probably only every other child will be affected.

Amniocentesis

This is carried out to obtain a sample of amniotic fluid for the estimation of pigment content. The concentration of pigment varies with the severity of the disease.

RHESUS INCOMPATIBILITY

Rhesus negative pregnant women can be divided into five groups.

1. No antibodies are present in the maternal blood.
2. Antibodies developing in the first affected pregnancy. This is the largest group, 60% of all affected pregnancies. The risk of stillbirth is 8% but all occur after 37 weeks.
3. The patient has already had an affected baby but no treatment was required. 10% of affected pregnancies occur in this group. The risk of stillbirth is the same as in the general population.
4. The patient has already had an affected baby who required treatment. This group constitutes 20% of affected pregnancies. The risk of stillbirth is 20% (50% if the previous child was severely affected). 40% occur before 37 weeks.
5. The patient has already had a stillbirth or a live born child suffering from hydrops. 10% of affected pregnancies are in this group. The risk of stillbirth is 70% and intra-uterine death occurs in half of the cases before 35 weeks.

Amniocentesis should only be carried out in groups 4 and 5. The fluid obtained is examined in a spectrophotometer and the optical density measured with light of wavelength varying from 400 mμ to 700 mμ. In normal pregnancy the density values at these various wavelengths form a straight line graph. In pregnancies affected by Rhesus incompatibility the fluid contains bile pigments and these cause a peak at 450 mμ. The difference in optical density between the normal and the abnormal at this wavelength is an indication of the severity of the disease.

The placenta must be localised before amniocentesis is attempted. Apart from the risk of haemorrhage, there is a very real danger that foetal red cells will escape into the maternal circulation with consequent increased stimulation of antibody formation, and the conversion of a pregnancy from group 2 or 3 to group 4 or 5.

In an affected pregnancy the optical density of the amniotic fluid diminishes with increasing maturity of the pregnancy and allowance must be made for this in interpretation.

| | Optical Density | |
Duration of Pregnancy	Mild to Moderate Disease	Severe Disease
28 weeks	0.06 – 0.28	> 0.28
32 weeks	0.04 – 0.18	> 0.18
36 weeks	0.03 – 0.12	> 0.12

RHESUS INCOMPATIBILITY

POST NATAL

The prognosis after birth is based on clinical examination of the baby and a full examination of the cord blood.

The following tests require to be carried out.

a. Coombs test.
b. Blood grouping and Rhesus typing.
c. Haemoglobin estimation
d. Bilirubin concentration.

A positive Coombs test indicates an affected baby. It is important to make this test since in some instances when a previous pregnancy has resulted in a baby suffering from erythroblastosis, the serum of the Rhesus negative mother may show a rising titre of antibody in a subsequent pregnancy even if the foetus is Rhesus negative and therefore incapable of stimulating an antibody response.

The reasons for the other tests are obvious:-

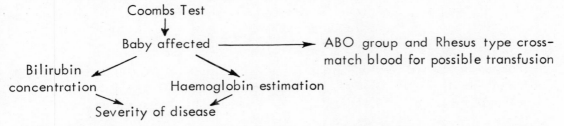

Rapidly increasing anaemia and rapid onset of jaundice indicate a severe form of the disease and the subsequent prognosis depends on efficient treatment.

TREATMENT

If treatment is prompt 95% of live born affected infants can be saved.

If the disease is mild no treatment may be required. Haemoglobin estimations should be carried out daily and if the level falls below 9 g per 100 ml. transfusion should be given.

In severe forms of the disease exchange transfusion should be carried out via the umbilical vein. The indications are:-

RHESUS INCOMPATIBILITY

1. Birth weight below 2.4 kilogrammes (5.5 lbs).
2. History of previously affected infant.
3. Cord haemoglobin less than 15.5 g per 100 ml.
4. Cord bilirubin greater than 3 mg per 100 ml.
5. Development of jaundice in first 24 hours.

During the five days following birth a close watch is kept on the infant. It is particularly important to estimate the indirect bilirubin. If the value for this rises above 20 mg per 100 ml. there is danger of KERNICTERUS developing. Should the bilirubin approach this level further exchange transfusions will be required.

Subsequently it is not uncommon for anaemia to develop. If the haemoglobin falls below 9 g per 100 ml. boost transfusions at the rate of 20 ml. per kilogram of body weight are given.

INTRA-UTERINE TRANSFUSION

This treatment is used when it seems likely that pregnancy will end in intra-uterine death. It is therefore the treatment of choice when there is a history of previous stillbirth or hydrops due to Rhesus incompatability.

Packed cells, generally Group O Rhesus negative, are injected into the peritoneal cavity of the foetus. The treatment may be repeated with the object of maintaining the foetus until at least 35 weeks when delivery is effected.

PREVENTION OF RHESUS HAEMOLYTIC DISEASE

Study has shown that the initiation of antibody formation starts in the first Rhesus incompatible pregnancy. Many women are found to have antibodies in their blood in the late puerperium in these instances. Although small numbers of foetal red cells escape into the maternal circulation during pregnancy the important immunising dose is received by the mother at the time of the delivery when the placenta is compressed and separated. If the foetal cells are ABO incompatible they are destroyed rapidly and Rhesus immunisation does not take place, but if they are ABO compatible they survive and the D factor stimulates the maternal antibody mechanism.

158

RHESUS INCOMPATIBILITY

The theory behind the attempt to prevent Rhesus iso-immunisation is that if the D factor is blocked the maternal cells will have no means of recognising the foreign nature of the foetal cells and antibody will not be formed

Immediately after birth of the baby the cord blood is tested for ABO and Rhesus groups. If the blood is Rhesus positive and ABO compatible with that of the mother, then the mother's blood is examined for the presence of foetal red cells. If they are present the mother is given an injection of anti-D hyper-immune globulin. This will coat the foetal cells and block the D factor. Antibody formation will be averted and the subsequent pregnancy will not be affected. The treatment, of course, has to be repeated at the end of each pregnancy thereafter.

KERNICTERUS

This condition arises in any form of neonatal jaundice when the 'indirect' bilirubin rises above 20 mg per cent. The bilirubin is able to enter brain tissue and cause necrosis of neurons especially in the basal ganglia. The infant becomes lethargic and refuses to suck. Convulsions, rolling of eyes and head retraction develop. Death may occur but if the infant survives there are permanent mental and physical disabilities.

Erythroblastosis due to Rhesus incompatibility is the main cause, but the condition may occur in premature babies especially if they are given excessive doses of vitamin K, which has a haemolytic action. Sulphafurazole may also lead to kern icterus because of its ability to displace bilirubin from its carrier protein – albumin. Novobiocin interfers with glucuronidation and therefore prevents conversion of 'indirect' to 'direct' bilirubin. Occasionally cytomegalic inclusion disease may cause erythroblastosis and lead to kern icterus.

OTHER ANTIBODIES

Occasionally immune antibodies to the foetal ABO system may arise in the mother. The effect is usually mild. Similarly there are many other red cell genetic factors which may cause maternal antibody formation – Duffy, Luther, Kell.

Any gene in the foetus not possessed by the mother may induce antibodies. It is therefore important to remember that a Rhesus positive woman may give birth to an erythroblastotic infant.

HYPEREMESIS

Hyperemesis gravidarum is a progression from the sickness common in early pregnancy. The change is usually gradual and may be confused by the patient's impression that she is 'unable to keep anything in her stomach' yet her mucosae are moist, the skin normal and the breath and urine acetone free, and so she deteriorates till her statement is correct and she is seriously ill. There seems to be a neurotic element in the illness as removal to hospital can be curative in itself.

The illness is shown diagramatically [   ];   and the treatments [- - - -]

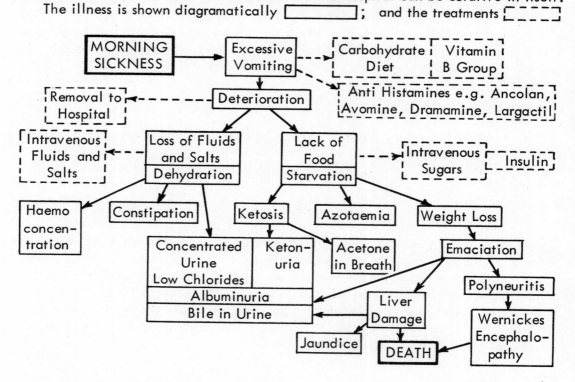

Removing the patient from her home surroundings often has a remarkable curative effect but dehydration and starvation may have to be overcome by intravenous fluids and sugars. Insulin will help the rapid utilisation of the carbohydrate. The B group of vitamins will aid the digestion of carbohydrates, protect the liver, and control polyneuritis. Hydatidiform mole is associated with hyperemesis gravidarum, and very rarely termination of pregnancy may have to be considered.

PRE-ECLAMPSIA

PRE-ECLAMPSIA

This is a disease which commonly appears in the last trimester, and is character-ised by the following signs:

1.   High Blood Pressure.

2.   Proteinuria.

3.   Pitting Oedema.

A definite diagnosis is considered to be possible when any two of the above signs are present, but generally considerable emphasis is placed on the presence of hypertension.

In normal pregnancy the blood pressure falls below non-pregnant levels in the second trimester.

The level at which hypertension may be diagnosed is lower than in the non-pregnant. By definition hypertension can be said to exist when the blood pressure reaches a level of 140 systolic/90 diastolic on two occasions more than 6 hours apart.

Similarly the levels of blood pressure used in clinical grading of severity are scaled down compared to the non-pregnant.

MILD PRE-ECLAMPSIA

This is characterised by:-

1.   Slight hypertension. The limits set by individual observers vary but the elevation does not exceed 150 - 155 mm. systolic and 90 - 95 mm. diastolic. For practical diagnosis there is no particular level at which pre-eclampsia can be said to exist.   The important feature is the detection of a sustained rise in pressure.

2.   Proteinuria - a trace.

3.   Oedema - slight or absent.

At this stage the disease is asymptomatic and all of the signs disappear rapidly in the puerperium.

PRE-ECLAMPSIA

SEVERE PRE-ECLAMPSIA

As the signs of the disease increase in severity symptoms tend to appear. In some cases the disease is of sudden onset and severe from the beginning.

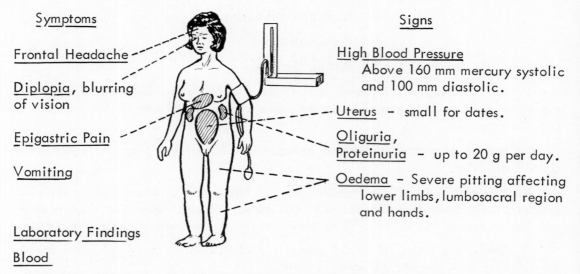

Symptoms

Frontal Headache

Diplopia, blurring of vision

Epigastric Pain

Vomiting

Signs

High Blood Pressure
Above 160 mm mercury systolic and 100 mm diastolic.

Uterus - small for dates.

Oliguria,
Proteinuria - up to 20 g per day.

Oedema - Severe pitting affecting lower limbs, lumbosacral region and hands.

Laboratory Findings

Blood

Haematocrit: In severe pre-eclampsia haemoconcentration occurs and the haematocrit rises.

Haemoglobin: The haemoglobin percentage will increase with the haemoconcentration. This may mislead the observer by masking an anaemia.

Proteins: Most plasma proteins fall progressively, especially albumen. Fibrinogen however increases but tends to fall in very severe cases.

Uric Acid. The blood uric acid is frequently increased in the later stages.

Hormone Changes

Urinary Gonadotrophin output increases so that the level may approach that found in early pregnancy.

Urinary Oestriol falls progressively as the clinical condition of the patient worsens.

Urinary Pregnanediol follows a pattern similar to oestriol.

PRE-ECLAMPSIA

PHYSIO-PATHOLOGY

Definite knowledge of this aspect of pre-eclampsia is scant. Three factors, oligaemia, arteriolar constriction and hypertension are possibly involved, and the following is a suggestion of some of the ways in which they may act.

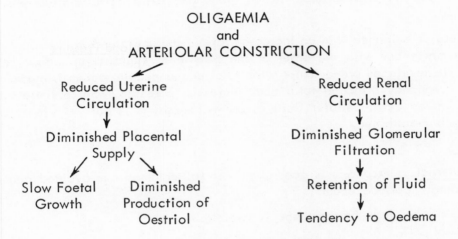

OLIGAEMIA
and
ARTERIOLAR CONSTRICTION

Reduced Uterine Circulation → Diminished Placental Supply → Slow Foetal Growth / Diminished Production of Oestriol

Reduced Renal Circulation → Diminished Glomerular Filtration → Retention of Fluid → Tendency to Oedema

Hypertension probably only affects the situation when the degree is severe.

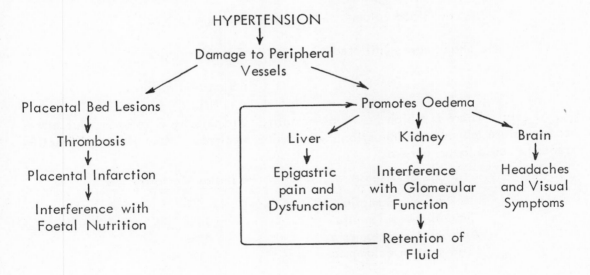

HYPERTENSION → Damage to Peripheral Vessels

Placental Bed Lesions → Thrombosis → Placental Infarction → Interference with Foetal Nutrition

Promotes Oedema → Liver → Epigastric pain and Dysfunction

Kidney → Interference with Glomerular Function → Retention of Fluid

Brain → Headaches and Visual Symptoms

PRE-ECLAMPSIA

SALT AND WATER METABOLISM

In established pre-eclampsia an apparently anomalous condition exists. The plasma volume is low but the extra-cellular fluid volume and total body water is increased. The retention of water is probably brought about by diminished glomerular filtration but the distribution between blood and extra-cellular fluid remains unexplained.

There is evidence that an increased rate of sodium retention is present prior to pre-eclampsia but with the onset of the disease a reduction in sodium retention occurs. In developed pre-eclampsia the total exchangeable sodium is the same as in normal pregnancy although total body water is increased. Since little protein is present in the extra-cellular fluid in pre-eclampsia it is not yet clear how isotonicity is maintained.

Prognosis

Maternal. Prognosis is good provided (a) eclampsia is avoided and (b) no haemorrhagic episode occurs.

The danger from haemorrhage is twofold:-

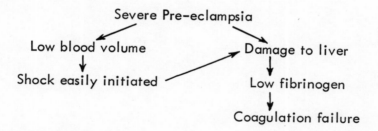

Foetal. There is a high perinatal mortality. Prematurity is common, due either to premature labour or to induction performed as treatment. Poor placental function tends to cause foetal anoxia.

Stage of Disease	Perinatal Mortality
Mild pre-eclampsia	5%
Severe pre-eclampsia	14%
Ante-partum eclampsia	47%
Intra-partum eclampsia	9%

PRE-ECLAMPSIA

Management

This is directed towards two ends.
1. To prevent eclampsia.
2. To reduce foetal wastage.

Ante-natal care plays an important part. The patient is weighed regularly, her blood pressure estimated, her urine tested for protein and a watch kept for oedema. These precautions do not prevent pre-eclampsia but lead to its early detection and treatment may keep it mild.

Bed rest is important —→ Reduces venous pressure in lower limbs —→ Increases circulating volume —→ Increase in placental blood flow.

If there is a gain of more than 2 lb per week in the last trimester a low salt diet is given and diuretics such as chlorothiazide prescribed. These cause electrolyte and water excretion. Regular estimations of blood electrolytes must be carried out.

If diastolic blood pressure rises the patient should be seen every week. Mild sedation in the form of phenobarbitone may be given and the patient advised to rest as much as possible.

If proteinuria appears rest in bed, preferably in hospital, should be advised. If there is no improvement after 2 or 3 weeks and the proteinuria is increasing the question of termination should be considered.

At this stage we are concerned with the health of the foetus. The time chosen to terminate the pregnancy will depend on the answers to a number of questions.
a) How quickly is the disease progressing?
b) What is the size of the uterus and is it growing?
c) Do tests such as oestriol excretion indicate a danger of foetal death?

The observer has to assess these factors and try to balance the danger of continued intra-uterine existence against those of prematurity.

Delivery

In pre-eclampsia the uterus is commonly hypersensitive. Induction of labour by puncture of membranes is usually successful and the labour is short. Caesarean section is only necessary if there is a delay in labour or if acute foetal distress should develop.

PRE-ECLAMPSIA

Severe Pre-Eclampsia

When this ensues the main concern is for the mother. Immediate hospitalisation is necessary. Treatment is directed towards:-

Central Nervous Sedation ⟶ to prevent eclamptic fits.

Hypotensive Therapy ⟶ to reduce blood pressure and prevent damage to blood vessels.

Diuretics ⟶ to reduce oedema on the basis that oedema of the organs is harmful and intra-cellular oedema may occur.

Sedation

Barbiturates are the most commonly used drugs, in the form of sodium amytal 180 mg or phenobarbitone 60 mg. These may be given orally twice daily or if eclampsia is thought imminent the intramuscular route may be chosen.

Hypotensive Drugs

Ganglionic Blocking Agents

These should be avoided. Although they inhibit vaso-constriction they cause pooling of blood with consequent reduction in venous return and cardiac output.

Noradrenaline Release Blocking Agents

Guanethidine is probably one of the most useful of this group. It is given in doses of 10 to 25 mg. The dose is increased at weekly intervals according to reaction up to a maximum of 150 mg per day.

Methyldopa inhibits noradrenaline and serotonin secretion but cardiac output is reduced and this affects renal and placental blood flow.

Protoveratrine. This is a useful hypotensive agent but the therapeutic dose is close to the emetic threshold and care must be taken in gauging the amount given.

Hydrallazine. This drug acts directly on vessels by relaxing smooth muscle. Cerebral, renal and uterine blood flow is increased. Unfortunately tolerance develops quickly.

All of these substances are only used to tide the patient over an acute condition for a short period of time. They have no place in the long term treatment.

ECLAMPSIA

Diuretics

Thiazide derivatives are effective but tend to cause retention of uric acid. Diabetes may be aggravated.

Spironolactone acts as a competitor of aldosterone and increases the excretion of sodium. There is no evidence that aldosterone output is increased in pre-eclampsia.

Triamterene acts directly on the distal renal tubule. This increases the excretion of sodium, bicarbonate and uric acid. Potassium excretion is reduced.

Treatment with diuretics does not reduce proteinuria.

In the majority of instances the measures mentioned above merely delay the inevitable induction of labour. This is carried out by puncture of membranes as already indicated.

ECLAMPSIA

This is commonly the terminal phase of a severe state of pre-eclampsia. The fits are preceded by a sharp rise in blood pressure, increase in proteinuria, and rapid extension of oedema. Symptoms increase in intensity and sudden blindness may supervene. There is a hypersensitivity to all stimuli and the reflexes are increased. Nursing should therefore be undertaken in a quiet darkened room.

The number of fits will depend on the efficacy of treatment. Three stages are recognised:

Premonitory Stage.

The patient rolls her eyes and there are twitchings of the hands and face.

Tonic Stage

Spasm of muscles spreads until the patient is rigid. Cyanosis is intense due to fixation of the chest and diaphragm.

Clonic Stage

The muscles now contract rapidly and spasmodically. The breathing is stertorous and 'bubbly'. This is followed by a period of coma.

ECLAMPSIA

Labour frequently starts shortly after a fit and with delivery the disease generally terminates. However the fits may continue and unless controlled may end in death of the patient.

Differential Diagnosis

A patient seen for the first time late in pregnancy suffering from fits and coma is almost certainly suffering from eclampsia. Other disease states may be the cause and must always be considered.

Epilepsy: This is not associated with hypertension or hyper-reflex action.

Cerebral Thrombosis: Proteinura is absent. Hypertension may be present.

Management

Fits must be controlled immediately. A gag is placed between the teeth and Morphine gr. $\frac{1}{4}$ (15 mg) is given when the patient is first seen. This drug is a respiratory depressant and should not be repeated.

The most useful drug is tribromethol (Avertin) given rectally, 0.09 ml/kg diluted 40 times is given initially. A second dose is given 3 hours later and repeated at 6 hourly intervals.

Rectal Paraldehyde, 30 - 40 ml every 6 hours may be used in the same way.

More recently 'lytic cocktails' have been used. They are anti-convulsant, hypotensive, hypothermic and inhibit salivary and laryngeal secretion. One recipe is as follows:-

Chlorpromazine 50 mg
Promethazine 50 mg } Mixed in 250 ml of 5% dextrose.
Pethidine hydrochloride 50 mg

Half of this is given rapidly by intravenous injection, the remainder by drip infusion, 200 drops per minute.

A second solution of chlorpromazine 100 mg and pethidine hydrochloride 50 mg in 250 ml of 5% dextrose is given by infusion at 40 drops per minute.

Following this 50 mg chlorpromazine and 50 mg pethidine are given intramuscularly every 6 hours, if required.

ECLAMPSIA

Magnesium sulphate may be given along with any of the preceding drugs. It has a general depressant effect on the central nervous system and acts synergistically with other sedatives. It is given intravenously 20 ml of a 20% solution every 4 hours for no more than 24 hours. Overdose can result in respiratory failure. Calcium gluconate is an antidote.

Post-Convulsive Stage

When the acute convulsive phase has been controlled induction of labour is carried out by rupture of membranes and if necessary a syntocinon drip is given. Hypotensive therapy is begun when the sedative effect of bromethol wears off.

During the convulsive phase oxygen should be given if cyanosis is at all prolonged. Digitalis is frequently employed to help sustain cardiac action. Atropine sulphate 0.4 mg is given if pulmonary oedema threatens.

Nursing

Good nursing is essential and must be done by a trained midwife constantly in attendance. Apart from general attention and helping with the administration of the treatment prescribed the following points are important.

1. The patient must be turned from side to side with reasonable frequency. This helps to prevent accumulation of oedema fluid in the lungs.
2. Frequent timing of the foetal heart should be carried out. The Doptone, utilising ultrasound, could be useful for this purpose.
3. A trained midwife will be able to detect the onset of labour.

Caesarean Section

Delivery by section is generally considered to be dangerous in eclampsia. This opinion is based on experience at a time when anaesthetics such as ether and chloroform were used. With the advent of muscle relaxants and 'lytic cocktails' the position of Caesarean section may require to be reviewed. In the British Isles antepartum eclampsia with numerous fits is becoming a rarity. The more usual case is one in which one or two fits occur during labour or soon after. With these changes a re-assessment of conventional attitudes to the disease may be necessary.

ECLAMPSIA

Prognosis

Foetal	Maternal	
	Overall mortality	4%
Mortality at least 40%	Ante-natal eclampsia	6%
	Post-partum eclampsia	2%

Causes of Death

Two factors operate in leading to death of the mother.

a)   Hypertension ⟶ Damage to blood vessels ⟨ Haemorrhage / Thrombosis

b)   Fits ⟨ Rise in venous pressure ⟶ Pulmonary oedema / Anoxia ⟶ Damage to organs especially heart

Death in the acute phase of eclampsia is usually due to cerebral haemorrhage and softening, or pulmonary oedema.

The patient may survive for a few days and then succumb to continuing pulmonary oedema with superimposed hypostatic pneumonia related to myocardial damage.

Very occasionally the patient may develop anuria due to renal cortical necrosis caused by damage to the renal vessels.

Pathology

The lesions in eclampsia are largely the result of hypertensive damage to vessels.
The most obvious lesions are found in the liver and brain. Microscopic lesions are present in the kidney.
Typically the liver shows subcapsular haemorrhages and tiny yellow or haemorrhagic areas of necrosis in its substance. Microscopically these are seen to be situated in the periportal region.
Brain lesions vary in extent. Large haemorrhages may be found in the region of the internal capsule. Sometimes a relatively large lesion may occur in the pons. Alternatively there may be scattered small lesions throughout the white and grey matter of the cerebrum.
Kidney lesions consist mainly of enlargement of glomeruli with swelling and occlusion of capillaries, casts in tubules and degeneration of some tubular cells.

PRE-ECLAMPSIA AND ECLAMPSIA—AETIOLOGY

The syndrome is commonly associated with the following:-

1. It is most common in the primigravida and patients are frequently short and rather obese.
2. The incidence is greater in multiple pregnancy, acute hydramnios and possibly diabetes.
3. It also tends to occur more frequently in patients carrying a hydropic foetus.
4. Its appearance early in pregnancy is associated with hydatidiform mole.
5. Primary hypertensive disease is often complicated by superadded pre-eclampsia.

The actual cause of pre-eclampsia is unknown, but various theories have been promulgated.

1. <u>Toxic Theories</u>. In this group a hypothetical toxin is supposed to be elaborated in the placenta or decidua. Various substances have been suggested – hysterotonin, thromboplastins.

2. <u>Tension Theories</u>. The manifestations of pre-eclampsia are said to be due to either general increase in intra-abdominal tension or increase in intra-uterine tension. These tensions lead to avascularity of the uterus and may also induce a utero-renal vascular reflex leading to hypertension.

3. <u>Endocrine Theories</u>. Pre-eclampsia is commonly associated with diminished levels of pregnanediol and oestriol and the disease is thought to be related to lack of these substances.
Equally it has been postulated that excess of posterior pituitary secretion is the cause. Excessive adrenal steroids have also been suggested as a cause.

4. <u>Dietary Deficiency</u>

Evidence is scant and ultimate proof lacking for all of these theories. The tension theory is favoured at present. One of the mechanisms suggested is as follows:-

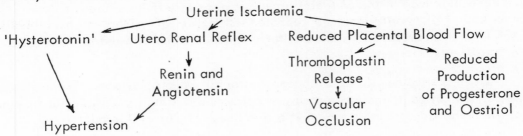

CHRONIC HYPERTENSION

This is a condition which becomes more common in the third and fourth decades. There is seldom danger to the mother and pregnancy does not appear to alter the prognosis. There is considerable hazard to the baby if the hypertension is severe and especially if pre-eclampsia supervenes.

	Foetal Loss %	Prematurity %	Underweight Babies %
Mild hypertension	1.7	8.0	5.4
Mild hypertension + pre-eclampsia	16.0	30.0	15.0
Severe hypertension	23.0	29.0	30.0
Severe hypertension + pre-eclampsia	41.0	63.0	44.0
Over-all incidence in population	2.0	7.0	

The table gives an indication of the kind of results reported in this condition.

Treatment

No special treatment is required for mild hypertension but a careful watch must be kept for signs of pre-eclampsia.

Provided a malignant phase does not arise the maternal prognosis is good in severe hyptertension. Regular examination of the retinal vessels should be carried out. Frequent monitoring of foetal growth is necessary if intra-uterine death is to be avoided. Ultrasonograms and repeated estimation of urinary oestriol levels are useful for this purpose. It is unusual for pregnancy to be allowed to continue to term in these cases.

When pre-eclamptic signs appear the foetal prognosis is poor. Treatment should be carried out as in uncomplicated pre-eclampsia but the indications for termination of the pregnancy are more urgent if a live baby is to be delivered.

172

CHAPTER 8

PLACENTAL INSUFFICIENCY
AND
FOETAL INVESTIGATIONS

PLACENTAL INSUFFICIENCY

If the foetus is not observed to be growing in size at the normal rate – the 'small-for-dates' or 'dysmature' foetus – placental insufficiency is suspected and there are various tests of placental function and foetal condition which may give warning of impending foetal death.

Measurement of Foetal Growth

The foetus gains about half a pound (0.25 kg) weekly during the last 6 weeks and this can be observed clinically. Even in the most experienced hands, assessment of maturity by this method carries an error of at least 1 week.

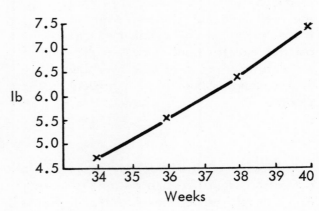

Cephalometry

A refinement is to observe the growth of the foetal biparietal diameter which increases by about 1 mm per week during the last few weeks. This measurement can now be made with accuracy by ultrasonic techniques and a decrease in the rate of growth would suggest that placental efficiency was waning.

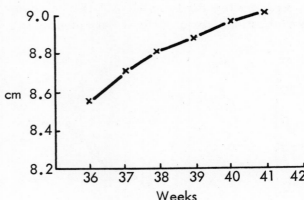

Radiology

Some information is given by the appearance of centres of ossification (distal femoral centre appears at 36 weeks, cuboid at 40 weeks) if these bones can be distinguished; and X-ray cephalometry will in experienced hands demonstrate growth of foetal biparietal diameter if repeated at intervals. Because of the technical difficulties and the need to avoid unnecessary irradiation, this method of assessment is not much used at the present day.

175

PLACENTAL INSUFFICIENCY

Oestriol Excretion Rate

Ninety per cent of urinary oestrogens in pregnancy are excreted as oestriol, produced by the placenta and probably by the foetal adrenal glands as well. There is a definite correlation between maternal oestriol excretion and foetal weight; and serial estimations over the last 10 weeks of pregnancy should show a gradual increase.

Week	Oestriol Excretion
20	4 mg/24 hr
24	7 "
28	11 "
32	14 "
36	18 "
40	24 "

Examples of oestriol excretion levels

Because of the wide day-to-day variations in excretion between individual patients it is difficult to define the normal limits of oestriol excretion and there is no definitely critical level, although values below 4 mg in 24 hours in the last trimester are regarded as serious. The important thing is to demonstrate an increase in serial estimations or at least not a continuing fall.

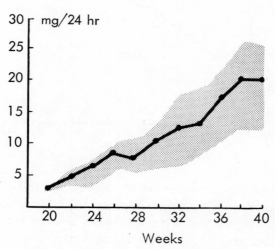

Average spread of oestriol excretion in pregnancy.

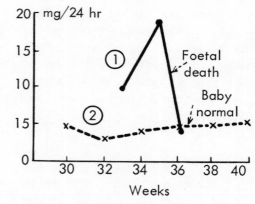

Graph ① showing fall in excretion rate after foetal death.

Graph ②. Low serial excretion rates with birth of a normal baby.

PLACENTAL INSUFFICIENCY

Amniotic Fluid Cytology

Cells in amniotic fluid are mainly epithelial whose cytoplasm stains blue with Nile blue dye. From about the 36th week another type of cell is seen which has no nucleus and is believed to be shed from foetal sebaceous glands. It contains droplets of fat which stain orange brown with Nile blue. They increase in number as a rule, as term approaches; and the presence of such cells would help to establish maturity of over 36 weeks in cases where the foetus is dysmature (small for dates).

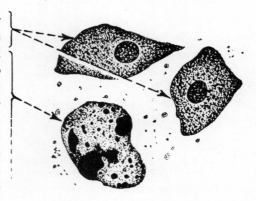

Vaginal Cytology

There is an association between pregnancy cytological appearances and placental function. In cases of marked insufficiency there is a decrease in the number of navicular ('pregnancy') cells relative to ordinary squamous cells, and an increase in the karyopyknotic index (see page 397). These changes are not really sufficiently clear cut or reliable to be clinically useful.

Indications for Applying Tests of Placental Function

There are a number of clinical conditions in which it is recognised that placental insufficiency may occur.

1. The small-for-dates foetus.
2. Postmaturity.
3. Pre-eclampsia and hypertensive disease.
4. The 'elderly' primigravida.
5. Mild antepartum haemorrhage.
6. Multiple pregnancy.
7. Bad obstetric history.
8. Diabetes mellitus.

PLACENTAL INSUFFICIENCY

Determination of Maturity and Postmaturity

It is generally accepted that postmaturity affects placental function, but it is often difficult to be sure that a particular patient is overdue. Ripeness of the cervix and descent of the presenting part are the most reliable indications of impending labour, but are not always present. In such situations the technique of amnioscopy may give some information about the state of the foetus. The tests of placental function already described are not sufficiently delicate to distinguish between maturity and postmaturity.

Amnioscopy

This means inspecting the lower pole of the amniotic sac by passing an illuminated speculum or endoscope through the cervix.

Technique
1. The patient is placed in the lithotomy psotion and cleaned and draped in the usual manner.
2. As large an endoscope as will enter the cervix is passed gently along the finger into the cervical canal. Alternatively this can be done under direct vision.
3. The obturator is removed and the endoscope adjusted to demonstrate the bag of waters.

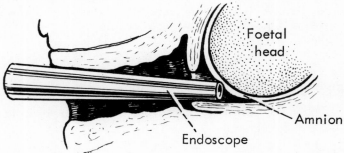

By this technique the obstetrician can learn without rupturing the membranes whether the liquor is meconium stained or clear. It is also possible to observe the yellow staining which appears with advanced erythroblastosis, and the brown stained liquor often associated with foetal abnormality.

Amnioscopy can only be done if the cervix is sufficiently dilated to admit at least a 12 mm diameter endoscope. This means in practice that the cervix must admit a finger, and attempts at forcible dilatation may cause pain and bleeding.

PLACENTAL INSUFFICIENCY

Foetal Blood Sampling in Labour

Estimation of the pH and acid-base state of foetal blood can be made on a sample of capillary blood obtained from the foetal scalp.   The pH is closely related to the degree of foetal oxygenation and should normally lie between 7.25 and 7.35 until shortly before delivery.

Technique

The patient is placed in the lith-otomy position and a special endo-scope is guided along the palm of the hand into the cervical canal, and pressed gently against the foetal scalp. Ethyl chloride is sprayed on the area and when reflex dilatation appears the scalp is smeared with silicone cream (to prevent spread of the blood) and a small cut is made in the scalp using a guarded blade which cannot penetrate more than 2 mm, thus avoiding the very vascular aponeurosis.   A blob of blood is sucked into a heparinised polyethylene tube, and about 0.18 ml will be required altogether if a full analysis is to be made using a Micro-Astrup apparatus.

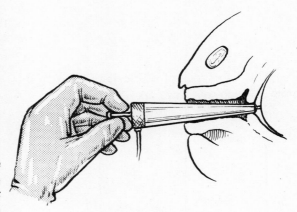

Complications

This examination especially if repeated may cause an increased discomfort to a woman in labour, but she should not otherwise be affected if the proper aseptic precuations are taken.   There may be some difficulty in getting the incision in the foetal scalp to stop bleeding, and the endoscope should not be removed until this is seen to have occurred.   Foetal exsanguination has been reported.

PLACENTAL INSUFFICIENCY

pH estimations are simply made by a pH meter which measures the electrical potential of the blood sample (this varies with H^+ ion concentration) and a low pH is called acidaemia - not the same as acidosis.

Respiratory Acidosis means a pCO_2 level above normal, and in the foetus is a direct result of inadequate oxygenation. But the body's first reaction is a slight increase in bicarbonate, so pH need not immediately fall.

Metabolic Acidosis means a reduction in the blood level of buffer base (bicarbonate, phosphate, protein) and results from the accumulation of lactic acid which is neutralised by buffer.

Some degree of metabolic acidosis is the rule in women in labour, and although transmitted to the foetus is usually harmless except that it reduces foetal reserves.

The two types of acidosis are easily distinguished on the Andersen-Engel nomogram. (Nomos: law. A nomogram is a sort of graphic ready reckoner.)

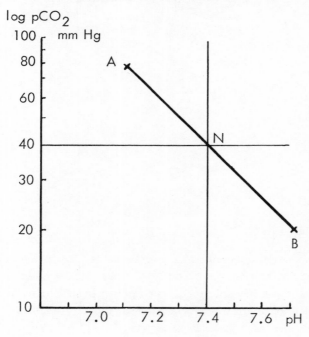

This nomogram is based on the fact that the relationship between pH and log pCO_2 is graphically a straight line within the clinical range. Thus if points A and B are determined by estimating the pH of samples of blood of known pCO_2 (easily done on a Micro-Astrup apparatus) all pH values for given pCO_2 levels will lie along the line AB. Point N on the graph is at pH 7.40, pCO_2 40 mm Hg. and is an arbitrary normal. A pCO_2 above 40 represents a respiratory acidosis.

PLACENTAL INSUFFICIENCY

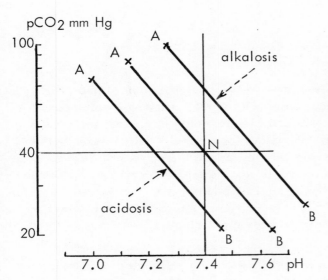

The placing of the line depends on the degree of metabolic acidosis. The further the line moves to the left of point N, the lower the level of buffer base and the greater the acidosis.

The actual levels of buffer base are read off from curves plotted on the nomogram and derived from values experimentally obtained. The upper curve shows actual levels of buffer base in mEq/l of blood. The lower curve shows at a glance the actual deficit from normal. In the example shown, the line has been drawn after establishing points A and B. The buffer base level is 40/mEq/l and the base deficit is –6 (i.e. the normal buffer base is around 46). A buffer base deficit of –6 is a degree of metabolic acidosis often met with in labour.

(In the foregoing explanation, the effects of oxygen saturation and haemoglobin concentration have been excluded).

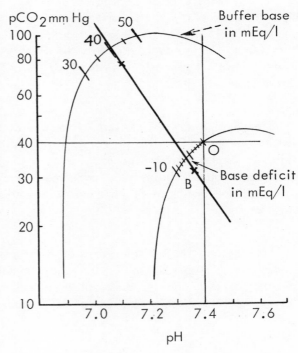

PLACENTAL INSUFFICIENCY

Interpretations of pH Estimations on Foetal Blood

The classical signs of foetal asphyxia – irregularity of the foetal heart and the passage of meconium – are not always easy to interpret. They may accompany the birth of a vigorous infant, or fail to give sufficient warning to prevent intra-uterine death. It is hoped that the monitoring of foetal blood pH will help towards the correct interpretation of clinical signs and perhaps reduce the number of deliveries by section which are performed unnecessarily. A significant fall in pH may be demonstrated before clinical signs of asphyxia have appeared, and this should help to reduce the perinatal mortality especially in conditions such as postmaturity and pre-eclampsia in which placental insufficiency may be anticipated.

There is still some argument as to whether the greater reliance should be placed on pH estimations or on degrees of acidosis. An exclusively respiratory acidosis of short duration (as in the second stage) is not of great danger to the foetus, but prolongation will lead to the formation of excessive amounts of lactic acid. On the other hand the foetus is normally in a state of metabolic acidosis (following the mother) which it seems to withstand well provided oxygen-carbon dioxide exchange is adequate.

Reliance on pH estimations alone can be misleading. Estimations refer only to the instant at which the blood sample was taken, and pCO_2 levels can change rapidly. Experience is necessary in carrying out the estimations, which like all micro-techniques require some practice. Monitoring of the foetal heart and observation of the presence or absence of meconium are still the most important signs of foetal asphyxia.

Present experience suggests that if the pH is over 7.25 then foetal oxygenation is adequate. A pH under 7.15 suggests definite asphyxia; and values inbetween these figures are regarded as 'suspicious' especially in the presence of other adverse factors, and would be an indication for further monitoring.

ULTRASOUND IN OBSTETRICS

Ultrasound is the name given to sound waves with a frequency over 20,000 cycles per second, the upper limit of the human ear.

The source of these waves is called a 'pulse generator', an apparatus which passes high voltage current through a crystal, causing it to vibrate at very high frequencies and emit ultrasonic pulses at rates between 200 and 1,000 per second. These are formed into a beam which is directed into the abdomen and reflected back to the crystal (the transducer) whenever it meets two apposed surfaces of different density (an interface). This reflected wave or echo is converted by the transducer into electrical energy and represented on a cathode ray tube, either by a vertical deflection of a horizontal line (known as A-scanning) or by a bright spot (B-scanning).

In B-scanning, the bright spot indicates the position of the echo as the probe is moved across the surface of the abdomen. These spots coalesce to give an anatomical outline of the plane of scan, and the probe is rocked mechanically through an arc of 30 or 60 degrees as it travels so as to pick up as many interfaces as possible (a compound sector scan).

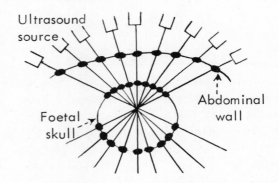

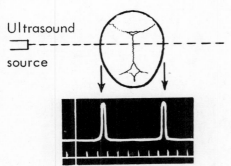

A-scan. Echoes from the two sides of the foetal skull show as blips on the cathode ray screen. If the positioning is correct the bi-parietal diameter can be calculated.

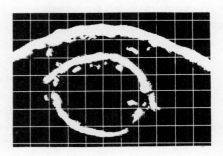

Transverse sonogram showing abdominal wall and foetal head

ULTRASOUND IN OBSTETRICS

Ultrasound can be of help in the diagnosis at an early stage of foetal abnormalities and malpresentations, and is the best way of diagnosing hydatidiform mole. It can also distinguish between pregnancy and non-pregnancy, or pregnancy and tumour; and it can help in locating the placenta.

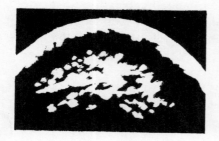

Hydatidiform Mole

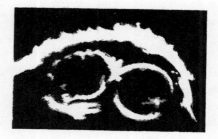

Twin pregnancy at level of thoraces.

Detection of the Foetal Heartbeat

An apparatus called the Doppler Flowmeter directs a continuous ultrasonic beam into the abdomen. The beam is reflected from interfaces at the same frequency until a moving interface (the foetal heart) is encountered. The frequency of the echo alters in the same way as a train whistle appears to alter – rising as it approaches the observer and falling as it leaves him. When amplified this alteration in frequency will be audible at the same rate as the foetal heart.

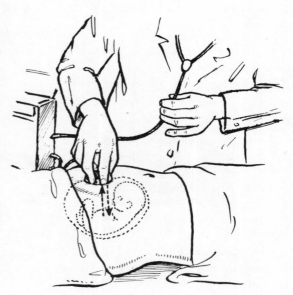

The particular usefulness of this technique is in diagnosing continuing pregnancy as early as the 12th week in cases of threatened abortion. A negative result after the 14th week suggests that the foetus has died.

CHAPTER 9

NORMAL LABOUR

NORMAL MECHANISM

LABOUR is the PROCESS of BIRTH.

The MOST COMMON PRESENTATION and POSITION is LEFT OCCIPITO-TRANSVERSE (L.O.T.). 95% of presentations are by the head and 40% of these are L.O.T. Therefore 38% of all births are L.O.T. to start. The presenting part is the VERTEX, the area bounded by the bregma, the parietal eminences and the posterior fontanelle. The DENOMINATOR is the OCCIPUT.

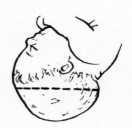

THE MECHANISM OF LABOUR

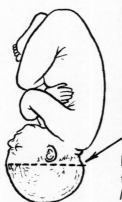

The HEAD is presenting in the TRANSVERSE diameter of the pelvic brim with the OCCIPUT to the LEFT. There is often ASYNCLITISM prior to engagement, i.e. when one or other parietal bone is the leading part.

The diagram shows the posterior parietal bone leading – this is posterior asynclitism. (If the anterior parietal bone is leading there is anterior asynclitism.)

At the BEGINNING of LABOUR the foetus is in an attitude of FLEXION but the neck is not yet fully flexed so the OCCIPITO-FRONTAL is the PRESENTING diameter.

As LABOUR PROGRESSES the foetus becomes compact. The neck is fully flexed and the SUBOCCIPITO-BREGMATIC becomes the PRESENTING diameter.

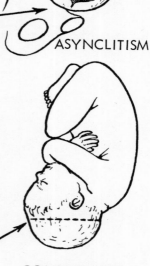

ASYNCLITISM

FLEXION

COMPACTION

186

NORMAL MECHANISM

DESCENT and ENGAGEMENT occur.

Engagement is descent of presenting diameters through pelvic brim.

The leading part – the vertex – is now near the level of the ischial spines.

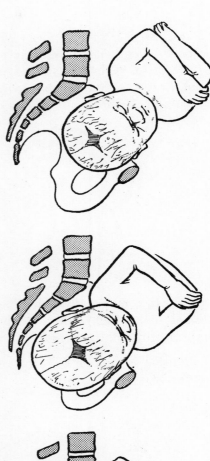

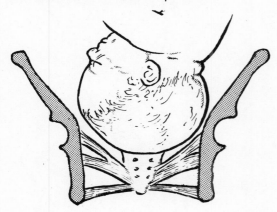

DESCENT CONTINUES and occiput rotates in cavity of pelvis anteriorly to the right oblique diameter bringing occiput to the left obturator foramen anteriorly.

Now in left occipito-anterior (L.O.A.) position.

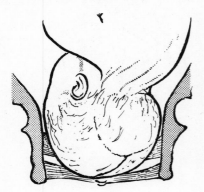

The L.O.A. position is partly attributed to the presence of the sigmoid colon in the left posterior quadrant of the pelvis.

Note how the neck is twisting.

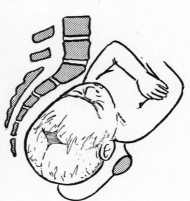

NORMAL MECHANISM

DESCENT CONTINUES and occiput reaches pelvic floor. Occiput now rotates to the front. This is INTERNAL ROTATION. The head is now occipito-anterior (O.A.).   Note twisting of the head and shoulders.   The shoulders are in the left oblique of the brim.

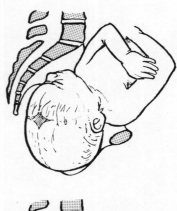

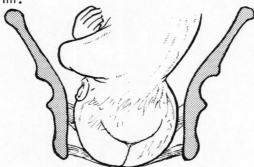

It is a maxim that the foetal part which first comes in contact with the pelvic floor rotates anteriorly (Internal rotation).

Rotation is through 45° from oblique and is called Anterior or Short rotation.

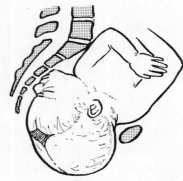

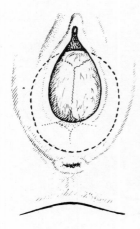

Occiput is now below the symphysis.   A further descent of the foetus pushes head forwards with a move-ment of extension and the occiput is delivered. Increasing extension round the pubis delivers the Bregma, Brow and Face.

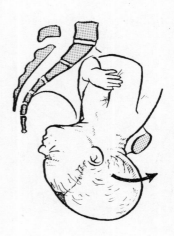

NORMAL MECHANISM

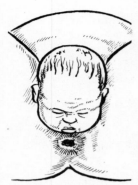

Delivery of Head

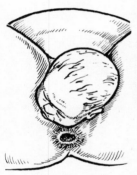

Restitution

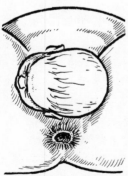

External Rotation

DESCENT and DELIVERY of the head has brought the shoulders into the pelvic cavity.

The head on delivery is oblique to the line of the shoulders. The bisacromial diameter is in left oblique diameter of the cavity.

The bisacromial diameter is the distance between the acromion processes and is 11 cm ($4\frac{1}{2}$ in.).

The head now rotates to the natural position relative to the shoulders.
This movement is known as RESTITUTION.

Descent continues and the shoulders rotate to bring the bisacromial diameter into the antero-posterior diameter of the pelvic outlet.

This descent and rotation causes the head to rotate so that the occiput lies next to the left maternal thigh. This is EXTERNAL ROTATION.

The anterior shoulder now slips under the pubis and with lateral flexion of the foetal body the posterior shoulder is born. The rest of the body follows easily.

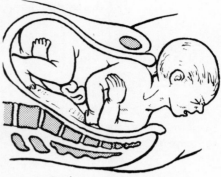

Delivery of Head

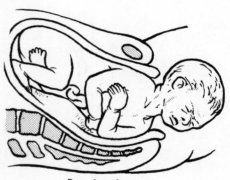

Restitution

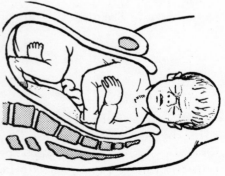

External Rotation

189

SOFT TISSUE CHANGES

The fibres of the myometrium CONTRACT and RELAX like all muscle.

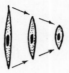

In LABOUR when the muscle fibres relax they do not return to their former length but become progressively shorter.   This is RETRACTION.

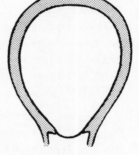

Retraction

The UTERINE CAPACITY is thus progressively REDUCED.

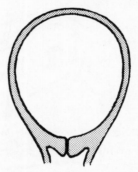

Before labour starts   After labour starts

In labour UTERINE CONTRACTIONS are Regular and Intermittent.   They tend to increase in Frequency, Duration and Intensity till the baby is delivered.

The thickness of the Uterine Wall is $\frac{1}{4}$ inch (6 mm) at the Start of Labour and 1 in. (25 mm) at the End of Labour.

The Lower Pole of the uterus (the Isthmus) and the Cervix contain little muscle tissue but mainly consist of fibrous connective tissue. This region stretches and forms the Lower Uterine Segment. The part of the uterus which is contracting and retracting forms the Upper Uterine Segment.

FORMATION OF LOWER UTERINE SEGMENT

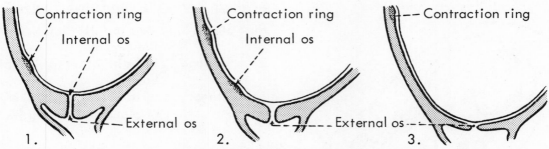

The formation of the lower uterine segment causes 'thinning', 'taking up' or effacement of the cervix. Effacement is found most commonly in the Primigravida.

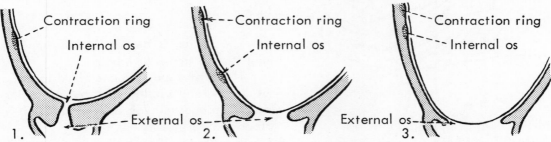

In the Parous patient dilatation and effacement of the cervix usually occur together.

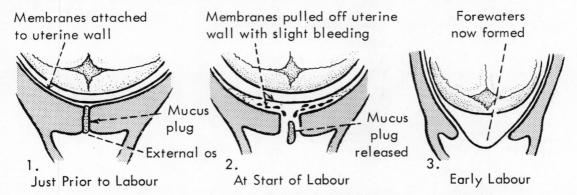

Membranes attached to uterine wall — 1. **Just Prior to Labour**

Membranes pulled off uterine wall with slight bleeding — 2. **At Start of Labour**

Forewaters now formed — 3. **Early Labour**

The effacement and dilatation of the cervix loosens the membranes from the region of the internal os with slight bleeding and sets free the mucus plug or operculum. This constitutes the 'Show' and allows the formation of the forewaters.

CHANGES IN BIRTH CANAL IN LABOUR

At BEGINNING of LABOUR

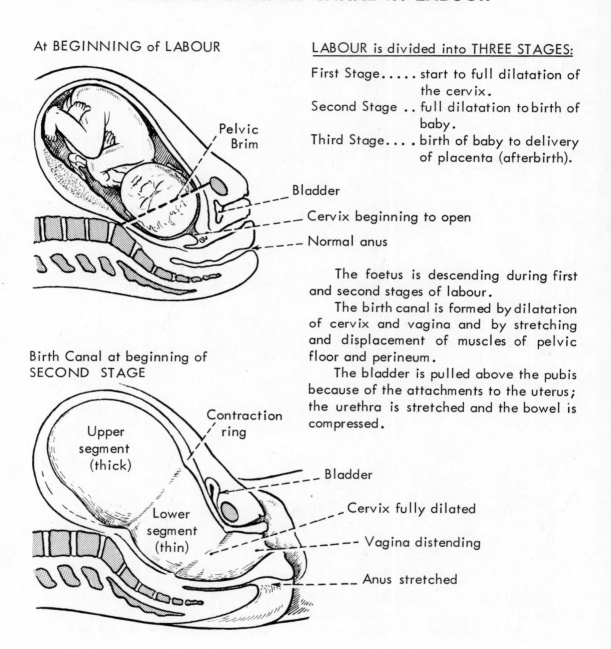

Pelvic Brim

Bladder

Cervix beginning to open

Normal anus

LABOUR is divided into THREE STAGES:

First Stage..... start to full dilatation of the cervix.

Second Stage .. full dilatation to birth of baby.

Third Stage.... birth of baby to delivery of placenta (afterbirth).

The foetus is descending during first and second stages of labour.

The birth canal is formed by dilatation of cervix and vagina and by stretching and displacement of muscles of pelvic floor and perineum.

The bladder is pulled above the pubis because of the attachments to the uterus; the urethra is stretched and the bowel is compressed.

Birth Canal at beginning of SECOND STAGE

Upper segment (thick)

Contraction ring

Lower segment (thin)

Bladder

Cervix fully dilated

Vagina distending

Anus stretched

CHANGES IN BIRTH CANAL IN LABOUR

At the END of the SECOND STAGE the birth canal has been fully formed. The outlet of the canal is at right angles to the inlet. This angulation is called the Curve of Carus.

Urethra

Constrictor vaginae muscle

Puborectalis m.

Iliococcygeus m.

Ischiococcygeus m.

Anus

(These diagrams emphasise how stretching and displacement have brought the vulva below its normal position.)

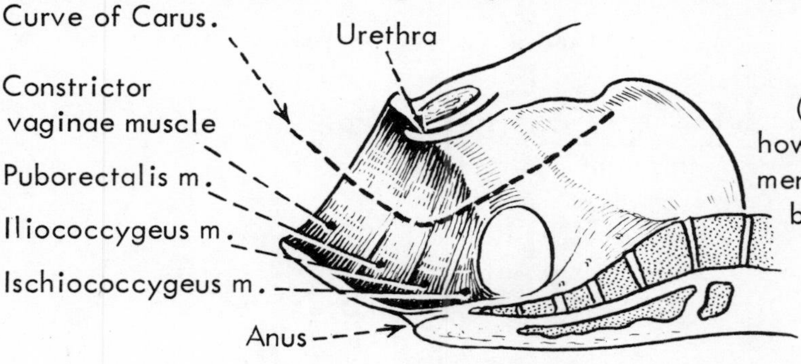

Dilated Birth Canal

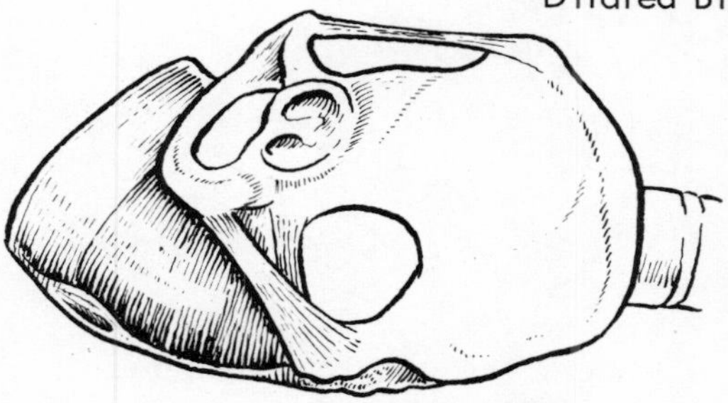

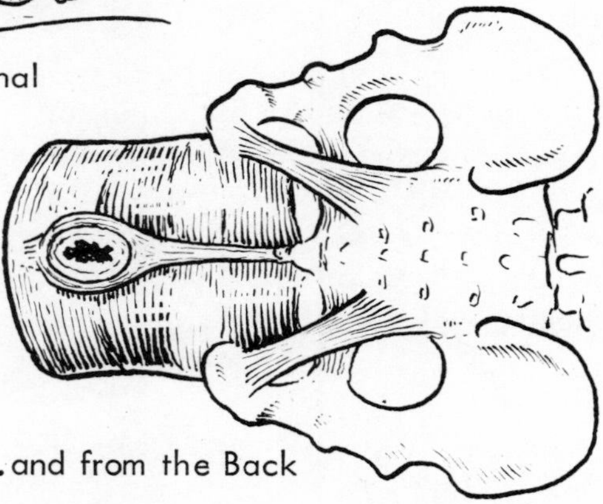

The canal from Outside the pelvis............and from the Back

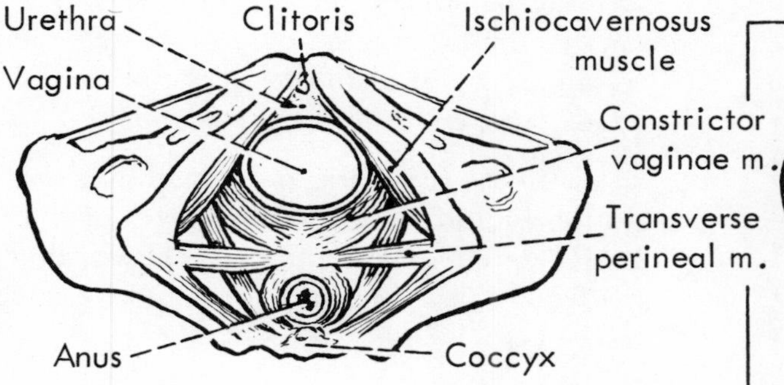

Urethra   Clitoris   Ischiocavernosus muscle

Vagina

Constrictor vaginae m.

Transverse perineal m.

Anus   Coccyx

Stretching and displacement viewed from below (after delivery)

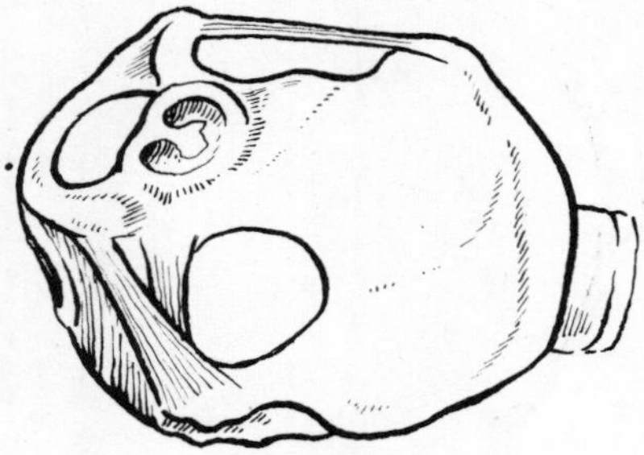

Normal at beginning of labour

DIAGNOSIS OF LABOUR

Onset of labour may be uncertain as dilatation and effacement of the cervix may be present before labour.

'Show' may not be apparent and observation over a period of time will be needed to establish the diagnosis.

<u>TRUE LABOUR</u>	<u>FALSE or SPURIOUS LABOUR</u>
Regular contractions.	Irregular contractions.
'Show'.	No ' show!
Progressive dilatation	No progressive dilatation or
and effacement of cervix.	effacement of cervix.

The altered abdominal contour shown on page 195 is due to the rising forward of the uterus so that it approximates to the direction of the pelvic birth canal. This movement is easier if the patient is upright.   Ambulation may therefore give mechanical advantage.

Pelvic brim

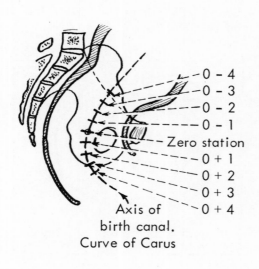

0 – 4
0 – 3
0 – 2
0 – 1
Zero station
0 + 1
0 + 2
0 + 3
0 + 4

Axis of birth canal.
Curve of Carus

Descent of the presenting part is judged by descent of the engaging diameters (suboccipito-bregmatic and bi-parietal in normal vertex) through pelvis: e.g. at the brim, high pelvic cavity, mid pelvic cavity or at the level of the ischial spines, low cavity or at the outlet.

Descent may also be judged by Zero Station Notation. Zero is the level of the ischial spines, that is the mid pelvis, and estimations are in centimetres above and below zero.

The leading part at zero = just engaged.

DIAGNOSIS OF LABOUR

LABOUR is RECOGNISED by:-

    (1)   PALPABLE UTERINE CONTRACTIONS which are Regular in Frequency and Intermittent in Character.

Intervals may be 10 minutes or even 30 minutes and each contraction may last half a minute or longer.

In labour the uterus becomes FIRM and RISES altering the abdominal contour.

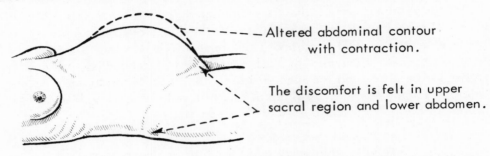

— Altered abdominal contour with contraction.

The discomfort is felt in upper sacral region and lower abdomen.

    (2)   "SHOW" – a little blood and mucus discharged from the vagina. This is from separation of the membranes at the lower pole causing bleeding which mixes with the operculum of the cervix.

    (3)   DILATATION of the CERVIX.   This is accompanied by the formation of Forewaters or Bag of Waters.

Cervical dilatation is gauged by vaginal or rectal examination and is expressed in the diameter across the cervix or by proportions of dilatation.

  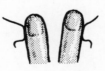 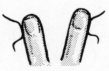

1 Finger
$\frac{3}{4}$ in. (2 cm)

2 Fingers
$1\frac{1}{2}$ in. (3.5 cm)
$\frac{1}{3}$ DILATED

3 Fingers
$2\frac{1}{4}$ in. (5.5 cm)
$\frac{1}{2}$ DILATED

4 Fingers
3 in. (7.5 cm)
$\frac{3}{4}$ DILATED

(These are Clinical Estimations)

DIAGNOSIS OF LABOUR

When labour is diagnosed the abdomen is palpated to determine the position of foetus. The level of the presenting part in relationship to the pelvic brim is noted and the foetal heart is checked.

The pudendal hair is shaved off to allow easy cleansing of the skin. An enema, unless the bowel has moved very recently, is given to reduce the risk of soiling by bowel contents in late labour. A shower or bath is given to cleanse the skin and to 'freshen' the patient.

In early labour ambulation is encouraged but some patients prefer to sit or lie down. If labour starts in the evening or following a restless night with little sleep, then the patient is put to bed and a simple sedative is given, e.g. butobarbitone or, if much discomfort, omnopon. Rest is important. Labour is work and the greatest physical effort is during the second stage. As far as is practicable an endeavour to maintain normal rhythms, by sleep at night, should be made. A light diet should be offered to the patient and plenty of fluids given.

Progress is noted and recorded:-
1. Strength, frequency and length of contractions.
2. Maternal Pulse Rate, Blood Pressure and Temperature.
3. Foetal Heart Rate. (Uterine contractions depress the foetal heart rate but it should be normal within 30 seconds.)

Progress is estimated by descent of the head on abdominal palpation.......and by changing foetal heart positions

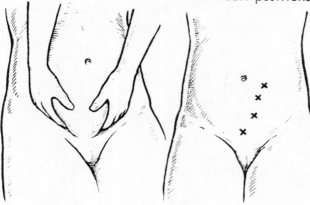

Progress also estimated by rectal examination giving dilatation of cervix and descent of head.

N.B. Remember that the sacral promontory is about 3 in.(7.5 cm) above the symphysis pubis and the pelvic cavity is downwards and backwards from the brim.

VAGINAL EXAMINATION IN LABOUR

Vaginal examination is a STERILE procedure. The examiner is masked, gowned and gloved. The patient is lying on her back with knees bent up and legs abducted.

The labia are parted with the left hand (A), allowing inspection of vulva and vaginal introitus, and the vulva is swabbed with antiseptic lotion from above downwards. Each swab is used once only.

A sterile or antiseptic lubricant is now applied to the right hand and the first and second fingers introduced into the vagina (B).

The wrist is now depressed and the fingers directed upwards behind the pubis to assess the conditions (C).

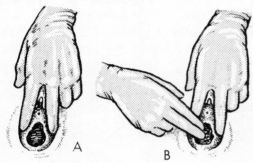

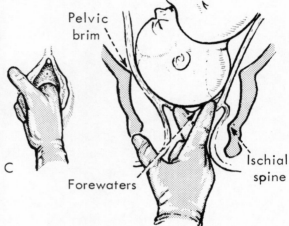

The assessment is:-

a. The state of the vagina (moist, free of abnormality).

b. Dilatation and effacement of cervix.

c. Presence or absence of forewaters. The forewaters tense and may bulge with each contraction.

d. Position of presenting part..determined by feeling suture lines and fontanelles in relationship to the pelvic diameters.

e. Level of presenting part.

Are major presenting diameters through the pelvic brim? If so how deep into the pelvis have they descended? This is judged by relationship to pelvic brim or to ischial spines.

The diagram shows a well flexed head in the L.O.T. position which is almost engaged (the suboccipito-bregmatic diameter is just above the brim), the cervix is about 3 fingers dilated and the forewaters are present.

RECTAL EXAMINATION is not a sterile procedure and will give almost as much information. The upper vagina and rectum lie close to each other. Only one finger can be introduced and the layers of rectum and vagina may mask fine detail. (See page 196).

MANAGEMENT—PROGRESS

The FIRST STAGE of labour in a Primigravida lasts about 12 to 16 hours and in a Parous woman usually 6 to 8 hours.

Progress is noted and recorded throughout......Frequency and length of contractions, maternal pulse rate and temperature, foetal heart rate, complaints of pain or distress, fluid intake, urine passed, presence or absence of acetone, blood pressure, results of examinations. Sedatives and/or Analgesics are given, if needed, to encourage rest between contractions. Sedatives - may be Barbiturates. Analgesics to relieve pain - such as Pethidine, or Omnopon - to relieve pain and encourage sleep. Tranquillising drugs such as Sparine and Largactil are useful. (It is remarkable how well a woman manages in labour without sedation in the presence of sympathetic company.. Sedation should not be withheld if thought necessary.)

The bladder may be full and cause pain and should be emptied by catheter if need be.

The SECOND STAGE of labour in a Primigravida lasts 1 to 2 hours and is shorter in the Parous. Gaseous analgesics are often used in this stage.

The second stage of labour is recognised by a change in the character of the contractions. They become more powerful and become expulsive with a desire to 'bear down', and the 'secondary forces' now come into action. The diaphragm is fixed, the patient holds her breath and the abdominal muscles contract.

At the transition to full dilatation of the cervix there is an increase in pain, there may be a desire to be sick and vomiting may occur. There may be bleeding.

Frequently the membranes rupture early in the second stage.

The patient may have the feeling that the bowel is about to move, due to pressure on the rectum, and this may have an inhibiting effect on her till the reason is explained.

The head now descends deep in the pelvis to the pelvic floor where rotation occurs.

Palpation of the perineal region by a finger on each side of the mid-line will indicate descent of head and often give impression of degree of rotation.

MANAGEMENT—DELIVERY

With the further descent and rotation of the head the perineum distends, the anus dilates and the vagina opens with contractions. There is regression between contractions but each contraction gives further progress and delivery is imminent.

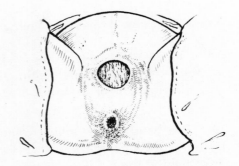

DELIVERY IS A STERILE AND ANTISEPTIC PROCEDURE

Delivery of the baby may be conducted in the left lateral or in the dorsal position.

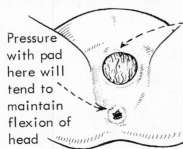

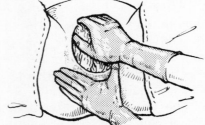

In the left lateral position the right leg is supported.

In the dorsal position the anal region is not so well seen.

A sterile pad soaked in antiseptic lotion is placed over anus. The synciput may be felt behind the anus at the tip of the sacrum.

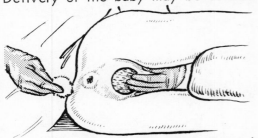

Pressure with pad here will tend to maintain flexion of head

⌐ Pressure downwards on head will promote flexion and allow occiput to slip under pubis. The distending diameter is usually the occipito-frontal.

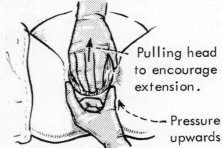

Pulling head to encourage extension.

– – Pressure upwards

Crowning of the head is when there is no recession between contractions and is due to the biparietal diameter having passed through the bony pelvis.

When occiput is free extension is encouraged and head is delivered. The neck region is now explored and if the cord is felt it is pulled to give some slack. The baby's eyes are wiped.

MANAGEMENT—DELIVERY

Restitution now occurs and then external rotation as the shoulders descend in pelvis.

The head is now grasped – fingers of the left hand beneath chin and jaw and the right fingers below the occiput.

The head is now taken towards the anus to dislodge the anterior shoulder from behind the pubis.

After the birth of the anterior shoulder the head is now lifted up over the pubis. This allows the posterior shoulder to slip over the perineum and be delivered. Traction should not be necessary, just guidance.

The perineum is often torn by the birth of the shoulders especially if the delivery is hurried and not allowed to occur with uterine contraction.

The shoulders are now gripped and the trunk delivered by lifting up over pubis. This can sometimes be aided by taking the shoulders posteriorly first and then upwards. The trunk and legs are thus delivered.

The baby's mouth and nose are drained by posture or some mechanical method and soon cries. The baby is now laid between the mother's legs and when the cord stops pulsating it is divided between clamps or ligatures.

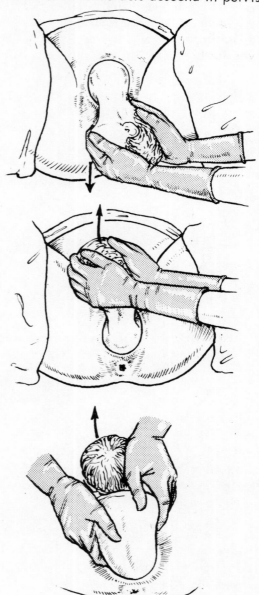

MANAGEMENT—THIRD STAGE

The first and second stages of labour are now complete and the THIRD stage has started.

It is useful to put a ligature on the cord at the vulva thus descent of the placenta will cause the ligature to move away from the vulva. A bowl is placed against the perineum to collect any blood.

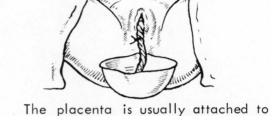

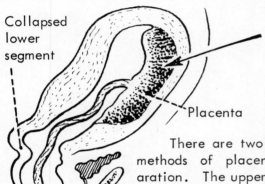

Collapsed lower segment

Placenta

There are two classical methods of placental separation. The upper segment contracts and separates the placenta and there is usually a little bleeding at this time.

Cord

The placenta is usually attached to fundus and anteriorly. The lower segment has been stretched and has no tone so it is collapsed. The upper segment is firm and the fundus is just below the umbilicus.

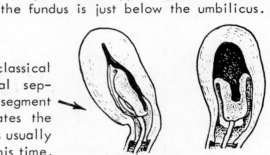
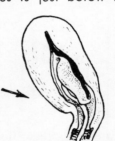

Matthews Duncan

Schultze

The placenta now descends into the lower segment and gives it form. The fundus thus rises above the umbilicus, is hard and, no longer containing the placenta, is narrower and often displaced laterally.

The placenta is then expelled, usually with the aid of the secondary powers, and as the lower segment is again empty it collapses and the fundus is now narrow, hard and found halfway between the pubis and umbilicus.

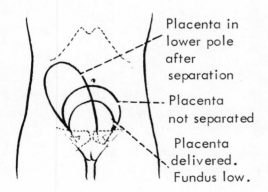

Placenta in lower pole after separation

Placenta not separated

Placenta delivered. Fundus low.

MANAGEMENT—THIRD STAGE

The management of the third stage is now explained in the light of this physiological description.

The guiding principle is to watch and wait and not to interfere. The third stage lasts about 30 minutes. Rubbing the fundus may cause irregular uterine activity which partly separates the placenta and allows bleeding.

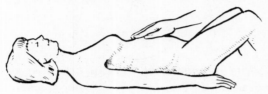

The fundal position may be seen or a hand may be placed gently on the fundus. Separation of the placenta causes the fundus to rise, a little bleeding and possible lengthening of the cord.

The third stage is conducted in the dorsal position. After separation the placenta lies in the upper vagina and lower uterine segment and is finally expelled by the patient bearing down.

When the placenta is being delivered it is cradled by both hands and then the membranes are twisted gently to allow them to peel off completely.

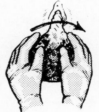

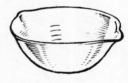

Murdoch's bowl

A bowl placed against the perineum allows blood loss to be assessed. The Murdoch's bowl is ideally suited for this as the blood loss is measured all the time. The normal loss is about 10 ounces (0.25 litres).

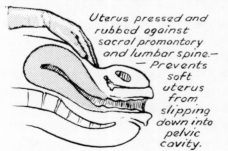

Uterus pressed and rubbed against sacral promontory and lumbar spine. — Prevents soft uterus from slipping down into pelvic cavity.

The uterine fundus is now rubbed up to assure firm contraction and then an oxytocic can be given e.g. Ergometrine, 0.5 mg intramuscularly.

The vagina, labia and perineum are inspected for tears or other injuries. The vulva is swabbed down and a sterile pad placed over it to collect the lochial discharges.

The placenta is now examined:- It is suspended by the cord to show the extent of the membranes and deficiencies, if any, and then placed on the hand (maternal side uppermost) to see if it is complete.

202

MANAGEMENT—PATIENT CARE

Each labour is an individual problem. The management and care can only be outlined.

Glucose sweets sucked in labour may prevent ketosis. If ketosis or dehydration develops, intravenous fluids and sugars are given but this restricts the patient to bed.

Drugs may be used to relieve pain or fear, to promote sleep or for a combination of these actions. Some patients need much sedation, others little.

The periods of maximum pain are towards the end of the first and second stages of labour. Temporary relief may be found with inhalant analgesics.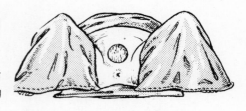

The first stage of labour ideally should consist of periods of rest, in chairs or bed, periods of ambulation and periods of sleep.

The second stage of labour is short and the patient should be taken to the delivery room as soon as this stage is recognised (full cervical dilatation).

Sterile drapes clothe the mother's legs and abdomen. She lies on an absorbent pad.

The patient is encouraged to 'bear down'. It may in fact be difficult to prevent her pressing down.

Inhalant analgesics are given. Perineal infiltration may be needed to permit incision of the perineum (Episiotomy, page 426) and to prevent ragged tearing.

Imminent tearing is recognised by:-

1. Fresh bleeding from the vagina – due to mucosal tearing.
2. Blanching and glazing of perineal skin.

MANAGEMENT—DELIVERY ROOM

The patient should be in pleasant friendly surroundings – her home provides these; however, few are confined at home and therefore the place of confinement should, wherever practicable, achieve as near as possible a domestic atmosphere.

The FIRST STAGE room should be in two parts: –

A. A Lounge furnished with comfortable chairs of various heights and types. Radio and television may provide entertainment and distraction.
The patient's husband or mother may give comfort and company.
The care by the staff should be unobtrusive, effective and sympathetic.

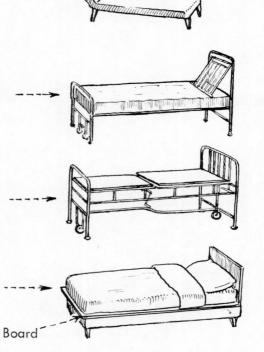

B. There should be a separate Bed Area. The beds should be firm but not rigid and of a size and height suitable for delivery in emergency.

The SECOND STAGE

The Delivery Room bed should be rigid with a thin waterproof mattress. There are many beds designed for the purpose, some made to tilt.

For HOME CONFINEMENT boards placed under the mattress are an advantage.

Board

In the delivery room all that is necessary for the birth of the baby, care and resuscitation of baby and mother are present.

MANAGEMENT—DELIVERY ROOM

FOR MOTHER
Sterile drapes for legs and thighs.
Sterile sheet and pad to go below
  buttocks and on bed.
Sterile towel to cover abdomen.

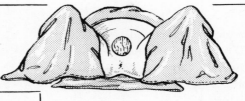

FOR EPISIOTOMY and REPAIR of PERINEAL WOUNDS
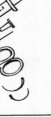
Local anaesthetic
syringe and needles.
Scissors – for cutting
perineum (episiotomy).
Sutures and needles
for repair.

FOR SWABBING and WIPING CLEAN
Bowls with lotions.
Swabs and cotton wool.
Gamgee pads.

COTTON WOOL FOR WIPING BABY'S EYES

FOR CARE of CORD
Pressure forceps to
clamp cord,
or cord clamp or
cord ligatures.
Scissors to cut cord.

FOR REPLACING SOILED ARTICLES
Spare sterile towels
and sheets.

FOR BABY CARE (see Care of New-born and Asphyxia.)
Sterile towel – for reception.
Mucus suction catheter.
Oxygen.
Laryngoscope.
Warm cot.
Syringes, needles and
ampoules of:-
Amiphenazole (Daptazole),
Nalorphine (Lethidrone),
Levallorphan (Lorfan),
Nikethamide (Coramine).

FOR CONTROLLING BLEEDING
Syringe and needles.
Pressure forceps for
bleeding points
in perineum.
Bowl to collect and
measure third stage
blood loss and to
receive placenta.

FOR ATTENDANTS CONDUCTING DELIVERY.
Sterile masks, caps,
gowns and gloves.

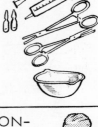

MANAGEMENT—DRUGS

HYPNOTICS

Amytal (Amylobarbitone) 90 – 180 mg
Nembutal (Pentobarbitone) 90 – 180 mg
Seconal (Quinalbarbitone) 90 – 180 mg

This group is short acting and useful in early labour.

They do not relieve pain but calm the mother and give rest or sleep.

Barbiturates have a depressant effect on the foetal respiratory centres and may also make the mother confused. The long acting Barbiturates are therefore undesirable. Welldorm (Dichlorophenazone), 650 – 1,300 mg, is an effective non-barbiturate hypnotic.

INHALANT ANALGESICS

These are used towards the end of the first stage of labour either alone or as an adjuvant to drugs and again for the birth. The apparatus is designed to give a fixed amount of Nitrous Oxide and Oxygen or Trilene and Air. They are self administered and work on demand so overdose is avoided.

NARCOTICS

Morphine 10 – 15 mg. For pain relief and sleep.

Pethidine 50 – 200 mg. 150 mg ≡ 15 mg morphine.

Pethidine is not so sedative as morphine. Both drugs depress the foetal respiratory centre and should not be given within 4 hours of birth. If the birth is unexpectedly soon then the depressant effect can be neutralised before birth by giving the mother Lorfan (Levallorphan) 5 ml, or Lethidrone (Nalorphine) 5 – 10 mg. The baby can be given 0.25 – 1 mg Lethidrone at birth.

Labour should be well established before giving Morphine or Pethidine as early administration may arrest labour.

Pethidine 50 mg given slowly intravenously gives quick relief.

Sparine (Promazine) 25 – 50 mg potentiates Morphine and Pethidine.

Scopolamine 0.4 mg will also potentiate but may make the patient unco-operative.

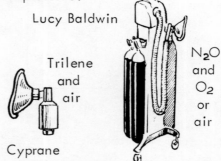

Lucy Baldwin

Trilene and air

N_2O and O_2 or air

Cyprane

The proportions can be varied with this type of apparatus

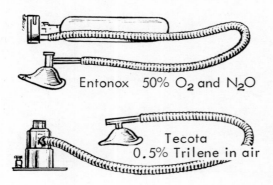

Entonox 50% O_2 and N_2O

Tecota 0.5% Trilene in air

CHAPTER 10

MALPOSITION AND MALPRESENTATION

MALPOSITION AND MALPRESENTATION

Malposition and malpresentation have ill fitting presenting parts compared to a well flexed vertex presentation in a normal pelvis.

Well fitting vertex

Breech

Flat pelvis

Shoulder

Face

Occipito posterior

Normal uterine polarity (see page 210) is disturbed. The ill-fitting presenting part will apply unequal pressures in the lower uterine pole. The contractions tend to be ill-sustained and irregular but become more normal as compaction of the foetus occurs, moulding takes place and caput forms.

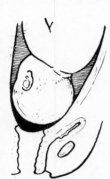
Well-fitting

An ill-fitting presenting part does not shield the forewaters from the pressures of uterine contractions.

The forewaters and membranes are stretched through the incompletely dilated cervix into the vagina. The membranes rupture early and the umbilical cord may be swept out by the outrush of liquor past the presenting part.

Prior to rupture the membranes are described as finger-like or sausage shaped and are found in the vagina with small dilatation of the cervix.

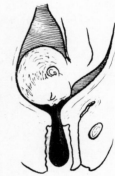
Ill-fitting

When the membranes rupture there is often a pause in labour as the lower segment pressure is suddenly reduced, and uterine polarity is again disturbed. Incoordinate labour follows till more normal polarity is again established.

Inco-ordinate uterine contractions are more painful than normal.

An ill-fitting presenting part is therefore associated with:-
1. Slow, erratic, shortlived contractions.
2. Early rupture of membranes with risk of cord prolapse (a vaginal examination to check for cord is advisable).
3. Pause in labour after rupture of membranes often leading to inco-ordinate and excessively painful labour.

UTERINE ACTION

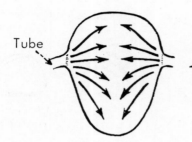

Tube

Uterine action in labour has been studied by tocodynamometers and intra-uterine catheters. Each contraction is initiated in the region of the tubes and round ligaments and spreads over the uterus.

The contractions show a gradient pattern with fundal dominance and the lower uterine segment least active.
This is <u>NORMAL UTERINE POLARITY</u>.

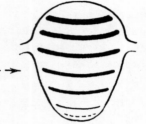

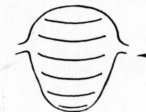

Prior to labour and in false labour there is no polarity of action.

With normal uterine action the contraction is palpable before there is complaint of discomfort or pain.

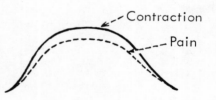

Contraction

Pain

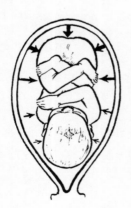

Normal uterine polarity in labour is encouraged by a well flexed foetus and a well fitting presenting part pressing on the lower pole of a normal uterus and with a normal pelvis. Normal polarity allows stretching and relative relaxation of the lower segment under dominant action of upper segment, and lower segment thins as upper segment thickens.

ABNORMAL UTERINE ACTION

NORMAL POLARITY

Weak Contractions

Primary inertia or Hypotonic inertia. → Normal type of action but poor performance. 'Lazy uterus'. → Long labour but not exhausting. Foetus not usually at risk. Treat with sedatives, and 'time' while uterus is 'playing in'. Usually settles down to more normal action.

Secondary inertia or Exhaustion. → Cessation of action. Find cause. May be obstructive. → Potentially dangerous because of cause. Treat cause – if not obstructive, rest with strong sedatives and fluids may relieve.

Excessively Strong Contractions

Obstructed labour. → Uterus trying to overcome obstruction. → 1. Obstruction being overcome. or 2. Uterine exhaustion. or 3. Uterine rupture.

No obstruction. → Precipitate labour. → Foetal distress due to persistent pressures on placental site and rapid moulding of head.

ABNORMAL POLARITY

Pain

Contraction

Disordered Uterine Action —— 96% are primigravid labours
or
Inco-ordinate Uterine Action → Painful and unproductive. Pain before and after palpable contraction.

Hypertonic Lower Uterine Segment or Reversed Polarity → Internal 'Battle of Forces'. No progress.

Localised Tonic Contraction or Contraction Ring → Grips round narrow part of foetus usually between head and shoulders.

Generalised Tonic Contraction → Squeezing child and placenta

All of these abnormal actions cause foetal distress by compression of foetus and placenta.

Cervical Rigidity... A form of obstructed labour. May be due to old trauma of cervix or failure of elasticity of cervix.

DIAGNOSIS OF MALPRESENTATION

The Mouth and Anus may be mistaken.

MOUTH

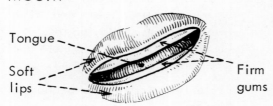

Tongue

Soft lips

Firm gums

The mouth may be mistaken for the anus because of oedema masking laxity of the orifice.

ANUS

 ← Nodules of sacral spines.

Grip on finger.

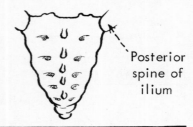

The breech may be mistaken for the face.

If in doubt do not use force as other tissues such as eyes or genitalia may be damaged.

SACRUM

The sacrum is recognised by the shape, nodular ridge of the spines and possibly the foramina and the posterior portion of iliac crest. The spine nodules are continuous with the vertebrae above.

Posterior spine of ilium

SUPRA-ORBITAL RIDGES

Supra-orbital ridges are recognised by double curve, root of nose, orbits and frontal suture. All may be partly obscured by caput.

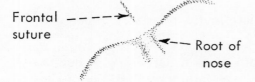

Frontal suture

Root of nose

NOSE

The nose is recognised by the 'saddle', and its firm elasticity.

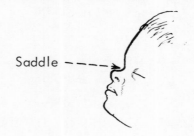

Saddle

DIAGNOSIS OF MALPRESENTATION

The Foot and Hand may be mistaken.

FOOT

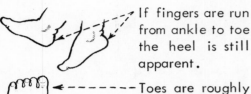

If fingers are run from ankle to toe the heel is still apparent.

Toes are roughly equal in length.

HAND

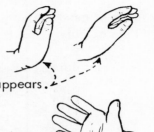

If fingers are run from wrist to palm then the 'heel' disappears.

Fingers are not equal and the thumb is separate.

Right from left is identifiable by the position of the great toe or thumb.

SHOULDER

The shoulder is identified by the humerus, scapula, acromion process, coracoid process, clavicle and ribs. All of these cannot be palpated at once.

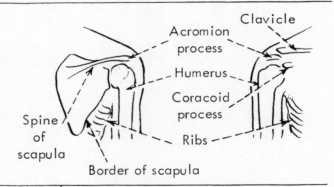

Clavicle

Acromion process

Humerus

Coracoid process

Ribs

Spine of scapula

Border of scapula

The Knee and Elbow may be mistaken.

KNEE

The knee has a hollow as the knee cap is not yet formed.

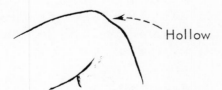

Hollow

ELBOW

The elbow has the point of the olecranon process.

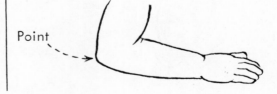

Point

OCCIPITO-POSTERIOR PRESENTATION

Occipito-posterior presentation is a malpresentation of the head and occurs in 13% of head presentations. The presenting part is the vertex and the denominator is the occiput. R.O.P. is three times as common as L.O.P.

Postulated causes of O.P.

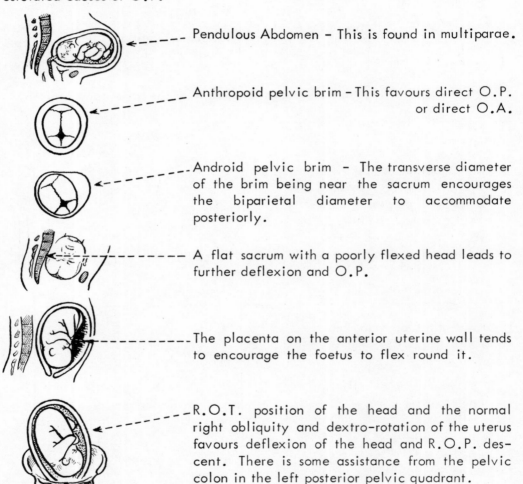

Pendulous Abdomen – This is found in multiparae.

Anthropoid pelvic brim – This favours direct O.P. or direct O.A.

Android pelvic brim – The transverse diameter of the brim being near the sacrum encourages the biparietal diameter to accommodate posteriorly.

A flat sacrum with a poorly flexed head leads to further deflexion and O.P.

The placenta on the anterior uterine wall tends to encourage the foetus to flex round it.

R.O.T. position of the head and the normal right obliquity and dextro-rotation of the uterus favours deflexion of the head and R.O.P. descent. There is some assistance from the pelvic colon in the left posterior pelvic quadrant.

Chance also is an apparent cause.

OCCIPITO-POSTERIOR PRESENTATION

Occipito-posterior labour is frequently straightforward and just as speedy as occipito-anterior. Sixty-five per cent deliver spontaneously as O.A.

PALPATION

A. The foetal back is found to one side in early labour before descent of head.

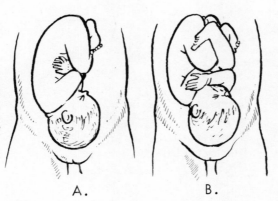

A.　　　B.

B. The foetal head is postero-lateral in early labour in android pelvis and with descent of head.

The limbs are to the front and give hollowing above the head.

Particularly noticeable after rupture of the membranes.

Check if the head is engaged or not.

AUSCULTATION

The foetal heart is heard best well out in the flank but descends to just above the pubis as the head rotates and descends.

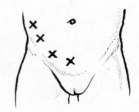

VAGINAL EXAMINATION

The membranes tend to rupture early, often before labour is established. If the membranes are intact they may protrude through the cervix giving finger-like forewaters, or may fill the upper vagina and obscure the presenting part. The presenting part is the vertex, but there is deflexion (incomplete flexion) so the anterior

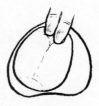

fontanelle is readily felt in the anterior part of the pelvis near the ileo-pectineal eminence. The sagittal suture aims towards the right sacro-iliac joint. The posterior fontanelle is not readily felt till the head is in lower pelvic cavity.

O.P. PRESENTATION—MECHANISM

Two types of occipito-posterior (O.P.) are described.

A Flexed O.P. with suboccipito-frontal and biparietal diameter engaging 4 in. (10 cm) x $3\frac{3}{4}$ in. ($9\frac{1}{2}$ cm).

B Deflexed O.P. with occipito-frontal and biparietal diameters engaging $4\frac{1}{2}$ in. ($11\frac{1}{2}$ cm) x $3\frac{3}{4}$ in. ($9\frac{1}{2}$ cm).

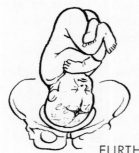

Engagement occurs in the transverse or the right oblique diameter of the brim. Descent occurs in the right oblique diameter of pelvis giving the right occipito-posterior position (R.O.P.). Descent continues to pelvic floor.

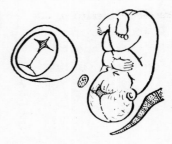

FURTHER PROGRESS DEPENDS ON FLEXION OF HEAD

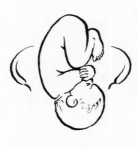

A If flexion of head increases in descent then occiput strikes pelvic floor first and rotates anteriorly through the right occipito-transverse (R.O.T.) position – and then to the R.O.A. position and to the direct O.A. position.

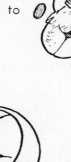

135°

The occiput has thus rotated through the angle of 135° to bring the occiput to the symphysis pubis. This is known as LONG rotation.

The mechanism is thereafter the same as for the occipito-anterior position.

O.P. PRESENTATION—MECHANISM

B If flexion of head remains incomplete in descent then rotation of the occiput anteriorly on the pelvic floor may not occur; but rotation of the occiput posteriorly may occur bringing the occiput into the hollow of the sacrum. This is known as SHORT rotation (45°) and gives the persistent occipito-posterior (P.O.P.) position or direct O.P. position.

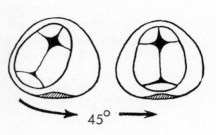

45°

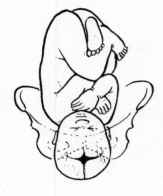

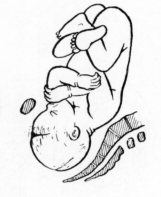

The mechanism now is difficult for flexion of the head is restricted by the foetal chest though the brow is pressed to the pubis and some flexion occurs. The soft tissues are stretched more than in O.A. and the foetus is delivered face to pubis.

If this does not occur then an impasse is reached and there is obstructed labour.

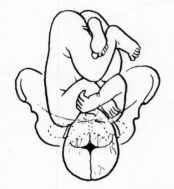

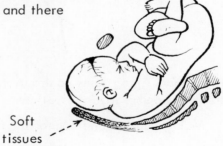

Soft tissues

Sometimes the long rotation of the O.P. is arrested and the head is left in the occipito-transverse position in the cavity of the pelvis. This is one form of transverse arrest of the head.

O.P. PRESENTATION—MANAGEMENT

O.P. may lead to a disorganised labour, especially in the primigravid patient. Initially the contractions are ill-sustained and irregular, with marked bachache. Sedation is advisable – morphine, 10 – 15 mg, will ease discomfort, allay anxiety and promote sleep. Pethidine, 100 – 150 mg, will act similarly but has not such a hypnotic effect.

Sleeping on the side which the head faces may be an advantage.

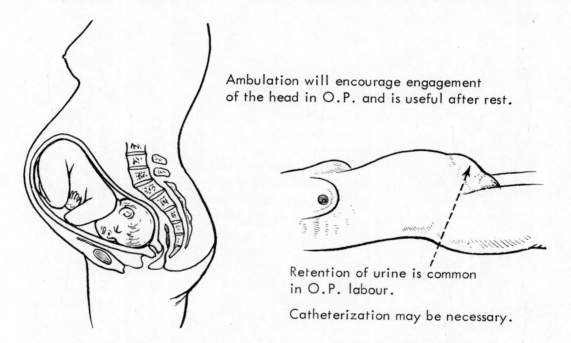

Ambulation will encourage engagement of the head in O.P. and is useful after rest.

Retention of urine is common in O.P. labour.

Catheterization may be necessary.

As labour progresses contractions become more normal, but severe bachache may persist and demoralise the patient.

Much sedation and comforting may be needed.

The patient may feel the need to bear down before the first stage of labour is complete. This may be due to pressure on sacrum and rectum so the cervical dilatation must be checked in O.P. labour, if the patient has an urge to bear down.

O.P. PRESENTATION—MANAGEMENT

Twelve per cent of cases will be delivered spontaneously in persistent occipito-posterior position (face to pubis). This is favoured by the anthropoid pelvis. An extensive episiotomy may be required to avoid laceration of the perineum by the greater diameters of the head which distend the perineum (occipito-frontal $4\frac{1}{2}$ in, $11\frac{1}{2}$ cm compared with suboccipito-frontal 4 in, 10 cm in O.A.).

Internal rotation of the occiput may be disturbed by:-

   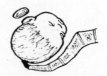 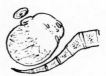

Prominent ischial spines   Inturned coccyx   Long narrow
                                                           sacrum

or other restriction of space in the cavity as in the android pelvis

or Deflection of the
head .... gives
equal moments.

Rotation is incomplete and there
is transverse arrest of the head.

This is an impasse and delivery must be completed by manipulation.

To complete delivery with a transverse arrest of the head the patient is anaesthetised and a gloved hand inserted into the vagina and the foetal brow and temples are grasped (in the R.O.T. position the right hand is more convenient). The other hand is placed at the pelvic brim to prevent displacement of the head from the pelvis and then the abdominal hand pushes the shoulder forward while the vaginal hand turns the brow towards the sacrum to bring the occiput to the pubis. (See page 438). The forceps are applied and delivery completed or Kielland's forceps are applied to rotate and deliver the head.

If forceps delivery of a persistent occipito-posterior head has to be undertaken then manipulation as described can be used but if the outlet is wide as in an anthropoid pelvis then delivery can be completed face to pubis.

Sometimes occipito-posterior labour is terminated by Caesarean section because of foetal distress. This is specially common in primigravid in the first stage of labour. Lack of progress may also justify Caesarean section.

BREECH PRESENTATION—MECHANISM

The breech is a malpresentation and occurs once in about 40 cases of labour. The presenting part is the breech and the denominator is the sacrum.

Aetiology: The breech is the presenting part in 25% of cases before 30 weeks therefore prematurity is an important factor.

The legs of the foetus may be extended and interfere with flexion of the body so breech with extended legs is common especially in primigravida.

Multiple pregnancy will interfere with spontaneous version.

Other related factors are:– Foetal malformation, hydramnios, lax uterus and pendulous abdomen, abnormal shape of pelvic brim or uterus, placenta praevia.

Three types of breech presentation are described:–

Fully flexed
foetus

Not fully flexed foetus
and with knee joints extended

One or both thighs
extended

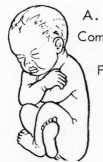

A.
Complete breech
or
Full breech

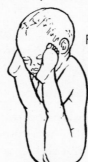

B.
Frank breech
or
Breech with
extended legs

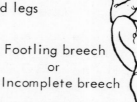

C.

Footling breech
or
Incomplete breech

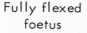

Mechanism

The denominator is the sacrum; the leading part the anterior buttock.

The bitrochanteric diameter (transverse diameter between the great trochanters of the foetus) is 4 in.(10 cm).   The most common position is the left sacro-anterior (L.S.A.). With labour there is compaction, descent and engagement of the breech (bisiliac diameter).

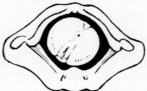

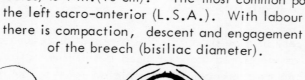

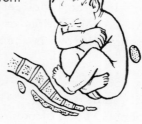

BREECH PRESENTATION—MECHANISM

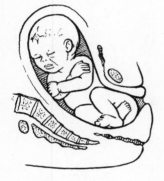

Descent continues till breech reaches pelvic floor. The anterior buttock rotates forward under the pubis (internal rotation).

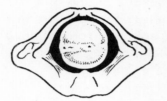

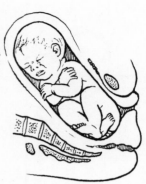

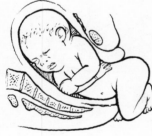

Lateral flexion of the foetal body round the pubis allows the anterior buttock to slip forward under the pubis and the posterior buttock to slip over the perineum. The breech is delivered followed by the legs. A movement of restitution of the hips takes place.

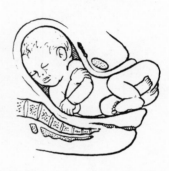

The shoulders now engage in the same pelvic diameter as the hips – the left oblique. (The bisacromial diameter of the shoulders is $4\frac{1}{4}$ in. – 11 cm.)

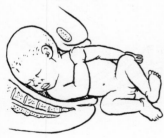

As descent continues internal rotation of the shoulders occurs in the pelvic cavity bringing one shoulder beneath the pubis and the other into the hollow of the sacrum. The anterior shoulder and arm are born first.

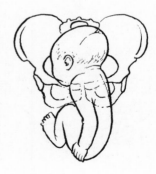

BREECH PRESENTATION—MECHANISM

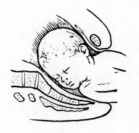

As the shoulders are being born the head enters the pelvic brim either in the transverse or left oblique of the brim.
The engaging diameters of the head are the biparietal and the suboccipito-bregmatic or sub-occipito-frontal.

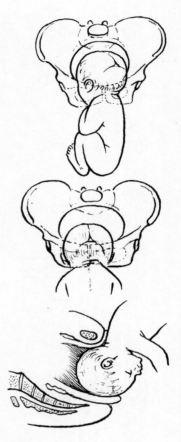

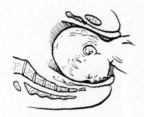

The head descends into the pelvic cavity and rotates to bring the occiput under the pubis.

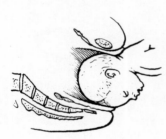

The occiput is arrested at the pubis and the head is born by flexion.   The chin, face and brow are born first, and then the occiput.

Sometimes the occiput rotates posteriorly.

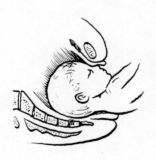

If the head is flexed the root of the nose is arrested behind the pubis and the occiput and vertex are born first followed by the face.
If the head is extended the chin is arrested above the pubis and the occiput and vertex are delivered and the face follows.

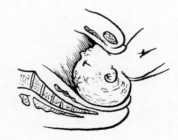

BREECH PRESENTATION—MANAGEMENT

PALPATION
1. Longitudinal lie.
2. Firm lower pole.
3. Limbs to one side.
4. Hard head at fun-
   dus. (Head may
   not be palpable
   at fundus because
   it is under the
   ribs – always con-
   firm by pelvic
   examination.)

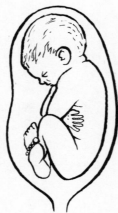

Full breech

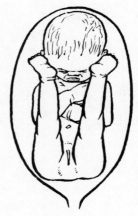

Frank breech

AUCULTATION
     The foetal heart (F.H.) is best heard above the umbilicus.

VAGINAL EXAMINATION
     No head in pelvis. Soft buttocks felt and hard irregular sacrum. Feet may be in pelvis as leading part. Meconium is often present in the vagina. This is the only time that passage of meconium may be considered normal.

The breech with extended legs (frank breech) forms a well fitting presenting part and labour proceeds normally at first. Frank breech gives little worry until the pelvic floor is reached. Delivery will only progress with lateral flexion of the trunk. This may not occur despite distension of the perineum as the legs splint the body. An episiotomy may allow delivery of the buttocks. However progress may only be slight after episiotomy because of the legs splinting. Groin traction with pains will help the breech descent. Delivery of a foot will relieve the splint effect.

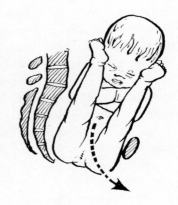

BREECH PRESENTATION—MANAGEMENT

Delivery of Legs

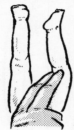
Pressure to the popliteal space to flex the knee and displace it to the side of the trunk.

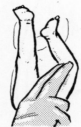
Fingers are worked along leg towards ankle to encourage further flexion of knee.

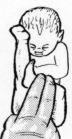
The ankle is grasped and the foot swept down over the other leg.

A loop of cord is pulled down as soon as is practicable to prevent possible tearing of it later.

Delivery is conducted in the lithotomy position at the end of the bed to allow room for the foetus to hang over the perineum.

When delivery of one leg is complete the delivery of the second follows quickly.

The delivery proceeds spontaneously and as the anterior shoulder blade appears the arm is delivered (1) by placing two fingers of the appropriate hand (right if right shoulder) over the clavicle and sweeping them round the point of the shoulder and down the humerous to the elbow and carrying the forearm free. (2) The ankles are then grasped and swung upwards. This permits the posterior arm being freed in a similar way. (3) The body is now allowed to hang till the head descends into the pelvis and the hair line shows (the Burns–Marshall method).

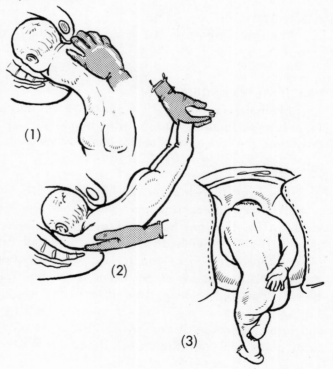

(1)

(2)

(3)

BREECH PRESENTATION—MANAGEMENT

The feet are then grasped (4) and with gentle traction are swept in an arc over the maternal abdomen (5) (the method of the Prague seizure). Thus the mouth is freed and a pause is made while the mouth is cleansed. The delivery is then completed slowly by further swinging over the abdomen (6).

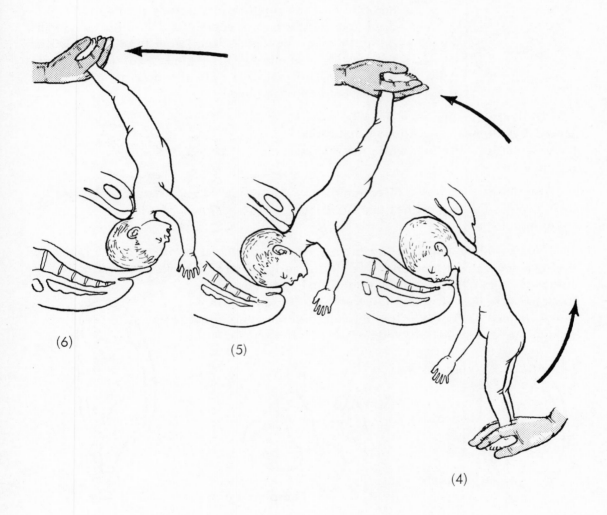

(6)

(5)

(4)

BREECH PRESENTATION—MANAGEMENT

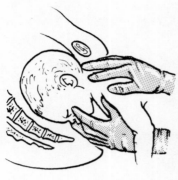

The head may be delivered by the Mauriceau-Smellie-Veit grip.

The child is laid along the left arm and the middle finger is placed in the mouth, the index and ring fingers catch the malar processes. Traction by these fingers will tend to promote flexion of the head. The index finger and thumb of the right hand grasp one shoulder, the middle finger presses on the occiput and the other two fingers grasp the other shoulder. Traction of the two hands will deliver the head and keep it flexed. Supra pubic pressure by an assistant will help the delivery and control rapid moulding of the head.

Delivery of the head may be completed by forceps. An assistant holds the baby upwards by the feet while the blades are applied.

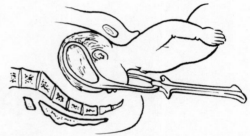

Traction is then in the direction of the birth canal. Forceps control and limit the moulding of the head.

The complete and footling breech have a slow and erratic start to labour as they are not well fitting, and have risk of early rupture of membranes and prolapsed cord. Sedation till labour is established is an advantage. Labour is speeded, if when the cervix is sufficiently dilated (3 – 4 fingers), a foot is pulled through into the vagina thus making the half breech the leading part and so reduce bulk.

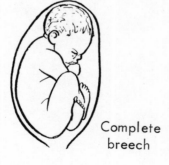

Complete breech

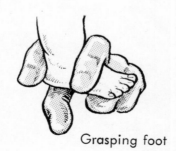

Grasping foot

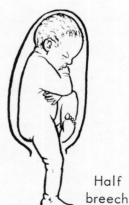

Half breech

BREECH PRESENTATION—MANAGEMENT

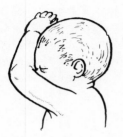

An extended arm has the same effect as increasing the diameter of the head and as a rule makes delivery impossible.

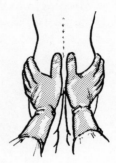

If manipulation is required the foetus is grasped by the pelvis with thumbs along spine to prevent crushing of viscus.

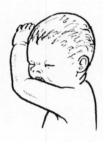

The trunk is turned so that the face comes to the arm. (Left arm – clockwise turn, right arm – anticlockwise). Then a hand is inserted up the foetal abdomen to reach the arm in the region of the elbow, flexes it and sweeps it down over the foetal chest.

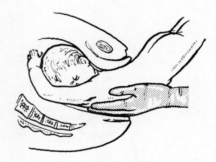

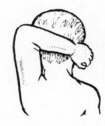

If the hand is displaced behind the head the condition is one of nuchal or dorsal displacement, and the same rotation as described above is used but must be greater to bring the arm to the face.

Malrotation may dislocate the shoulder or fracture the humerus. If both arms are displaced it is usually easier to free the posterior arm first because of the space in the sacral bay. After one arm is freed the opposite rotation permits the other arm to be dealt with.

BREECH PRESENTATION—MANAGEMENT

Løvset's manoeuvre for the delivery of arms which are extended or for nuchal displacement makes use of the inclination of the pelvic brim, the short anterior wall and the long posterior wall of the cavity. The anterior shoulder is above the symphysis while the posterior is below the promontory and if these are now reversed in position, the posterior shoulder will keep below the brim and be just below the symphysis and can be easily delivered.

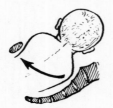 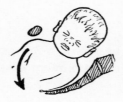 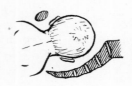

The Løvset manoeuvre is done by grasping the foetus by the pelvis and pulling gently while rotating to bring the posterior shoulder to the front. The direction of rotation is so that the posterior arm trails towards the chest (anti-clockwise rotation with back to mother's left and clockwise rotation with back to mother's right).

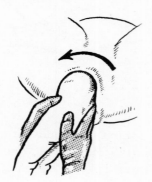 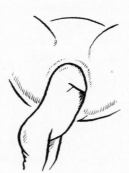 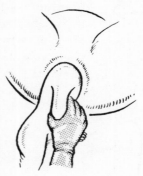

The arm is then lifted out and the rotation reversed, using the delivery arm for traction, so that the original anterior arm, which became posterior below the promontory is now swept round in the cavity to be easily picked out below the symphysis. (Often the second arm can be extracted easily without further rotation when the first arm has been delivered.)

BREECH PRESENTATION—MANAGEMENT

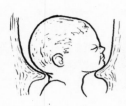

The breech in footling or full breech presentation and especially in prematurity may slip through an incompletely dilated cervix. The chin may arrest on this and cause extension of the head. A hand is passed up the foetal abdomen and a finger inserted into the mouth. Traction on the jaw promotes flexion and passage through the cervix.

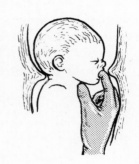

Suprapubic pressure   Traction on jaw

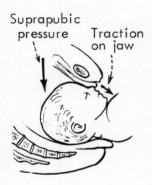

The head may rotate to bring the occiput to the sacrum. Delivery is completed by traction on jaw to maintain head flexion and supra pubic pressure to encourage descent. If the chin is above the pubis the foetal body is rotated up over the maternal abdomen as in the Prague seizure to allow the head to rotate around the pubis and so deliver.

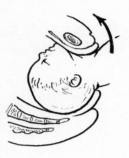

The obstetric forceps will help delivery in either case of occiput posterior.

Summary

In the antenatal period every effort is made to reduce the number of breech presentations by external version (see page 428).

If breech presentation is present at term then the question of a breech labour and delivery versus Caesarean section must be considered.

A working rule is that if there is a breech presentation and any other complicating factor then Caesarean section is probably the method of choice.

BREECH PRESENTATION—RISKS TO FOETUS

Manual breech extraction (operative delivery with the breech in high cavity or not engaged) is not used now. The foetal mortality is high, Caesarean section is the alternative method of choice.

Breech delivery is associated with a risk of injury to the child.

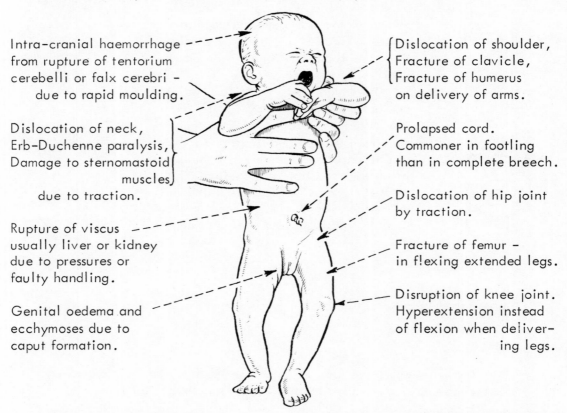

Intra-cranial haemorrhage from rupture of tentorium cerebelli or falx cerebri - due to rapid moulding.

Dislocation of neck, Erb-Duchenne paralysis, Damage to sternomastoid muscles due to traction.

Rupture of viscus usually liver or kidney due to pressures or faulty handling.

Genital oedema and ecchymoses due to caput formation.

Dislocation of shoulder, Fracture of clavicle, Fracture of humerus on delivery of arms.

Prolapsed cord. Commoner in footling than in complete breech.

Dislocation of hip joint by traction.

Fracture of femur - in flexing extended legs.

Disruption of knee joint. Hyperextension instead of flexion when delivering legs.

The placenta **separates** frequently in the second stage of labour as the active uterus contracts and the foetal head is in the pelvis. Asphyxia is therefore a danger.

Manual assistance to complete delivery of baby is essential and may be a sudden need. Episiotomy is desirable to permit sudden interference, or complete perineal tear may result.

FACE PRESENTATION

Face presentation is a malpresentation and occurs once in about 300 cases. The presenting part is the face and the denominator is the mentum or chin.

<u>Aetiology</u>. Lax uterus and pendulous abdomen, flat pelvis, multiple pregnancy, prematurity, obliquity of uterus, brow, thyroid enlargement or tumour of neck, anencephaly, spasm of the muscles of the back of the neck, dead foetus, dolichocephalic foetal skull (dolichocephalic = long headed – where breadth is less than 4/5 of length).

The face may be a primary presentation, i.e. it is present before labour, but secondary face presentation is more common, i.e. it develops in labour.

Incomplete flexion with occipito-posterior vertex and marked uterine obliquity can promote extension.

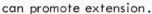

Parietal
eminence

Bitemporal
diameter

The action of the uterine forces, which normally tends to cause compaction, is in fact promoting extension of the head at the atlanto-occipito joint because the back of the foetus is in the same direction as the uterine obliquity.

Uterine obliquity is commonly to the right. A head presenting R.O.T. with some deflexion may also convert to a face presentation if for example in a flat pelvis there is partial arrest of the biparietal diameter but an easier passage for the bitemporal diameter.
[Note that the brow is an intermediate presentation in these conversions to face.]

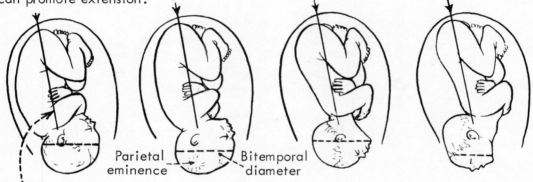

– If the foetus has its back to the opposite side the same forces would cause compaction and further flexion.

FACE PRESENTATION—MECHANISM

The engaging diameters in a face presentation are the submento-bregmatic followed by the biparietal.

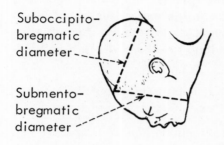

Suboccipito-bregmatic diameter

Submento-bregmatic diameter

The submento-bregmatic and suboccipito-bregmatic diameters are the same size ($3\frac{3}{4}$ in., $9\frac{1}{2}$ cm). Therefore the engaging diameters are the same size as in a normal vertex presentation.

In a normal vertex the suboccipito-bregmatic and the biparietal diameters are in the same plane.

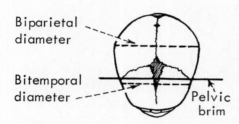

Biparietal diameter

Bitemporal diameter

Pelvic brim

In a face presentation the submento-bregmatic and the biparietal diameters are in different planes. The submento-bregmatic and bitemporal diameters engage together.

In a normal vertex presentation the engaging diameters enter the plane of the brim together.

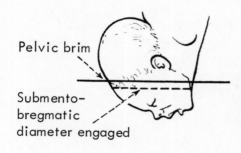

Pelvic brim

Submento-bregmatic diameter engaged

In a face presentation the submento-bregmatic diameter enters the plane of the brim and is followed by the other engaging diameter.

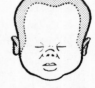

The pale areas engage first followed by the shaded areas.

Engagement is usually in the transverse diameter of the brim giving a right or left mento-transverse position. Left mento-transverse (L.M.T.) is the more common.

FACE PRESENTATION—MECHANISM

Descent continues till the pelvic floor is reached and rotation occurs.

A Most commonly the mentum leads and rotates forward (internal rotation) to the oblique diameter - left mento-anterior (L.M.A.).

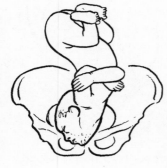

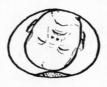

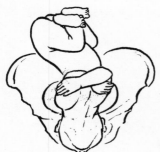

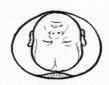

With further descent the rotation is completed to bring the mentum to the symphysis. This is the mechanism in 75% of face presentations.

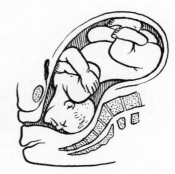

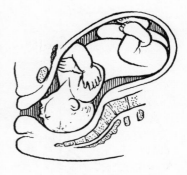

Descent continues and chin escapes from under pubis and progressive flexion allows the birth of the head.

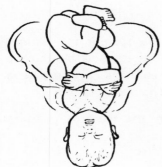

Thereafter restitution and external rotation take place and further descent delivers the baby as in a persistent occipito-posterior delivery.

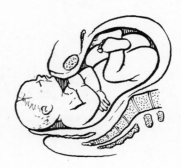

233

FACE PRESENTATION—MECHANISM

B   If the sinciput leads and rotates forward the mentum is carried to the hollow of the sacrum.

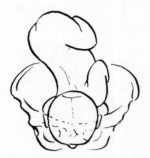

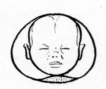

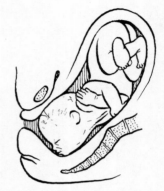

This is now a difficult mechanism because further extension of the head is necessary to negotiate the lower birth canal – and the shoulders must engage too.

A normal pelvis cannot accommodate a normal foetus because the bregmatic – sternal diameter is 7 inches (18 cm). Obstruction therefore occurs.

A small foetus in a roomy pelvis may permit birth.

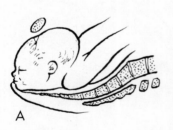

A

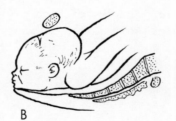

B

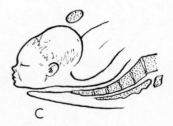

C

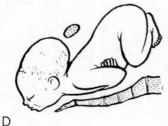

D

Descent continues and the occiput crushes into the shoulders till the occipital bone is behind the pubis, the perineum slips beneath the chin, the head starts to flex and the occiput is free.

The mechanism is then the same as occipito anterior.

234

FACE PRESENTATION—MANAGEMENT

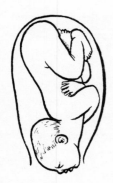

PALPATION
1. Longitudinal lie.
2. Head in lower pole.
3. Groove between head and back (best felt after membranes rupture).
4. Lack of head prominence on ventral side.

Diagnosis is difficult by palpation.
(X-ray will confirm.)

AUSCULTATION

Foetal heart best heard at front of foetus.

VAGINAL EXAMINATION

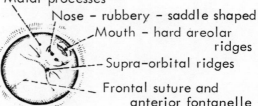

Malar processes

Nose – rubbery – saddle shaped

Mouth – hard areolar ridges

Supra-orbital ridges

Frontal suture and anterior fontanelle

The face is ill fitting at first, so contractions are poor and irregular and early rupture of membranes occurs with risk of prolapsed cord.

Labour may proceed normally thereafter when caput has formed. Engagement of biparietal diameter occurs only when mentum is deep in the pelvis.

If the chin rotates anteriorly spontaneous delivery can occur. Rotation occurs very deep in pelvis.

If the chin rotates posteriorly interference is required to procure delivery unless in exceptional circumstances (the head very small or anencephaly).

The head may be arrested in the transverse position.

Manual rotation of mento-posterior

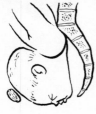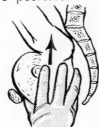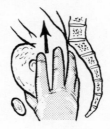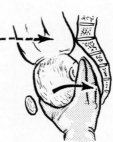

When chin is posterior the face and chin are gripped and displaced upwards to free the shoulders from the pelvis and then the head is rotated in the cavity, the other hand used to apply pressure to the shoulders. The mentum is thus brought to the front and forceps are then applied or, alternatively, manual rotation may be only to the transverse and Kielland's forceps applied.

FACE PRESENTATION—MANAGEMENT

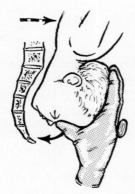

It may be possible to convert the face presentation to a vertex. Full dilatation of the cervix is necessary and liquor should be present. A hand grasps the cranial vault and promotes flexion of the neck. This is assisted by pressure on the chest, and pressure on the buttocks will help too. This manoeuvre can only be accomplished above the brim. Maintenance of the corrected position may be difficult or impossible.

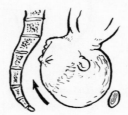

Internal version may also be used to convert to a breech. Full dilatation of the cervix and the presence of liquor are essential for success. A hand is passed into the uterus till a foot can be grasped and gently pulled towards the vagina as the head is displaced towards the fundus by the other hand working through the abdominal wall.

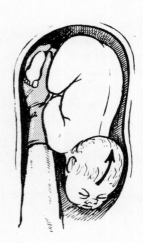

These manipulations require deep anaesthesia.

Caesarean section may be the method of choice for a difficult face labour. Remember that foetal abnormality incompatible with life can cause the face to present. X-ray examination therefore, is important. If there is gross abnormality then a destructive operation may permit vaginal delivery.

BROW PRESENTATION

A brow presentation is unstable and tends to convert to an occipital or face presentation.

The aetiology is similar to that of face.

There is no mechanism for brow presentation given a normal sized foetus and pelvis, because the engaging diameters are the mento-vertical and biparietal.

The mento-vertical diameter is $5\frac{1}{2}$ inches (14 cm.) and the largest pelvic diameter is 5 inches ($12\frac{1}{2}$ cm.)

If the head is small or the pelvis roomy moulding takes place and engagement occurs with descent.

The uterine forces thrust down. The head is roughly equal in size in front of and behind the brow. Thus the leverage to encourage flexion or extension is equal.

Unequal resistance of the pelvic parts or oblique direction of thrust will tend to create flexion or extension of the head.

Oblique thrust and
equal resistance will tend to cause flexion.
Thrust in the other oblique would cause extension.

Straight thrust and
unequal resistance will tend to cause extension.
Opposite inequalities of resistance would cause flexion.

Oblique thrust and unequal resistance may augment or neutralise each other.

If conversion to an occipital or face presentation does not occur then moulding reduces the occipito-mental and increases the occipito-frontal diameters.

BROW PRESENTATION—MECHANISM

Moulding

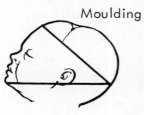

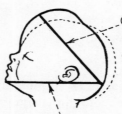

Occipito-frontal diameter increases

Occipito-mental diameter decreases

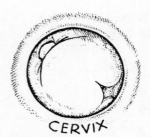

CERVIX

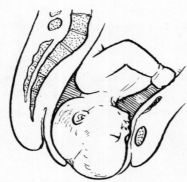

The brow slowly descends to pelvic floor and turns forward under the symphysis.

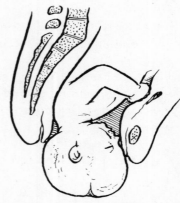

Flexion then follows and the brow,. vault of the skull and occiput are born.

The head drops back over the perineum and the face and chin are born.

The mechanism thereafter is the same as O.P.

BROW PRESENTATION—MANAGEMENT

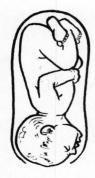

PALPATION

This feels like normal vertex except that the head feels unduly large, due to palpation across the mento-vertical diameter. Head appears disproportionate.

AUSCULTATION Foetal heart site not significant.

VAGINAL EXAMINATION Head is high because of disproportion. Membranes rupture early in labour. Brow is palpated through cervix and is identified by:-
1. Anterior fontanelle and frontal suture leading to
2. Supra-orbital ridge and root of nose.

The brow is ill fitting so membranes rupture early and labour is poor at the beginning. There is risk of cord prolapse. With a normal baby and pelvis labour is impossible. Brow is an unstable presentation and may convert to vertex or face, but moulding and caput formation help to stabilise the malpresentation.

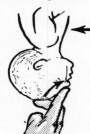

If the presentation is seen and recognised in early labour an attempt by vaginal and abdominal manipulation to correct it should be made - somewhat as in face - under general anaesthesia. One or two fingers through the cervix displace the head and encourage flexion while the other hand applies pressure on the foetal chest towards its back - an assistant pressing on the breech will help. The brow may be altered to a face presentation.

Caesarean section is the treatment of choice, but bipolar version to breech may be attempted where the facilities are limited.

If the foetus is small in relation to the pelvis then a normal type of labour and delivery will ensue.

A BROW PRESENTATION SHOULD BE SUSPECTED WHEN A PAROUS WOMAN HAS UNEXPECTED DYSTOCIA.

COMPOUND PRESENTATION

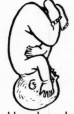

Head and hand

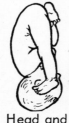

Head and foot

A compound presentation is when two or more parts of the foetus present. If the head and foot or hand engage together, the pelvis should be adequate for labour. The limb however is usually held back at the brim.

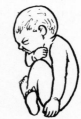

Breech and hand

PARIETAL PRESENTATION

Parietal presentation is rare and only found in platypelloid or flat pelvis. The head is partly flexed bringing anterior and posterior fontanelles to same level and is in the transverse diameter of the brim.

 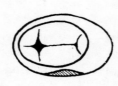 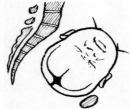

Compaction of the foetus occurs and lateral displacement of the head towards the occiput brings the bitemporal diameter ($3\frac{1}{4}$ inches, 8.25 cm) nearer the conjugate of the brim and the biparietal diameter ($3\frac{3}{4}$ inches, 9.5 cm) into the bay thus gaining advantage.

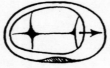 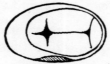

The head also rolls adopting the attitude of asynclitism with advantage too as the biparietal diameter is substituted by the subparietal-supraparietal diameter ($3\frac{1}{4}$ inches, 8.25 cm).

The presentation is described as (1) an anterior parietal presentation (anterior asynclitism) or (2) a posterior parietal presentation (posterior asynclitism).

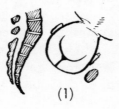 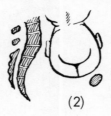

(1)   (2)

240

PARIETAL PRESENTATION—MECHANISM

Anterior asynclitism is more favourable as the anterior parietal bone has passed the depth of the pubis and the posterior parietal bone has to pass the shallow promontory of the sacrum. In posterior asynclitism the posterior parietal bone has passed the sacral promontory but the anterior parietal bone has still to descend past the symphysis pubis.

Anterior asynclitism – the head engages (1) and then the anterior parietal bone descends into the pelvis increasing the asynclitism (2) till the anterior parietal eminence is behind and just below the pubis and the sagittal suture is close to the sacrum; then the head descends further by decreasing the asynclitism (3) and pushing the posterior parietal eminence past the sacral promontory (4). The pelvic cavity and outlet are relatively roomy and further descent causes flexion of the head and the final mechanism is that of O.A. or O.P.

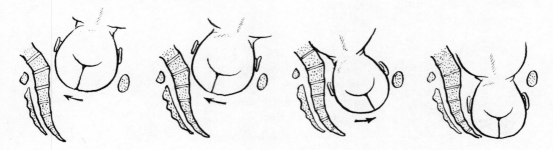

The mechanism of posterior asynclitism is similar but the positions are reversed. Difficulty is found, and thus delay, in pushing the parietal eminence past the pubis.

In these circumstances Caesarean section is advisable because the head is not engaged.

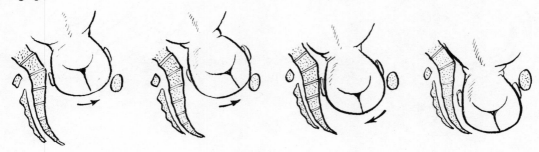

SHOULDER PRESENTATION—MECHANISM

Shoulder presentation is a malpresentation and occurs in 1 out of 250 – 300 cases. It is more common in multipara than in primipara and in premature than in mature labours.

Aetiology. Similar to other malpresentations. Twins, hydramnios, placenta praevia, contracted pelvis, anything preventing engagement of the head in the pelvis, undue mobility of the foetus or unusual shape of the foetus, abnormal shape of uterus – e.g. subseptate uterus.

The Lie is transverse or oblique.
The Denominator is the Shoulder.
The head may be to right or left and the back may be anterior or posterior.
When the foetus is of normal size and the pelvis is of normal size there is obstruction and no mechanism.

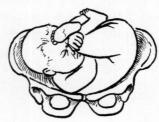

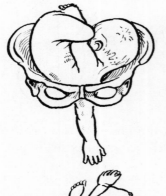

If the pelvis is large and the foetus small then the mechanism of spontaneous evolution takes place. The head remains above the pubis and the arm and shoulder descend behind the symphysis.

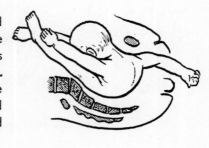

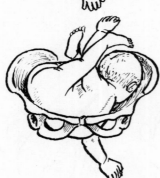

The chest then descends into the pelvis.

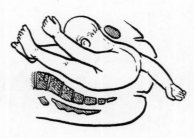

SHOULDER PRESENTATION—MECHANISM

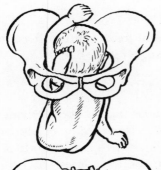

The breech follows.

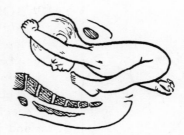

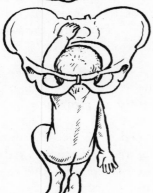

The birth is then that of breech with one arm extended.

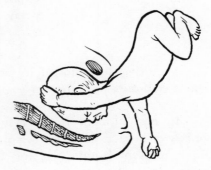

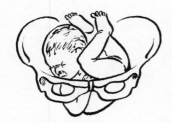

Occasionally, when the child is dead, it may be expelled with shoulder leading and the rest of the baby doubled up and following (corpore conduplicato). This is spontaneous expulsion.

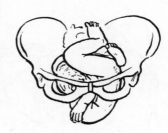

There are two other mechanisms.

1. <u>Spontaneous Rectification</u> – The head or breech may displace the shoulder and the mechanism is that appropriate to the presenting part.

2. <u>Spontaneous Version</u> – The head is held high in the iliac fossa of one side and the breech drives into the pelvis. The mechanism then is that of breech.

SHOULDER PRESENTATION—MANGEMENT

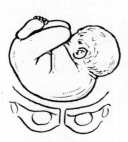

PALPATION

1. Fundal height is less than expected.
2. Uterine breadth is greater than expected.
3. Head in one flank and breech in opposite side.
4. Lie may be transverse or oblique.

AUSCULTATION

Site of foetal heart not significant (best heard through foetal back).

VAGINAL EXAMINATION

Prior to labour and in early labour, pelvis is empty. Hand, arm or elbow may be in pelvis, or ribs may be felt or tip of shoulder or iliac crest or trochanter of foetus. Placenta praevia may be a cause of transverse lie.

Shoulder presentation is an impossible labour unless the foetus is very small. The membranes rupture early in labour and the cord frequently is prolapsed.

In early labour if the membranes are intact external version (page 428) to a vertex or breech can be attempted. If the membranes have ruptured and there is still liquor present bipolar version (page 429) to a breech may be performed. This requires general anaesthesia. Caesarean section is preferable.

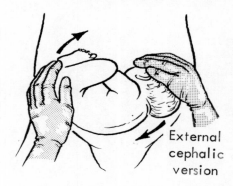

External cephalic version

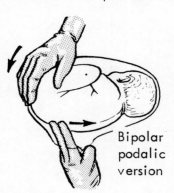

Bipolar podalic version

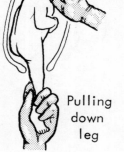

Pulling down leg

If the liquor has drained away the uterus wraps round the foetus and manipulation even under deep anaesthesia may cause uterine rupture. If the foetus is alive Caesarean section is the method of choice. If the foetus is dead then decapitation or exenteration is preferable.

MULTIPLE PREGNANCY

Multiple pregnancy is the term used when more than one foetus is present in the uterus.

Twins are found once in about 80 pregnancies.

Hellin's Rule (a mathematical approximation) gives triplets as 1 in 80^2 (6,400) pregnancies and quadruplets as 1 in 80^3 (512,000) pregnancies.

Twins may be monovular (monozygotic or monochorionic) - from one ovum; or binovular (dizygotic or dichorionic) - from two ova.

Binovular twins are 3 or 4 times as common as monovular twins.

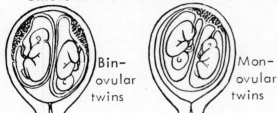

Bin-ovular twins

Mon-ovular twins

Monovular more common in ages 20 - 35 years. Binovular more common in older mothers twinning at maximum ages 35 - 40 years. Monovular twins more common in primigravidae and secundigravidae.

The incidence of binovular but not monovular twins is influenced by age, parity and heredity. Heredity is both maternal and paternal.

Twin pregnancy occurs more commonly in Negroid peoples than in Caucasian and is least frequent in Mongol races. The difference is due to variation in binovular twinning, the incidence of monovular twins being the same in all races.

Hydramnios is present in 10% of multiple pregnancies, is commoner in monovular than in binovular twins and usually affects the upper sac. Foetal abnormality is twice as common in twin as in single pregnancy.

Multiple pregnancy is suspected by finding that the uterus is progressively bigger than the dates suggest.

Repeated examinations give the impression of an accelerating pregnancy.

Actual

Expected

MULTIPLE PREGNANCY

Other possible causes of apparently abnormal uterine enlargement in early pregnancy are:-

1. <u>Mistaken Dates</u> - bleeding after conception being considered as a period.
2. <u>Hydramnios</u> - rare in early pregnancy.
3. <u>Fibroids</u>
   These tend to
   flatten and soften
   in pregnancy but
   may be irregular.

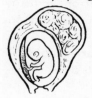

4. <u>Abdominal Cyst</u>
   It is usually pos-
   sible to differ-
   entiate two masses.

5. <u>Hydatidiform Mole</u>
   Usually accom-
   panied by staining.
   The pregnancy test
   will be positive in
   dilution.

6. <u>Retention of Urine</u>
   'Catheter will cure'.
   It may be associated
   with retroversion and
   incarceration of the
   uterus.

Ultrasound will differentiate all these conditions and also diagnose a multiple pregnancy. X-ray or ultrasound is the only sure way of diagnosing multiple pregnancy especially if more than twins. X-ray is diagnostic but is undesirable in early weeks.

In later pregnancy the uterus is more globular and larger than normal for the dates.

The conceptus is not as easy to define as a single foetus, but two heads may be identified and a third pole (breech) must be found to be sure.

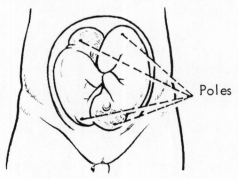

Poles

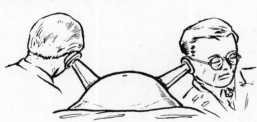

Two foetal hearts may be heard but they must be heard at the same time and differ in rate by 10 beats.

MULTIPLE PREGNANCY

Twins may present in various ways:—

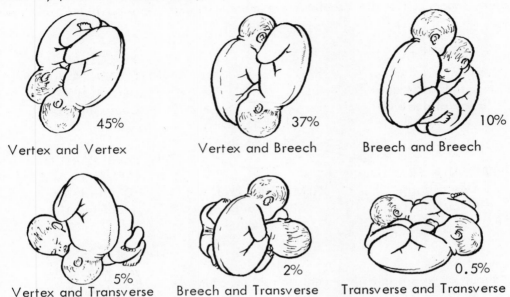

45%	37%	10%
Vertex and Vertex	Vertex and Breech	Breech and Breech
5%	2%	0.5%
Vertex and Transverse	Breech and Transverse	Transverse and Transverse

Double vertex is commonest and in three quarters of cases the first presentation is by the vertex. The first foetus as a transverse lie is very rare and it must be corrected in early labour by bipolar version to a breech. The lie of the second is unimportant till the first is born as the second then tends to adopt a longitudinal lie. If not, the lie is corrected by external version and if that is not possible, by internal podalic version.

The birth of the second twin is usually rapid when contractions restart as the birth canal is already dilated.

Twins tend to be premature about 32 – 34 weeks gestation – therefore there is considerable foetal loss due to prematurity. The second foetus is at greater risk than the first.

There is greater nutritional demand on the mother in multiple pregnancy, and the burdens of pregnancy increase more quickly. A high protein and mineral diet should be prescribed and folic acid should be given because of the foetal demand.

MULTIPLE PREGNANCY

Much rest should be taken especially from 30 – 36 weeks because of the risk of premature labour. Certain problems are more prone to develop in multiple pregnancy.

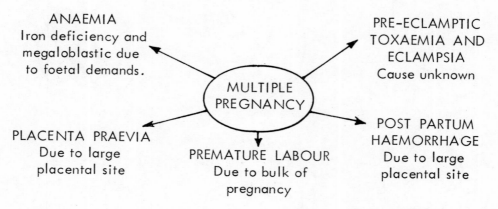

ANAEMIA
Iron deficiency and megaloblastic due to foetal demands.

PRE-ECLAMPTIC TOXAEMIA AND ECLAMPSIA
Cause unknown

MULTIPLE PREGNANCY

PLACENTA PRAEVIA
Due to large placental site

PREMATURE LABOUR
Due to bulk of pregnancy

POST PARTUM HAEMORRHAGE
Due to large placental site

Labour often starts with premature rupture of membranes. Prolapse of the cord should be considered and the presentation checked. There is often a considerable delay before contractions start.

Collision or jostling of the leading parts occasionally occurs as they each try to enter the brim. External manipulation will usually displace one. Normally the left twin tends to be a little lower and enters the brim first.

Labour is usually straightforward though assistance may be necessary for the actual delivery especially if very premature. Episiotomy should be used to relieve pressure on the foetal head, or delivery completed by forceps.

The cord is double clamped in case there are monovular twins and a risk of the second bleeding from the cord of the first.

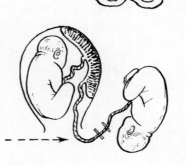

MULTIPLE PREGNANCY

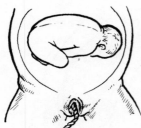

When the first baby is delivered the position of the second is checked and if necessary corrected by external version to a vertex or a breech; if that is not possible then internal podalic version is performed.

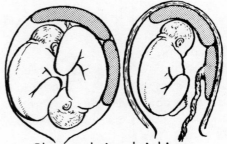

Delay in the birth of the second twin gives risk of foetal loss as the placental site shrinks with the birth of the first and the reduction in uterine size also alters the uterine vascular system.

Placental site shrinking

Before contractions restart after the birth of the first twin there is some delay and this may be dangerous if prolonged. To avoid this the second sac is ruptured and the mother asked to bear down. This often stimulates contractions. Oxytocin may also be used.

If the delivery of the first has occurred under general anaesthesia it is usual to deliver the second baby as soon as practicable. It is usually the smaller and the head may be pushed into the brim and then delivered by forceps, or podalic version can be followed by breech extraction.

If the second twin is bigger than the first there is delay while the birth canal is further dilated.

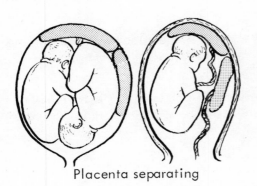

Placenta separating

Rarely the first placenta is born before the second baby. Bleeding is not usually severe. The uterus is actively contracting and the reduction in size of the placental site and the pressure of the foetus on it helps to control the blood loss.

The second birth should be completed without delay, and the placenta delivered as quickly as possible – manually if need be – and an oxytocic drug given.

MULTIPLE PREGNANCY

Locked twins is a very rare condition in which parts of one interlock with the other causing an impasse. It most commonly occurs with the first as breech and the second as a vertex. The head of the second slips down with the shoulders of the first and prevents the engagement of the head of the first in the pelvis.

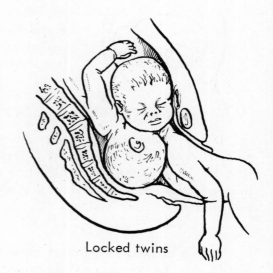

Locked twins

Early recognition is essential as the condition has a high foetal mortality. The treatment is to push the lower head out of the pelvis to free the head of the first foetus and allow delivery. If displacement is not possible the head of the first is cut from its body and then the second twin is delivered and finally the head of the first twin.

Other forms of locking are dealt with similarly - displace out of pelvis - free and then deliver.

Conjoined twins are due to imperfect separation of monovular twins and delivery is not possible vaginally except in rare instances or with marked prematurity.

Triplets and quadruplets have similar problems and difficulties. Premature labour is much commoner because of the increased bulk and perinatal mortality higher.

MULTIPLE PREGNANCY

The placentae may be separate or appear as one so that the diagnosis of monovular or binovular twins is uncertain. The membranes between the sacs are examined.

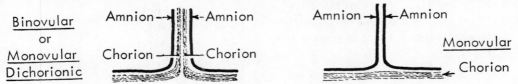

Binovular
or
Monovular
Dichorionic

Amnion → ← Amnion

Chorion → ← Chorion

Amnion → ← Amnion

Monovular

← Chorion

Binovular twins have two amnions sandwiching one or two chorions (the two chorions sometimes fuse), but sometimes monovular twins may be dichorionic if division of the embryonic disc has occurred before the formation of the amnion. Monovular monochorionic twins may have one or two amniotic sacs. Genotyping may be necessary to determine whether like-sex dichorionic twins are binovular or monovular.

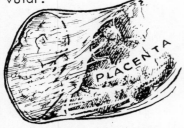

Foetus papyraceous

Sometimes a twin does not develop but becomes amorphous or shrivelled and flattened. This is called foetus papyraceous or compressus. It may be readily apparent or may be found wrapped in the membranes of the placenta.

Monovular twins may not develop normally as the more vigorous heart and circulation of one takes over the function of the other and an acardiac monster develops. This usually has no head, little thorax but fairly well developed abdomen and legs.

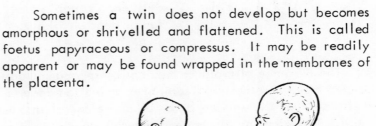

The 'transfusion syndrome' is sometimes found with monovular twins. This is dependent on a placental arterio-venous shunt. The arterial system of one leads closely to the venous system of the other and the arterial twin pumps some of its blood into the other circulation starving itself and making the other bulky, plethoric and polycythaemic.

PROLAPSE AND PRESENTATION OF THE CORD

Prolapse occurs after rupture of the membranes when the presenting part is ill-fitting or abnormal. It is associated with multiparity and prematurity, disproportion and malpresentation, foetal abnormality and hydramnios.

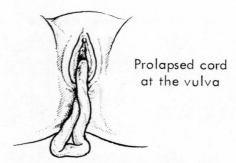

Prolapsed cord at the vulva

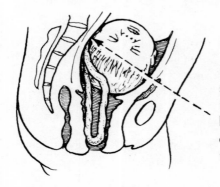

Once the cord is out of the uterus, and especially when out of the vagina, the foetal blood supply is obstructed, either because of the drop in temperature, or spasm of the vessels, or compression between the pelvic brim and the presenting part. If delivery is not effected within about 40 minutes, foetal death is likely.

The presence of prolapse may not be recognised until cord appears at the vulva; or cord may be palpated on vaginal examination done to assess progress of the labour or because of the sudden onset of acute foetal distress. It is essential to make a vaginal examination as soon as the membranes rupture in all patients who display an ill-fitting or non-engaged presenting part.

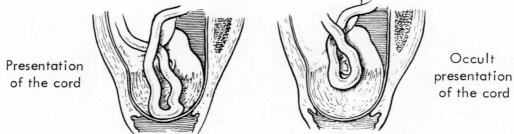

Presentation of the cord

Occult presentation of the cord

Presentation of the cord means that the cord is palpable at the cervix through intact membranes. Occult presentation means that the cord is lying alongside the presenting part but will not be palpable on vaginal examination. It is a particularly dangerous condition and may be a cause of unexpected foetal distress.

TREATMENT OF PROLAPSED CORD

Treatment of Prolapsed Cord

1. Determine the presence or absence of cord pulsation and foetal heart sounds. If the foetus is dead the labour may be left to proceed normally (if no other complication is present).
2. If the foetus is still alive, Caesarean section must be carried out as soon as possible unless vaginal delivery by forceps or breech extraction is likely to be straightforward.
3. While arrangements are being made for operation, the cord should be pushed back into the vagina and kept up with a gauze pack or by hand. An attempt is made to prevent compression of the cord between the presenting part and the pelvis by getting the mother to adopt a suitable position. The foot of the bed should be raised.

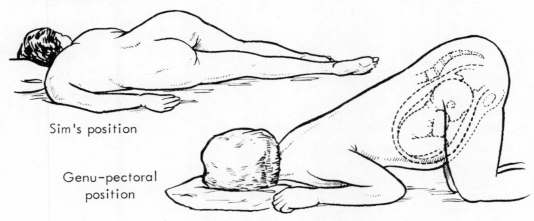

Sim's position

Genu-pectoral
position

4. If delivery cannot be carried out at once, an attempt should be made to replace the cord in the uterus. The prolapsed loop is wrapped round with thick sterile gauze and pushed through the cervix.
5. Prolapse of the cord, although often fatal for the child, carries no risk for the mother unless proper precautions are neglected for the sake of saving time. However great the need for haste, the mother must be properly prepared, her stomach emptied, premedication given, and cross-matched blood made available.
6. Presentation of the cord when discovered by vaginal examination is an indication for section; but as the membranes are intact there is no immediate danger for the foetus, and more time is available.

CONTRACTED PELVIS

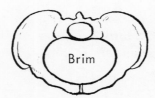 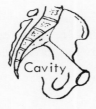 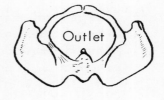

Gynaecoid Brim Cavity Outlet

A contracted pelvis is one in which an important diameter is $\frac{1}{2}$ in. (1.25 cm) less than that of the normal gynaecoid pelvis (page 64).

◄- - The anthropoid pelvis can be considered normal for clinical purposes as its measurements are equivalent to a gynaecoid pelvis turned through 90° (page 64).

The anthropoid pelvis is frequently found in association with a high assimilation of the sacrum - the fifth lumbar vertebra is incorporated in the sacrum making a sixth segment. The effect is to alter the angle of the pelvic brim so that it is about 75° rather than the normal 55° (page 62). This makes engagement more difficult and delayed. The long sacrum makes the pelvis deeper so that the head has further to travel in the confines of the pelvic cavity.

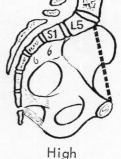

High assimilation

◄- - -The android pelvis (page 65) is a pelvis with decreasing capacity the deeper the head descends. The greatest difficulty is at the outlet. It is sometimes called the 'funnel' pelvis.

◄- -The flat pelvis is contracted at the brim levels (page 65) with a more capacious cavity and outlet. The difficulty is at the brim.

CONTRACTED PELVIS

The generally contracted (Justo-minor) pelvis is a miniature pelvis with all measurements reduced but all proportionate to each other. The mother is small but not deformed. The baby also tends to be small.

A Working Rule:- If the height of the mother is less than 61 in. (155 cm) suspect pelvic contraction. If the hands and feet are small then the pelvis is possibly justo-minor. If the hands and feet are more normal in size then pelvic distortion may be present.

REMEMBER THAT PELVIC SIZE AND CAPACITY MUST BE JUDGED BY PELVIC EXAMINATION.

A pelvis of pure type is not always found and many pelves have mixed characteristics. For example, an android brim has a normal diagonal conjugate diameter and if the rest of the pelvis has gynaecoid characteristics, the reduced brim capacity may not be noticed.

Causes of Contracted Pelvis

A. Genetic   1. with deformity (e.g. achondro-plasia. Naegele's pelvis – absence of one sacral ala).

                      2. without deformity (e.g. justo-minor).

B. Nutritional   e.g. rickets, osteomalacia. An extreme type of this deformity is illustrated.

C. Bony Disease e.g. tuberculosis, osteomyelitis.

D. Trauma   e.g. old fractures of pelvis.

CONTRACTED PELVIS

Routine pelvic examination is shown on page 88, but the following additional investigations should be undertaken where contraction is suspected.

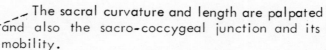

The sub-pubic angle is estimated by putting two fingers under the symphysis and spreading them.

The depth and thickness of the symphysis is assessed.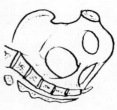

The angle of the pubis may also be demonstrated by placing fingers and thumb along the descending rami of the pubis.

The sacral curvature and length are palpated and also the sacro-coccygeal junction and its mobility.

The ischio-sacral ligaments of each side are located by feeling the ischial spine. Each ligament should accommodate two fingers easily. The thickness and prominence of the ischial spines are noted and especially any tendency to encroach on the cavity.

The posterior sagittal diameter of the outlet is measured — from the tip of the sacrum to the bituberous diameter. This can be measured by calipers or by putting a finger into the rectum to reach the sacral tip and measuring the finger length to the bituberous diameter. This measurement is important when the pubic arch is narrow as the head will be arrested unless the posterior sagittal diameter is large.

Posterior sagittal diameter too small – head arrested.

Adequate posterior sagittal diameter.

The bituberous diameter plus the posterior sagittal diameter should be 7.5 in. (20 cm). If the sum is 6 in. (15.25 cm) dystocia may result.

CONTRACTED PELVIS

. Disproportion arises when the presenting part is too big for the pelvis. The pelvic capacity can be assessed radiologically (page 106). The biparietal diameter may be measured by X-ray or ultrasound. The assessment of disproportion is a clinical judgement and is a comparison between the foetal head and the pelvic brim. There may be doubt till labour has been in progress for some time.

The method of clinical estimation is to try to push the head into the brim. If the patient sits up and leans forward the head may engage.

1. Head behind pubis — there should be no problem of disproportion.

2. Head flush with pubis — may or may not mould and engage.

3. Head over-riding pubis and will not enter brim. Caesarean section method of choice.

The unknown factors in labour are:-

1. Ability, quality and character of the contractions.
2. Moulding of foetal head and stamina of foetus.
3. Stamina of the mother.

The assessment of disproportion may be made by having an assistant push the head to the pelvic brim. The examiner feels whether or not the head descends by fingers in the vagina and with his other hand feels for overlap (Müller's Method). - - - - - -

The head may be pushed to the brim with one hand and the fingers of the other gauge descent while the thumb feels for overlap (Munro Kerr's Method). - - - - - -

Disproportion at the brim of an android pelvis is very serious and vaginal delivery should be avoided.

Gross pelvic contraction is nowadays uncommon – and therefore unsuspected minor contraction becomes more deceptive.

Remember that malpresentation of a normal-sized head can cause disproportion.

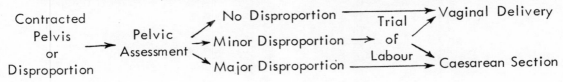

Contracted Pelvis or Disproportion → Pelvic Assessment → No Disproportion → Vaginal Delivery; Minor Disproportion → Trial of Labour; Major Disproportion → Caesarean Section

CONTRACTED PELVIS

'Trial of Labour' is the term used when there is doubt about the pelvic capacity, but when with good contractions and good moulding vaginal delivery is thought to be feasible.

Trial of labour may be undertaken by induction before term when the head is slightly smaller and more able to mould. On the other hand, the foetus is less robust and induction of labour may be difficult.

Labour can be left to occur spontaneously and the trial conducted then. If induction of labour is the choice, it can be done medically or surgically. Surgical induction is more certain, but if labour has not started in a reasonable time then Caesarean section is carried out (48 hours would be a maximum delay). If labour becomes established 12 hours of good contractions will determine the outcome. Foetal distress may bring the trial to an end.

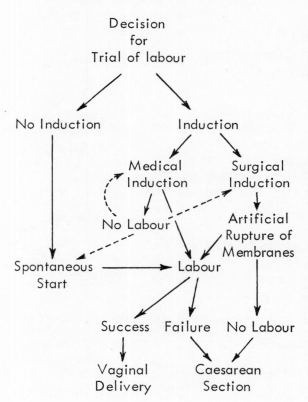

The conduct of a trial of labour necessitates constant vigilance, frequent checking of descent of the head, cervical dilatation and foetal heart rate.

Sedation is important to allay fears and encourage rest.

The possibility of immediate Caesarean section is always present so food and fluids should be reduced to a minimum.

In some ways we should consider every labour a trial of labour.

If the membranes have been ruptured for 24 hours and delivery has not occurred antibiotic cover should be given to reduce the risk of intra-uterine infection to foetus and mother.

Oxytocin may be given to stimulate contractions but it must be used with great care.

A trial of labour should not be carried on to the stage of obstruction or imminent uterine rupture.

HYDRAMNIOS

Amniotic fluid has normally a volume of 1 – 3 pints (550 – 1,300 cc) and if it is excessive it is called hydramnios. Four pints (1,900 cc) will be detectable clinically.

<u>Signs of Hydramnios</u>

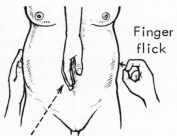

Finger flick

1. The uterus is bigger than expected.
2. Identification of the foetus and foetal parts is difficult.
3. The foetal heart is difficult to hear.
4. Ballottement of the foetus is easy.
5. A fluid thrill is detected.
6. Abdominal girth at umbilicus is more than 40 in. (100 cm) before term. The abdominal girth varies a little – an ebb and flow.

Hand on abdomen to cut transmission of impulse round abdominal wall

The source of amniotic fluid is uncertain. It may be a transudate through the membranes from the mother or a secretion from the amniotic epithelium. It is in a state of dynamic balance and there is a turnover of the water and salts. The rate of change varies with the factor studied. The water turnover takes 3 hours.

Foetal swallowing and urinary excretion make contributions to this change.

Excess liquor amnii is associated with foetal abnormality – especially anencephaly, spina bifida, oesophageal atresia, hydrops foetalis and monovular twins.

Haemangioma of the placenta is found on rare occasions with hydramnios.

Maternal conditions associated with hydramnios are diabetes and the more severe forms of heart disease and pre-eclamptic toxaemia.

The development of hydramnios is usually gradual and in the last trimester. The symptoms are due to the bulk and weight of the uterus.

1. Discomfort and dyspnoea.
2. Indigestion.
3. Oedema, increase of varicose veins and haemorrhoids.
4. There may be abdominal pain.

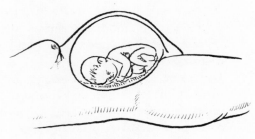

Hydramnios

HYDRAMNIOS

Hydramnios may be acute – developing quickly, usually 24 – 30 weeks. Acute **abdominal** pain and a feeling of bursting is often the presenting symptom. Frequently there is vomiting. The abdominal skin is glazed, sometimes oedematous and often with fresh striae. The uterus is tense and tender and may be mistaken for concealed accidental haemorrhage, but there is no shock.

Acute hydramnios leads to abortion or premature labour.

Treatment is by rest, sedation and paracentesis.

Treatment of chronic hydramnios is also by rest in bed and sedation: the foetus should be X-rayed.

One third diabetic pregnancies develop hydramnios.

One half anencephalic foetuses are associated with hydramnios.

One eighth multiple pregnancies have hydramnios.

The treatment of diabetes, heart failure and severe pre-eclampsia takes precedence. If the foetus appears normal by X-ray, then the aim is to conserve the pregnancy. Rest and sedation will help but paracentesis of the hydramnios may be desirable, if the patient becomes distressed.

A needle, Southey's tube or plastic catheter may be introduced into the uterine cavity.

1. The bladder is emptied.
2. A local anaesthetic is introduced into the skin of the abdomen over the lower left quadrant (to avoid placenta). If there are twins, the upper sac is more commonly affected and the chosen area is then just above the umbilicus.
3. The needle is pushed through into the uterus (if blood is obtained another site is chosen) and at least one pint (540 cc) of liquor is allowed to drain out slowly.

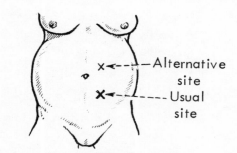

Paracentesis (amniocentesis) sites

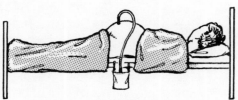

Paracentesis

HYDRAMNIOS

Alternatively, if the foetus is abnormal, hind water rupture will stimulate uterine activity and after the presenting part enters the brim the forewaters may also be ruptured if need be.

Too much fluid rushing out at once may cause separation of the placenta and the problems of accidental haemorrhage – hence hind water rupture.

The cord may prolapse with hydramnios but if the foetus is abnormal this is unimportant.

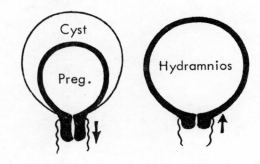

Differential <u>Diagnosis</u>

1. Multiple pregnancy – no fluid thrill.
2. Ovarian cyst – The cyst tends to press the pregnancy and cervix down into the pelvis.
   The hydramnios tends to lift the pregnancy out of the pelvis and the cervix is high.
3. Hydatidiform mole – noted in early pregnancy but usually accompanied by bleeding.
4. A full bladder – this is usually caused by the uterus being incarcerated in the pelvis.

Ultrasound will differentiate all these conditions if there is still doubt after clinical examination.

OLIGOHYDRAMNIOS

This is a rare condition. The liquor is reduced to a few ounces of milky fluid.

It may cause foetal abnormality or injury because of the lack of the amniotic fluid cushion and space, e.g. talipes, torticollis, skin deficiency.

The foetal skin is dry, leathery and scaly.

CHAPTER II

UTERINE DISPLACEMENTS AND ANOMALIES

RETROVERTED GRAVID UTERUS

This condition is probably a result of conception occurring in an already retroverted uterus. The commonest outcome is spontaneous correction between the 9th and 12th weeks, but sometimes the uterus becomes incarcerated in the pelvis as it grows, especially in the presence of some obstruction to correction such as adhesions or pelvic contraction.

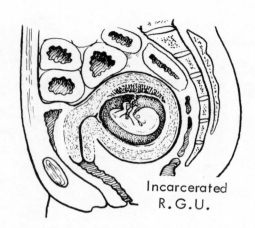

Incarcerated
R.G.U.

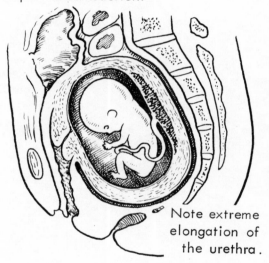

Note extreme elongation of the urethra.

The patient complains of pelvic pain and backache and defaecation is painful. The urethra is compressed and elongated causing frequency, retention overflow and infection, and sometimes acute retention and rupture of the bladder. In addition the vesical blood supply is obstructed and gangrene of the bladder has been reported.

The pregnancy usually aborts; but it can continue by a process of sacculation – hypertrophy and distension of the anterior wall of the uterus, which allows growth into the abdomen. If such a pregnancy reaches maturity delivery must be by section.

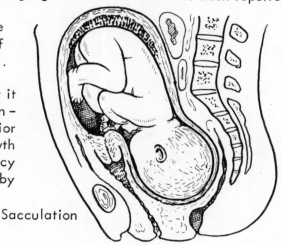

Sacculation

RETROVERTED GRAVID UTERUS

Diagnosis

Urinary frequency and incontinence in early pregnancy always call for pelvic examination. In retroversion the cervix is high behind the pelvis and difficult to reach, the bladder is pushed up, and the soft uterus is felt in the pouch of Douglas.

Differential Diagnosis

Urinary retention and Pouch of Douglas swelling may also be due to:-

Haematocoele from tubal pregnancy. Tenderness is extreme.

Fibroids are as a rule harder and more irregular.

An Ovarian Cyst may push the uterus up and forwards. Catheterisation should reveal this swelling as uterus rather than bladder.

Treatment

1. If a symptomless retroverted gravid uterus is detected, pelvic examination should be carried out every week until the uterus has emerged from the pelvis by the 12th or 13th week.

2. If urinary or other symptoms are present, the patient should be admitted and rested in bed for 48 hours with an indwelling catheter. A large watch-spring pessary may be inserted at the same time and the patient should lie more or less prone. If this simple treatment fails an attempt at correction by manipulation should be made with the patient under anaesthesia.

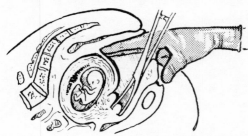

1. The cervix is pulled down with forceps with the patient in the knee elbow position. The fundus is pushed up through the posterior fornix.

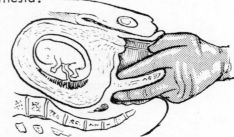

2. Another method is to use finger pressure alone, via rectum and vagina.

As a last resort the uterus may be lifted out of the pelvis after laparotomy. Abortion is particularly likely after this.

OTHER UTERINE DISPLACEMENTS

FORWARD DISPLACEMENT OF THE UTERUS ('PENDULOUS ABDOMEN')

If the pelvis is contracted and prevents descent, or if the abdominal muscles are weak (a consequence of repeated pregnancies) the uterus will project forward. A compensatory lordosis develops, and the woman suffers great discomfort from backache and the stretching of the abdominal muscles. The condition causes delay in engagement of the presenting part apart from any disproportion, and may contribute to uterine rupture. A corset should be worn during the pregnancy and a binder may help when labour begins.

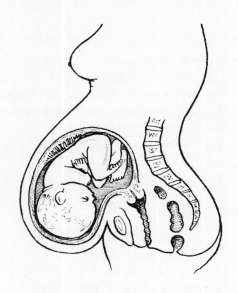

LATERAL DISPLACEMENT OF THE UTERUS

This may be discovered between the 6th and 10th weeks when the softening of the isthmus is at its maximum (see Hegar's sign, page 75). It is of no clinical significance except that it may be mistaken for a tubal pregnancy.

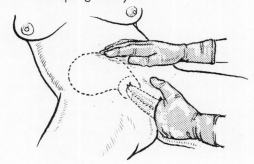

266

OTHER UTERINE DISPLACEMENTS

PROLAPSE OF THE UTERUS

This may co-exist with pregnancy and will be aggravated in the early months by the softening and stretching of the tissues. The cervix projects well beyond the vulva and becomes oedematous and ulcerated. A ring pessary will maintain the uterus in the correct position until it is too big to descend through the pelvis (usually about the 20th week).

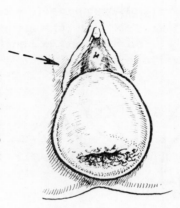

TORSION OF THE UTERUS

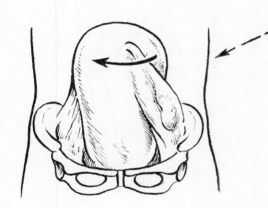

Some dextro-rotation is normal in pregnancy, probably because the pelvic colon takes up some of the space available in the left pelvis. Occasionally this rotation reaches $90°$ and if seen at Caesarean section care must be taken not to incise the left broad ligament and arteries. Torsion so severe as to interfere with the blood supply is unknown except as a complication of pregnancy in one horn of a double uterus when it is usually mistaken for concealed accidental haemorrhage.

HERNIA OF THE UTERUS

Inguinal hernia if present is aggravated in the early stages of pregnancy before the uterus fills the pelvis. A very rare complication is the herniation of the uterus through the dilated inguinal ring. A more common type of hernia is through a previous abdominal scar such as for Caesarean section. In later pregnancy the uterus will come to occupy a sac composed only of skin and peritoneum.

CONGENITAL ABNORMALITIES

These are the result of imperfect fusion of the two Müllerian ducts. The uterus, cervix and vagina, separately or together, can be single, double or intermediate; so classification is difficult and nomenclature confused. The anomalies described here are representative.

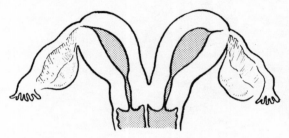

Double uterus, cervix and vagina
(Didelphys – 'double womb')

Torsion of one horn can occur more easily than in the normal uterus and may occur during version, causing foetal death and symptoms of accidental haemorrhage. The non-gravid horn develops its own decidua and hypertrophies, and has been known to occupy the pelvis and obstruct labour.

Uterus Didelphys

When both horns are well developed the pregnancy proceeds normally. Diagnosis is difficult but a double vagina and cervix may be observed, although easily missed at routine pelvic examination.

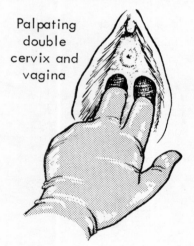

Palpating double cervix and vagina

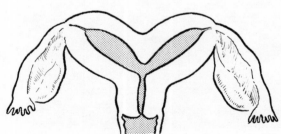

Uterus bicornis, unicollis, single vagina

Uterus Bicornis Unicollis

It is impossible to diagnose this condition except at laparotomy or perhaps during removal of a retained placenta which is more common with these abnormalities. This uterus encourages breech presentation – the head occupies one horn, the feet the other.

CONGENITAL ABNORMALITIES

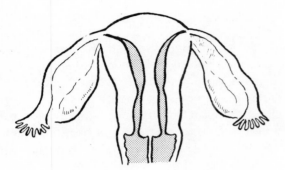

Uterus Septus

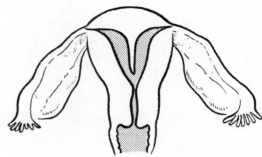

Uterus Subseptus

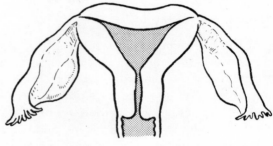

Uterus Arcuatus
('Cordiform Uterus')

This group can only be diagnosed when the uterus is opened at Caesarean section, although the arcuate uterus is often suspected on abdominal palpation through a thin abdominal wall. As a group they predispose to abortion, and to some complications of later pregnancy such as abnormal or unstable lie, and retained placenta.

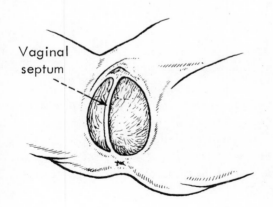

Vaginal septum

Vaginal Septa

These can occur on their own in otherwise normal genital tracts and are often incomplete. Sometimes the second stage may be delayed because of a septum preventing the advance of the head. The best treatment is to await this situation, and then when the septum is stretched, inject a little local anaesthetic, ligate, and divide with scissors.

269

CONGENITAL ABNORMALITIES

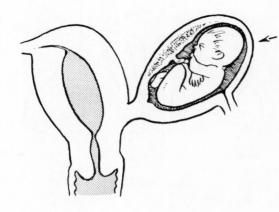

Pregnancy in Rudimentary Horn (Cornual Pregnancy).

Even though the horn has no access from the vagina, a 'wandering' sperm may fertilise an ovum on that side. Rupture with severe haemorrhage usually occurs at about the 4th month, but continuation to term has been reported. The non-pregnant horn hypertrophies, and the condition is usually (and fortunately) diagnosed as a tubal pregnancy, as the symptoms are similar. The treatment is excision of the gravid horn.

Angular Pregnancy

The ovum implants in the angle of the uterus near the tubal opening. The condition causes severe pain as the pregnancy progresses and the uterus enlarges asymmetrically. It may continue to term but there is a tendency to abortion, and tubal pregnancy may be diagnosed because of the patient's continual complaint of pain and the irregular swelling.

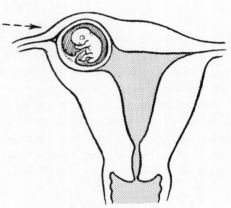

Interstitial Pregnancy

This is an ectopic implantation in the interstitial portion of the tube and is discussed under Ectopic Pregnancy on page 377. It is included here because of the similarity which it presents clinically and on palpation to angular and cornual pregnancies.

TUMOURS COMPLICATING PREGNANCY

The important ones are carcinoma of the cervix, fibroids and ovarian cysts.

FIBROIDS

Pregnancy in the presence of fibroids is rather rare. They contribute to infertility and are usually found in older women.

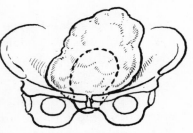

Multiple fibroids
at 12 weeks

Diagnosis: Fibroids are harder than any other pelvic mass likely to be met with and more likely to be multiple, but diagnosis is often presumptive. Twins, tubal pregnancy, ovarian cysts, salpingitis, cornual or angular pregnancies must all be considered. But fibroids are usually symptomless and can be left alone.

Degeneration: Fibroids are subject to 'red degeneration' during pregnancy, when they become tender and painful and cause symptoms of fever. Sedation only is required until the condition subsides in a few days; but sometimes laparotomy may have to be done to exclude appendicitis. Degeneration may also complicate the puerperium.

Pressure Symptoms: If the fibroids are very big or are impacted in the pelvis, dysuria, dyschezia, abdominal distension, varicose veins and even dyspnoea may be complained of. Treatment should always be conservative unless an obstruction develops. Myomectomy in pregnancy is a very haemorrhagic operation, and likely to be followed by abortion.

Management of Labour: If the fibroid appears to be obstructing descent and engagement, Caesarean section should be carried out, but if not the labour should proceed normally, although the patient is likely to develop some of the complications of the older age group. If there is doubt about obstruction the labour should be allowed to continue for a period to see if dilatation of the cervix causes the fibroid to be moved aside.

If delivery is by section, myomectomy should not be done at the same time. Fibroids regress considerably in the months following pregnancy and the uterine incision may be placed anywhere, through the fundus if necessary, to avoid interfering with the fibroids which will bleed excessively.

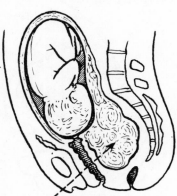

Fibroid obstructing
labour

TUMOURS COMPLICATING PREGNANCY

These tumours are generally removed at once because of their tendency to mechanical complications and the possibility of malignancy.

The commonest type is the simple cyst (70%) or the dermoid (25%). About 5% are malignant.

Diagnosis

Palpation is much easier in early pregnancy before the uterus occupies most of the pelvis. An ovarian cyst is more mobile than a hydro- or pyosalpinx, and less tender than a tubal pregnancy. In the later months if palpation is unsatisfactory, X-rays or ultrasonography may help. If the swelling is due to hydramnios postural X-ray will demonstrate gravitation of the foetus. This would not be seen if a cyst were present.

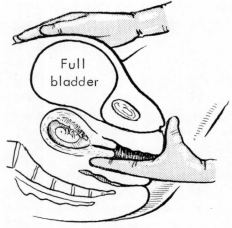

Palpating a full bladder

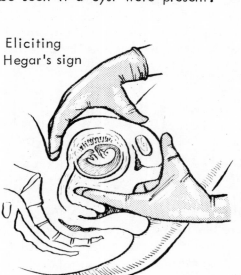

Eliciting Hegar's sign

Pitfalls in Diagnosis

1. A full bladder especially when dislodged from the pelvis by the gravid uterus, is often mistaken for a cyst.

2. A normal gravid uterus from the 2nd to the 4th month has a very soft isthmic region (see Hegar's sign, page 75) and it is easy to mistake the cervix for the uterus and the corpus for a cyst.

3. The cyst may be a large corpus luteum. It is a good working rule to observe rather than operate on any single cyst up to the size of say a tangerine orange. Even then a corpus luteum is occasionally removed.

272

TUMOURS COMPLICATING PREGNANCY

Complications in the Cyst

1. Torsion is the commonest and may lead to rupture. The symptoms are acute, with sudden onset of abdominal pain, vomiting and pyrexia. These subside, to occur again a few days later. Pelvic examination will reveal a tender cystic mass and the distinction from tubal pregnancy may be impossible.

2. Pressure symptoms may arise if the cyst becomes incarcerated in the pelvis or is of very large size. These will include dysuria, pain, abdominal distension, varicose veins, dyschezia.

3. Suppuration. This is most likely in the puerperium as a result of trauma sustained during delivery.

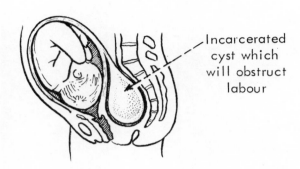

Incarcerated cyst which will obstruct labour

Complications in the Pregnancy

1. There is an increased tendency to spontaneous abortion if the cyst is large.

2. A cyst in the pelvis will obstruct labour, causing malpresentation or non-engagement of the head.

- -

Treatment

1. The principle is to remove the cyst as soon as its presence is detected and its nature diagnosed. The risk of abortion is not increased unless the uterus has to be handled to give access to the cyst, and this is more likely the later the pregnancy. Also a laparotomy scar must be given several months to heal before being subjected to the stress of labour.

2. If the pregnancy is at about 32 weeks and the tumour symptomless, delay for a few weeks is indicated in the interest of the foetus.

3. If the cyst is discovered at or near term, and is well clear of the pelvis, labour should be induced and the cyst removed a few days later. If there is any suggestion of obstruction Caesarean section and ovariotomy should be carried out forthwith.

4. If obstruction by a cyst is discovered only because of delay in the second stage of labour, the cyst should be incised or aspirated through the vaginal wall, delivery completed, and the cyst removed within 24 hours before suppuration and adhesions can develop.

CHAPTER 12

ABNORMALITIES OF THIRD STAGE
OF LABOUR
AND OF PLACENTA AND CORD

RETAINED PLACENTA

Retention of the placenta and haemorrhage are the chief complications.

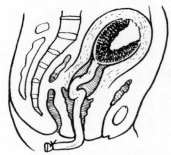

RETAINED PLACENTA

It may be completely separated, and all that is required is forcible expulsion by the mother or manual expression by the obstetrician.

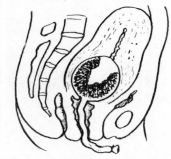

In such cases there have usually been signs of placental separation – bleeding, alteration of the shape of the uterus, lengthening of the cord.

Expression of the Separated Placenta.

When the placenta is separated and in the vagina or lower segment, manual expression should deliver it with very little force.

The uterus is gently rubbed up to stimulate a contraction, and then pressed down into the pelvis. At the same time gentle traction is applied to the cord.

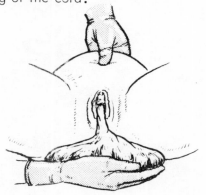

Brandt–Andrews Expression

If the placenta has separated but is still apparently in the upper segment, this method of expression may be of use. The cord is pulled gently, and the other hand presses the uterus upwards so as to prevent inversion. A slight see-sawing motion is imparted by both hands; and provided separation has occurred the placenta should be delivered.

RETAINED PLACENTA

Retention may be due to its being still partly or wholly attached, because of the absence of uterine contractions, the presence of an hour-glass constriction in the lower segment (often said to be a result of ergometrine) or because of some pathological adherence.

In such circumstances the signs of separation will be absent or equivocal, although bleeding may have occurred.

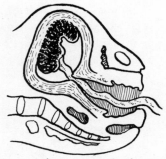

Hour-glass constriction

Treatment

It is usual to wait for up to 30 minutes for delivery of the placenta, provided there is no bleeding. It is a principle of third stage management to handle the uterus as little as possible so that irregular contractions do not produce partial separation, but after 30 minutes it is permissable to make one attempt at manual separation and expression. This is called Credé's Manoeuvre and its great disadvantage is that it often fails to separate the placenta and instead provokes haemorrhage and sometimes shock.

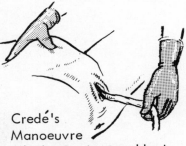

Credé's Manoeuvre
(1) The fundus is rubbed up to obtain a contraction.

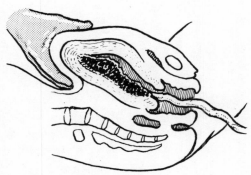

(2) The fundus is squeezed (to separate) and the uterus is pressed into pelvis (to express).

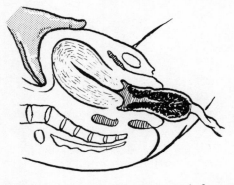

(3) The placenta is squeezed from the upper to the lower segment and pushed out.

277

RETAINED PLACENTA

If simple expression and Crede's Manoeuvre have failed, manual removal of the placenta should be resorted to. The longer the delay the greater the chance of haemorrhage. This procedure is carried out under general anaesthesia and the patient is cleaned and draped and the bladder emptied.

The hand covered with antiseptic cream is introduced into the vagina, following the cord.

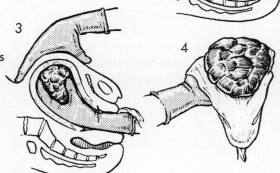

The fingers begin to separate the placenta from the uterine wall. Never grasp the placenta until it is separated.

Note that the abdominal hand presses the uterus into the placenta and prevents tearing of the lower segment.

The placenta is inspected at once to see that it is complete and, if there is any doubt, the uterus is re-explored. Ergometrine is then given.

Risks of Manual Removal

Infection. Unless strict aseptic and antiseptic precautions are observed, the hand will introduce infection into the uterus. Prophylactic antibiotic cover is justified if there is any doubt about this.

Trauma. Immediately after delivery the lower segment is very easily torn by clumsy internal manoeuvres.

Placenta Accreta. Abnormal adherence to the uterine wall due to a defect in the decidua. It may be partial or complete and is extremely rare. When complete there is no third stage bleeding at all and attempts at manual removal are unsuccessful. The usual treatment is hysterectomy, but in a patient wanting more babies, it might be permissable to leave the placenta to slough away provided the inevitable infection were controlled.

POSTPARTUM HAEMORRHAGE (PPH)

Blood loss from the birth canal in excess of 20 oz (560 ml) within 24 hours of delivery. After 24 hours it is classed as secondary PPH.

Immediate Causes

① Uterine Atony. For some reason the uterus fails to contract and control bleeding from the placental site. This is the commonest and potentially most dangerous cause.

② Partial failure of the placenta to separate. The uterus is prevented from contracting. (This is sometimes called third stage haemorrhage.)

③ Retention of placental fragments.

④ Cervical or vaginal tears (including episiotomy).

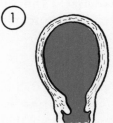

Uterus failing to contract

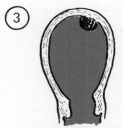

Incomplete separation

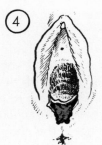

Retention of placental fragment

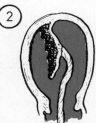

Vagino-perineal tear

Predisposing Causes

1. Excessive uterine distension (twins, hydramnios, large baby).
2. Multiparity and malnutrition.
3. Uterine exhaustion usually ending in operative delivery under general anaesthesia. Deep anaesthesia may be a contributory factor.
4. If vaginal delivery occurs with placenta praevia, the lower segment does not contract well enough to stop bleeding.
5. After accidental haemorrhage the 'Couvelaire' uterus may not contract. In addition the coagulation defect by itself causes haemorrhage.

Consequences of PPH

1. Bleeding may be very rapid causing circulatory collapse leading to shock and death.
2. Puerperal anaemia and morbidity.
3. (Very rarely) damage to the pituitary blood supply, leading to pituitary necrosis – Sheehan's syndrome.
4. Fear of further pregnancies. Haemorrage is terrifying for the mother.

279

POSTPARTUM HAEMORRHAGE—TREATMENT

Measurement of Blood Loss

Blood spilt on bed linen and dressings is ignored and only blood actually collected in a bowl is measured. The estimated loss is therefore always lower than the actual loss, and it is better to give plasma or plasma expanders before they appear to be needed.

Use of Oxytocic Drugs

Two are used: Ergometrine 0.5 mg and oxytocin 5 units. Syntometrine is a proprietary combination of both in these doses. Ergot alkaloids are vasoconstrictor, and ergot toxicity includes gangrene of the extremities. Oxytocin acts mainly on the uterus and the lactating breast but has very mild antidiuretic and vasoconstrictor effects (including bradycardia). However

Time between injection and action of oxytocic agents.

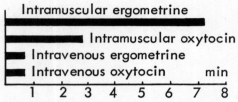

The earlier the drug is given the less the blood loss but the greater the chance of retained placenta.

the purified preparations used today have virtually no side effects unless given far in excess of the therapeutic dose. When given intramuscularly ergometrine takes 7 to 8 minutes to act and oxytocin 2 to 3 minutes: so in emergency either drug can be given intravenously with almost immediate effect. The earlier the drug is given the greater the chance of retained placenta.

Plan of Treatment

1. Give syntometrine intramuscularly, or ergometrine into a vein.
2. Raise the foot of the bed (or drop the head) and put up a plasma infusion.
3. Treat the Cause:

   a) If retention of a placental lobe is suspected from re-examination of the placenta, the uterus must be explored under anaesthesia.

   b) Damage to vagina or cervix must be dealt with. This should be suspected when the uterus is well contracted and bleeding continues.

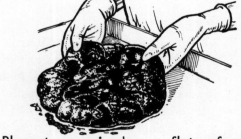

Placenta examined on a flat surface to demonstrate any missing lobe.

c) If neither of these causes is found uterine atony must be diagnosed and treated.

280

POSTPARTUM HAEMORRHAGE—TREATMENT

Treatment of Uterine Atony

    Oxytocic drugs must be given at once and at the same time the uterus is compressed between the hands to control bleeding and stimulate contraction. This can be done abdominally but more efficiently with the hand in the vagina.

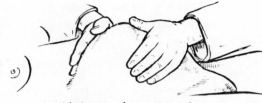

Abdominal compression
of uterus

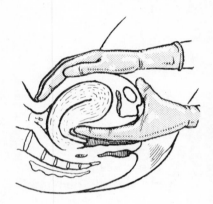

The fingers of one hand are pressed into the anterior fornix. If a good pressure is not obtained, and the vagina is lax, the whole fist can be inserted.

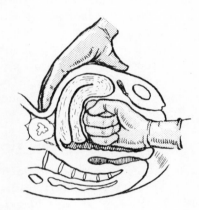

    As a last resort the patient can be anaesthetised and the uterus packed, using saline soaked gauze at 120° F (49° C). If contraction is still not obtained, hysterectomy must be carried out. By this time the patient is likely to be in a serious condition and the decision to operate, difficult as it is, must not be made too late.

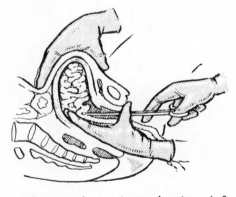

    In any postpartum haemorrhage, especially when prolonged, a clotting defect may be an additional complication, and the clotting time should always be estimated. (Coagulation defects are dealt with on page 410.)

ABNORMALITIES OF THE PLACENTA

The placenta develops from the chorion frondosum, the part in contact with the most vascular decidua. Any developmental abnormality may have a clinical significance.

Placenta Membranacea (syn: Diffusa)

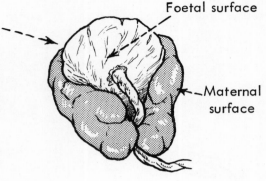

Foetal surface

Maternal surface

More or less the whole chorion develops functional villi and the placenta occupies the greater part of the uterine wall. This may cause retention in the third stage. Antepartum haemorrhage may also occur.

Another variety is placenta annularis in which the placenta surrounds the chorion like a wide ring. This is normal in the dog, while membranacea is normal in the pig.

Placenta Bipartita

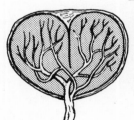

The placenta is partly divided into two lobes, with connecting vessels.

Placenta Duplex

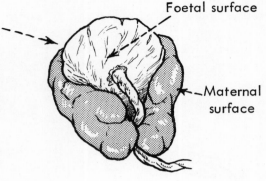

The placenta is completely divided into two lobes, with vessels uniting to form the cord.

Placenta Succenturiata ('substitute')

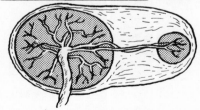

(A variant of Duplex)

Sometimes the placenta is partly or completely divided into two or more lobes (multipartita, multiplex). In placenta succenturiata there is a vascular connection between main and accessory lobes. This may be torn at delivery, and torn vessels may be seen at the edge of the membranes. In such cases the accessory lobe is retained and must be manually removed.

ABNORMALITIES OF THE PLACENTA

Placenta Circumvallata. The membranes appear to be attached internally to the placental edge, and on the periphery there is a ring of thick whitish tissue which is in fact a fold of infarcted chorion. This abnormality has an association with antepartum and postpartum haemorrhage.

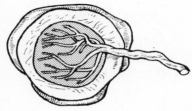

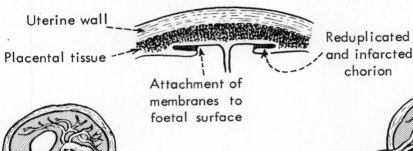

Uterine wall

Placental tissue

Attachment of membranes to foetal surface

Reduplicated and infarcted chorion

Placenta Fenestrata

A defective area appears in the middle of the placenta. It may be wrongly taken for the site of a missing lobe.

Battledore Placenta

Sometimes the cord has a marginal instead of a central insertion. This has no clinical significance.

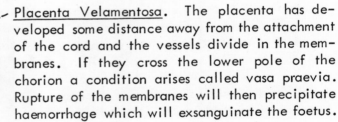

Placenta Velamentosa. The placenta has developed some distance away from the attachment of the cord and the vessels divide in the membranes. If they cross the lower pole of the chorion a condition arises called vasa praevia. Rupture of the membranes will then precipitate haemorrhage which will exsanguinate the foetus.

Placental Infarcts are areas of degeneration showing hyaline and often calcareous change. Their aetiology is unknown and they have no clinical significance unless so large as to interfere with foetal nutrition.

Placental Tumours are exceedingly rare and the haemangioma is the only one of any significance. It is often accompanied by hydramnios.

ABNORMALITIES OF THE CORD

Cord Round the Neck

One or two loops of cord are quite often seen round the baby's neck at vertex delivery and normally do no harm. As soon as the neck is visible at the vulva all the loops should be clamped and divided before delivery of the shoulders and trunk.

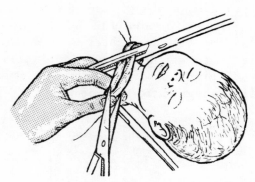

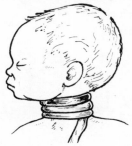

Much less frequently six or seven loops are drawn tightly round the neck. As the foetus descends the cord tightens, and the blood supply is interrupted and the baby is stillborn.

Abnormal Length of Cord

The average length is 20 in. (50 cm) but extremes of 6 in. and 60 in. have rarely occurred. Prolapse and looping round the neck seem more likely with lengthy cords, while delayed foetal descent and premature placental separation may occur with very short ones. A cord of normal length may become relatively short because of multiple looping round the neck.

Knots in the Cord

True knots are seen quite often, but Wharton's jelly usually prevents actual obstruction by kinking. False knots are protuberances of connective tissue matrix, sometimes containing varices.

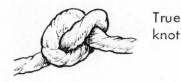

True knot

Single Umbilical Artery

This abnormality is frequently associated with other congenital abnormalities in the foetus.

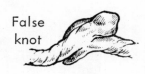

False knot

284

CHAPTER 13

THE PUERPERIUM

THE PUERPERIUM

The puerperium is the period following childbirth when the woman (now a 'puerpera') is returning as nearly as possible to her pre-gravid state.

For purposes of Notification of Infections the puerperium is defined, in law, as the 14 days (England and Wales) or 21 days (Scotland) following confinement.

The Midwives Board require their midwives to attend the puerpera for a period of not less than 10 days.

The uterus contains a raw bleeding surface - a wound. INFECTION must be prevented.

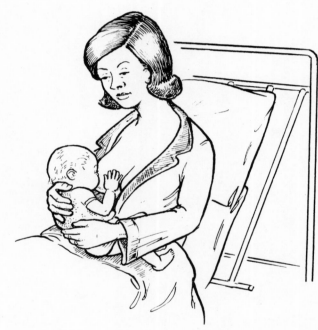

The newborn baby requires careful nursing and observation.

Breast feeding must be initiated (or lactation properly suppressed).

Muscles are of poor tone and ligaments slack after pregnancy and labour. Systematic exercises must be given to prevent chronic postural defects, hernia and prolapse.

The mother's mood is unstable: she must be given **sympathy and support**.

PHYSIOLOGICAL CHANGES

The process by which the uterus returns almost to its pre-gravid state is known as INVOLUTION – a dramatic example of atrophy due to withdrawal of hormonal support (in this case the placental oestrogens).

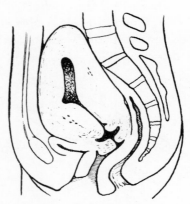

Uterus after delivery

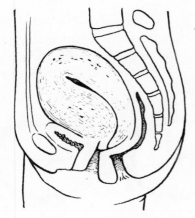

Uterus at 6th day

Involution is caused by the phenomenon of AUTOLYSIS – enzymatic digestion of excess cytoplasm – and thrombosis and hyaline degeneration of vessels; but traces of fibro-elastic tissue remain as evidence of pregnancy. The endometrium is re-generated by the 10th day, except at the placental site, where it takes 6 weeks.

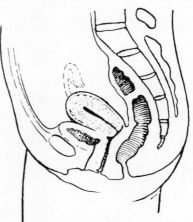

Non-gravid uterus

The LOCHIA (the discharges of child-birth) consist mainly of blood and necrotic decidua. It persists for about 2 weeks, gradually becoming colourless and scanty. It is sterile to begin with but by the 3rd – 4th days the inside of the uterus is said to be colonised by vaginal commensals (anaerobic streptococcus, B.coli, etc.).

PHYSIOLOGICAL CHANGES

The uterus reduces to about 1/25 of its size in about 6 weeks although it never returns exactly to its nulliparous proportions.

Muscle fibres from uterus

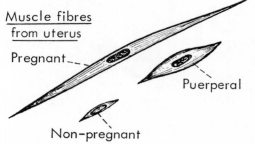

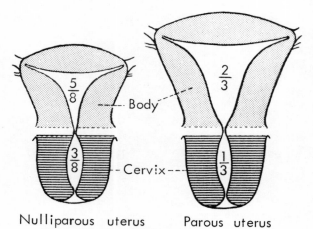

Nulliparous uterus   Parous uterus

This reduction in size is achieved partly by the removal of blood and blood vessels, and partly by digestion of a large part of the cell cytoplasm. The number of muscle cells is probably not much diminished, but the individual fibres are very much shorter and thinner than during the pregnancy.

Time post partum	Wt. of Uterus	Ht. of Uterus
post partum	2 lb. (1 kg)	7 in. (17 cm)
1 week	1 lb.	5 in.
2 weeks	12 oz.	3 in.
4 weeks	6 oz.	2½ in.
6 weeks	1½ oz. (40 g)	2 in. (5 cm)

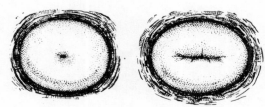

Nulliparous cervix   Parous cervix

The cervix never returns to its pristine appearance and although completely healed will always give evidence of parturition.

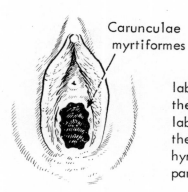

Carunculae myrtiformes

The vagina and vulva, considerably stretched during labour, have returned almost to their pre-gravid size by the 3rd week. Rugae appear in the vagina, and the labia regress to a less prominent and fleshy state than in the nulliparous condition. Only small sessile tags of hymen are left (carunculae myrtiformes) and, like the parous cervix, are evidence of previous pregnancy.

CLINICAL ASPECTS

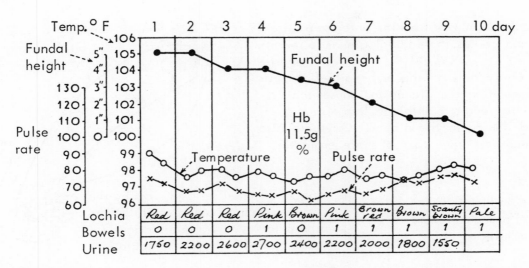

	1	2	3	4	5	6	7	8	9	10 day
Lochia	Red	Red	Red	Pink	Brown	Pink	Brown red	Brown	Scanty brown	Pale
Bowels	0	0	0	1	0	1	1	1	1	1
Urine	1750	2200	2600	2700	2400	2200	2000	1800	1550	

FUNDAL HEIGHT is measured each day. The bladder must be empty and the uterus in the mid-line. The uterus is rubbed up to contract and the height of the fundus above the symphysis is measured.

PULSE tends to be slower, about 60 – 70 per minute, probably because the woman is resting completely after the exertion of labour.

TEMPERATURE may be slightly elevated during the first 24 hours, but thereafter should remain within normal limits.

CONSTIPATION is the rule for some days. Oestrogens continue to inhibit smooth muscle motility.

URINE – There is a diuresis during the 2nd to 5th days and urinary nitrogen is much raised. The body is getting rid of the excess fluid retained during pregnancy, and the high nitrogen excretion is a direct result of the autolytic process at work in the uterus.

LOCHIA should gradually change colour from red to pale yellow over 10 days. There are great variations in this due to the fluctuations in the amount of blood being lost during this period.

BLOOD. The haemoglobin level is important and should be stable by the 5th day, when normal haemoconcentration is approached.

LACTATION AND BREAST FEEDING

PROLACTIN from the anterior pituitary gland causes the lacteal glands to secrete milk. OXYTOCIN from the posterior pituitary acts on the myo-epithelial cells surrounding the glands and causes the milk to be secreted into the lactiferous ducts and thence to the nipple. Oxytocin also stimulates the output of more prolactin.

Sensory stimuli to pituitary gland

Prolactin

Oxytocin

The 'milk let-down' reflex
The 'draught' reflex
The 'milk ejection' response

The conditioned reflex set off by the stimulus of the baby's mouth at the nipple (or even by preparations for feeding) which results in lactation.

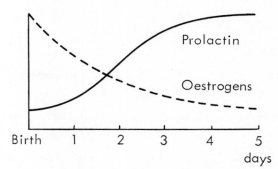

Prolactin

Oestrogens

Birth   1   2   3   4   5
days

PLACENTAL OESTROGENS inhibit the secretion of prolactin; and it takes 3 or 4 days for this effect to wear off completely. Normal milk is not being secreted until that time. While oestrogens still dominate (during pregnancy and immediately after delivery) COLOSTRUM is secreted.

COLOSTRUM is a yellowish fluid, containing a much greater quantity of protein than normal milk, plus quantities of desquamated endothelial cells. Its function is not known; but its high gamma-globulin content may be a provision for the supply of antibodies which the baby must acquire in the first months. Dairy farmers always feed the colostrum to their calves as a protection against disease.

	Colostrum	Human milk
Protein	6%	1%
Fat	2.5%	3.5%
Carbohydrate	3%	7%

LACTATION AND BREAST FEEDING

SUPPLEMENTARY FEED

A supplementary feed is given in place of a breast feed. It might be required when the breast is being rested because of cracked nipples; or in the case of twins taking turns at breast and bottle.

COMPLEMENTARY FEED

A complementary feed is given at the end of a breast feed if the baby is not contented or is not gaining weight. The time at the breast is shortened to 5 minutes at each breast (most of the milk is taken in that time) and the baby is offered an ounce or two of artificial feed.

SUPPRESSION of LACTATION

At present many mothers prefer the emancipation of artifical feeding from the beginning. The best time to suppress lactation is before it is properly established; and stilboestrol or its equivalent in doses of 15 mg thrice daily for 3 days must be given and a few minutes' expression with a breast pump will help to reduce discom—fort. Diuretics have no enhancing effect at this stage and it is not necessary to restrict fluids. The milk will probably not disappear until about the 10th day, but this dosage of stilboestrol will prevent the discomfort of engorgement. The course may have to be repeated in a fortnight or less if the breasts fill up again.

WEANING

Weaning is the gradual change from breast feeding to completely artificial feeding or mixed feeding (milk and semi-solids). Three months might reasonably be the recommended age for beginning. The mother should begin by giving a bottle instead of the 2 p.m. feed and continue over a week. The 6 a.m. feed will be the last to be given up as the breasts tend to be fullest at that time, after a night's rest.

Supply of milk should decrease step by step with demand; but if the weaning is done abruptly, oestrogens will be required.

SOME COMMON COMPLICATIONS

(Any pathological condition in the mother will affect breast feeding at once)

NOT ENOUGH MILK

The only way to prove this is by weighing the baby before and after each feed for 24 hours. If the mother is not producing at least 2 oz. per feed, and the baby is not gaining weight, she must eat and drink more and generally lead as placid an existence as possible. There are no drugs known to increase lactation.

TOO MUCH MILK

This is suspected if the baby passes undigested stools – bulky and offensive, sometimes bloodstained – or leaves the breast unemptied. It may also regurgitate milk and may even vomit during or immediately after a feed. Such babies are usually strong, voracious feeders and treatment is to reduce the time at the breast and give boiled water if the baby will not sleep. The milk remaining must be expressed.

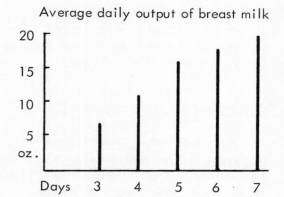

Average daily output of breast milk

PAINFUL NIPPLES

Cracks and fissures of the nipples are caused by too vigorous sucking by the baby in an effort to get the nipple properly into its mouth. It is because of this that nipple protraction should be encouraged in the antenatal period. Treatment is to use a nipple shield through which the baby sucks, or to rest the nipple for 24 hours using stilboestrol (15 mg thrice daily) and breast expression to prevent engorgement.

The nipple needs no special treatment other than washing and drying after each feed; but if tenderness is present, zinc and castor oil cream may help. It must be removed before the next feed.

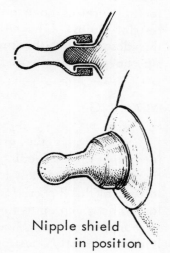

Nipple shield
in position

POSTNATAL EXAMINATION

Postnatal examination is usually made about 6 weeks postpartum.

Objects:- 1. To make sure that the genital tract has returned to normal; and to give treatment if necessary.

2. To make sure that lactation is satisfactory (or that it has been effectively suppressed) and that the baby is feeding well and gaining weight.

3. To deal with any other problems, and offer birth control advice if required.

RETURN OF MENSTRUATION

In the lactating woman menstruation is suppressed for about 3 months but after that there is a tendency for it to return.

The amenorrhoea of lactation is due to suppression of ovulation; and if menstruation is occurring, so probably is ovulation.

In the non-lactating woman bleeding is irregular, depending on the fluctuating oestrogen levels. The normal cycle should be restored at least by the third month.

Wide variations in these patterns are met with. On rare occasions, a new pregnancy may be diagnosed at the postnatal visit.

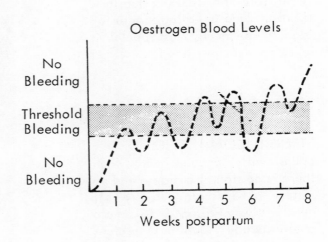

Oestrogen Blood Levels

Weeks postpartum

POSTNATAL EXAMINATION

Involution should be complete by 6 weeks. The size, shape and mobility of the uterus is noted, and vaginal and cervical lacerations palpated to make sure there is no potential source of dyspareunia.

A speculum is passed and the CERVIX examined. A cervical smear may conveniently be taken for cytology.

All parts of the squamo-columnar junction will provide cellular material which might be missed by a random biopsy.

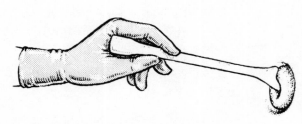

Taking a cervical smear.

Remember that a rubbing of cells is required, not a smear of cervical discharge.

DISCHARGE   Slight discharge is the rule at 6 weeks postpartum. If profuse and irritating, bacterio-logical specimens must be taken and treatment instituted.

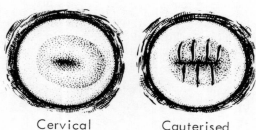

Cervical erosion   Cauterised cervix

STRESS INCONTINENCE occasionally occurs even when there is no sign of prolapse and no history of difficult delivery. It nearly always responds to simple physiotherapy (such as conscious contraction and relaxation of the levator ani muscles) but sometimes surgical treatment is needed.

The CERVIX may show an 'erosion' – an overgrowth of regenerating cervical endothelium. This should only be cauterised if badly in-fected, as squamous overgrowth tends to occur. Cautery 6 weeks postpartum usually causes a good deal of bleeding.

POSTNATAL EXAMINATION

Retroversion means posterior displacement of the uterus, with the corpus leaning backwards instead of forwards. It should be ignored unless causing backache or discomfort.

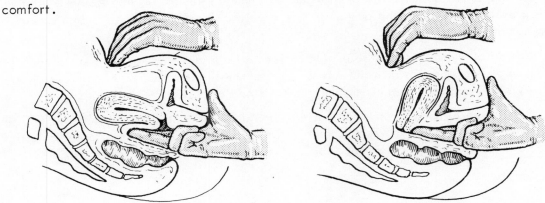

Correction of Retroversion is called 'Basculation': the manipulating hand 'rocks' the uterus forward. (Fr. bascule, a cradle.)

The corrected position is maintained with a Hodge pessary for a month. The pessary when in position cannot be felt by the patient and should not interfere with any pelvic function, including intercourse.

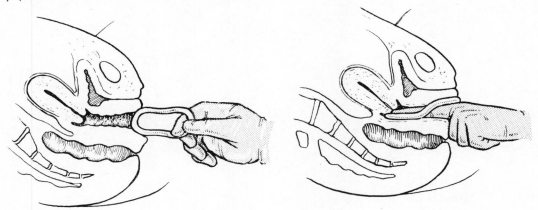

Inserting a Hodge pessary.

POSTNATAL EXERCISES

During the latter half of pregnancy ligaments are softened and slackened (probably a consequence of the fluid retention caused by placental hormones), muscles are stretched, posture changed to compensate for the increasing weight of the gravid uterus. During parturition, the pelvic floor is always stretched and may be damaged.

Postnatal exercises are given (1) to prevent the development of hernia, pelvic floor prolapse and postural defects such as sacro-iliac strain; (2) to prevent circulatory stasis and reduce the risk of thrombosis and embolism.

Besides early ambulation, the patient should be instructed in a systematic course of exercises designed to restore tone in the different muscle groups, especially the lumbo-dorsal, abdominal and perineal. The following are examples:-

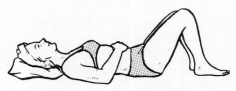

Patient's hands press on abdominal muscles. First, thoracic breathing is done, then abdominal.

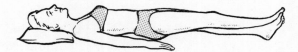

Both knees straight and legs crossed, buttocks and thighs are contracted and relaxed. Anus and perineum are drawn in as if trying to prevent micturition.

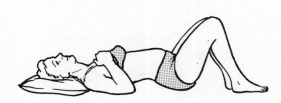

Lying on back with knees bent, rock abdomen and buttocks backward and forward.

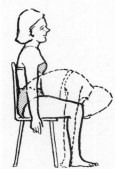

Sitting in a chair, slowly bend forward to touch toes, and slowly sit up and straighten shoulders.

CHAPTER 14

MATERNAL INJURIES
AND
PUERPERAL INFECTION

PERINEAL DAMAGE

DAMAGE to the PERINEAL BODY

This is more common in primigravidae who have more rigid perineums. Probably the most important factors are the width of the pubic arch (and hence the amount of room available) and the size and position of the foetal head. All malpresentations increase the amount of distension of the perineum.

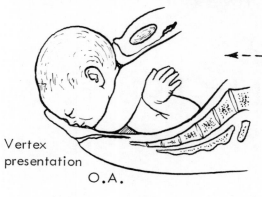

In the normal O.A. position the suboccipito-frontal diameter (4 inches) distends the vulva, and the widest part of the head is under the bony arch.

Vertex presentation
O.A.

When the position is O.P. the occipito-frontal diameter ($4\frac{1}{2}$ inches) distends the vulva, and the widest part of the head distends the perineum.

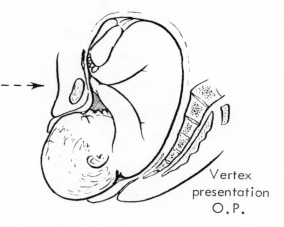

Vertex presentation
O.P.

Face presentation
M.A.

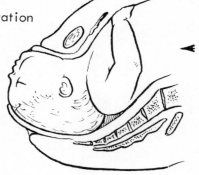

When the face is presenting, once the chin is delivered, the submento-vertical diameter ($5\frac{1}{4}$ inches) will distend the vulva, and again the widest part of the head passes over the perineum.

298

PERINEAL DAMAGE

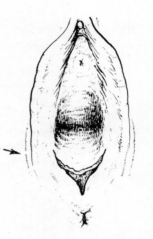

1st degree Perineal Tear

Vaginal and perineal skin are torn but the perineal muscles are intact.

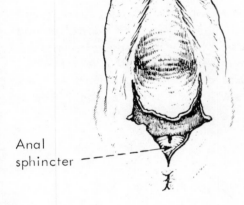

2nd degree Tear

The perineal body is torn right down to (and sometimes partly involving) the anal sphincter. The vaginal tears often extend up both sides of the vagina.

Anal sphincter

3rd degree Tear - "Complete Tear"

The whole anal sphincter is torn apart, and there may be a tear of the rectal wall. Note how the ends of the sphincter muscles tend to retract.

This injury, if not repaired, leaves the patient with faecal incontinence.

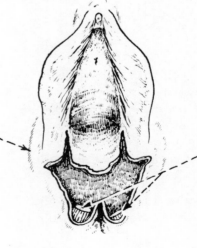

Torn ends of anal sphincter

PERINEAL DAMAGE—REPAIR

Perineal damage should be repaired very soon after delivery. Blood loss will be lessened, the chance of infection reduced, and the patient is usually relaxed and euphoric.

The repair is done under aseptic conditions with the patient in the lithotomy position under a good light. 20 – 30 ml. of 1% lignocaine are injected into the muscles and under the skin.

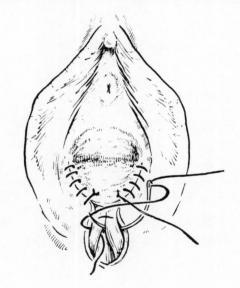

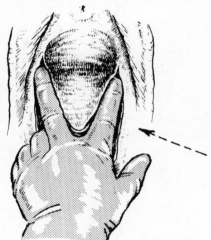

Correct anatomical apposition is essential. Bleeding must be controlled and swabs used freely to expose the tissues, and the upper limits of the tear must be demonstrated by stretching apart with the fingers so that suturing may begin there.

1. Close vaginal tears with continuous No. 1 catgut.
2. Suture perineal muscles together with interrupted No. 1 catgut.
3. Close skin over muscles with catgut or non-absorbable material.

Sutures tied too tight will cause pain. Be sure the vagina admits 2 fingers easily when the repair is completed.

PERINEAL DAMAGE—REPAIR

3rd degree Tears

Such tears heal much better if repaired at the time rather than months or years later. The operation is best performed with the patient under general anaesthesia.

1. The rectal wall is repaired with fine chromic catgut sutures, tied inside the rectum.
2. The two ends of the anal sphincter are picked up in tissue forceps and apposed with 2 or 3 No. 1 catgut sutures. (The anus should then accommodate the little finger).
3. The repair is continued as for a 2nd degree tear. The skin of the anal margin should be closed with fine catgut.

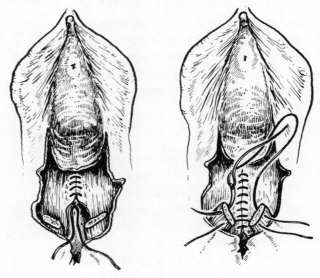

Post operative treatment

1. Low residue diet for a week.
2. No bowel movement for 5 days, then give Agarol 0.5 oz (14 ml.) twice daily until a soft stool is passed.
3. If no bowel movement, an olive oil enema may be given.

If the repair breaks down, it should be left for 3 months before a second repair is attempted.

If pregnancy follows a well-healed complete tear, section might be considered. Certainly a large episiotomy would be needed.

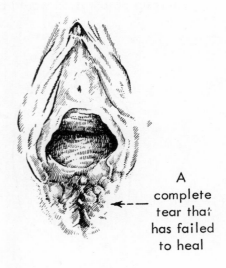

A complete tear that has failed to heal

INJURIES TO THE VULVA

HAEMATOMA of the VULVA

Rupture of vaginal veins (after prolonged or operative delivery) may produce a very large effusion of blood, extending downwards into the labium majus. If acute and extensive it causes great pain and this with blood loss soon causes shock.

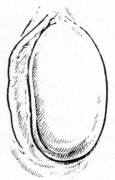

Treatment

1. Treat collapse with transfusion etc.
2. Under general anaesthesia, evacuate clot and pack and suture the cavity. If bleeding continues, a vaginal pack may be used for 12 hours to increase pressure.
3. Antibiotics should be given.
4. If infection and induration occur, healing will be delayed and an oral trypsin preparation would be justified.

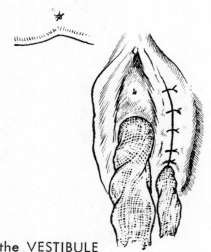

TEARS of the VESTIBULE

These are not common and arise from much the same causes as perineal tears. They may bleed freely, especially if the clitoral artery is approached, and should be sutured. If the tear passes close to the urethral meatus a catheter should be inserted and continuous drainage with antiseptic cover continued for 48 hours (see page 305).

INJURIES TO THE VAGINA—TEARS

COLPORRHEXIS (rupture of the vaginal vault). The commonest site is the posterior or lateral fornix and the cervix may be involved. Tearing may result from obstructed labour, but it is more often due to improper application of the forceps.

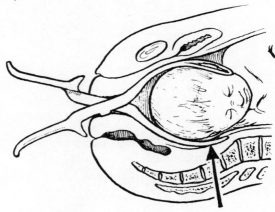

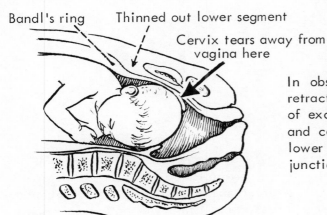

Bandl's ring

Thinned out lower segment

Cervix tears away from vagina here

In obstructed labour the pathological retraction ring (Bandl's ring) is a sign of excessive traction on lower segment and cervix. Rupture may occur in the lower segment or at the cervico-vaginal junction.

If the posterior blade of Kielland's forceps is not properly guided by the hand, the tip of the blade may perforate and tear the posterior fornix.

<u>Treatment</u>. If the examining finger passes completely through the vaginal tear, laparotomy is necessary to check on the extent of the damage. The symptoms are those of rupture of the uterus, and bleeding is usually considerable. A massive blood transfusion will be needed and hysterectomy will probably be the quickest and easiest way of stopping the haemorrhage.

INJURIES TO THE VAGINA—FISTULAE

Vaginal fistulae are uncommon injuries in present day obstetrics.

VESICOVAGINAL FISTULA

Caused by direct trauma (instruments, bony spicules) or by prolonged compression of vaginal wall and bladder between foetal head and maternal symphysis pubis.

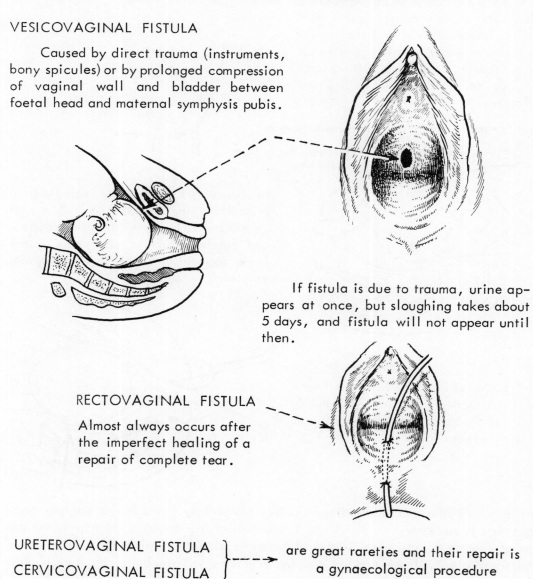

If fistula is due to trauma, urine appears at once, but sloughing takes about 5 days, and fistula will not appear until then.

RECTOVAGINAL FISTULA

Almost always occurs after the imperfect healing of a repair of complete tear.

URETEROVAGINAL FISTULA
CERVICOVAGINAL FISTULA } ⟶ are great rareties and their repair is a gynaecological procedure

REPAIR OF FISTULAE

REPAIR OF VESICOVAGINAL FISTULA

If observed at delivery it should be closed forthwith, using fine chromic catgut (interrupted through-and-through , then a continuous suture).

Continuous catheter drainage is instituted for 10 days, and antibiotic cover provided.

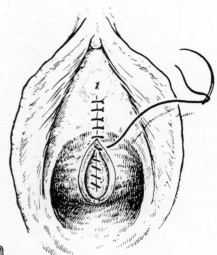

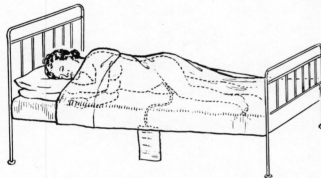

The patient should be encouraged to lie on her side or front as much as possible to keep urine from collecting on the bladder base.

If the fistula is a result of a sloughing wound and does not appear for 5 days after delivery, drainage must be prolonged for several weeks to allow every chance of spontaneous closure or at least shrinkage. Repair is then a gynaecological procedure.

REPAIR OF RECTOVAGINAL FISTULA. As has been said this nearly always results from imperfect healing of a repair of complete tear. No attempt at re-repair should be made for at least 3 months, and the operation is then performed in a gynaecological ward. It is usual to break down the perineum to some extent so that the rectum may be mobilised before suture.

INJURIES TO THE CERVIX

LACERATIONS of the CERVIX

The cervix is always torn to some extent during delivery, and severe tears may follow strong contractions on a rigid cervix, or arise from a previous cervical operation. The commonest cause is surgical trauma following forceps or breech delivery.

A tear is suspected when bleeding is heavy although the uterus is firmly contracted. The cervix must be examined and this may be difficult because of the bleeding and friability of the tissues.

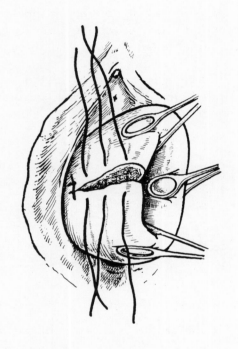

Several pairs of ring forceps and at least one assistant are needed and, once demonstrated, the tear should be sutured with interrupted catgut sutures. By the time the operation is completed, if not before, the patient may need a blood transfusion.

ANNULAR DETACHMENT of the CERVIX

This rare laceration usually occurs in a primigravida in whom strong contractions are driving the vertex against a rigid cervix. The vaginal cervix gradually develops a pressure necrosis, and the sloughed cervix separates and is delivered in front of the head. There is little bleeding and the cervical stump heals well.

306

RUPTURE OF THE UTERUS

A ruptured uterus is an uncommon injury, due nearly always to rupture of a previous section scar or to obstructed labour.

RUPTURE of CLASSICAL CAESAREAN SCAR – – –→

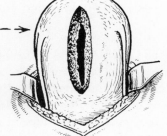

(Commonest cause of rupture): Occurs in late pregnancy or early labour. Bleeding is slight unless the placenta is lying underneath. There may be some vaginal 'show' and haematuria and the patient will think she is in labour.

RUPTURE of a LOWER SEGMENT SCAR

Usually caused by obstructed labour, it is said to be accompanied by a "tearing" pain, and bleeding may not be heavy. This type of rupture may not be perceived (and may not occur) until the third stage.

SPONTANEOUS RUPTURE   – – – – – – →

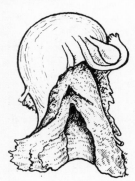

The patient is typically of high parity, and labour has been obstructed by malpresentation or disproportion. Contractions have been strong and rupture begins in the lower segment and is accompanied by pain, bleeding, haematuria and collapse.

RARE CAUSES

1. Previous trauma due to clumsy manual removal or curettage.   (Myomectomy scars withstand pregnancy well).
2. Trauma due to forceps or breech delivery or internal version late in labour.
3. Serious accidents: or simple accidents such as falling face downwards.
4. Induction of labour with oxytocin (buccal or intravenous) unless carefully controlled.
5. Congenital abnormalities such as uterus didelphys.
6. Severe accidental haemorrhage where extravasation of blood into the myometrium is excessive.

RUPTURE OF THE UTERUS

Diagnosis may be obvious and easy: or difficult and impossible without laparotomy.

INTRA-ABDOMINAL HAEMORRHAGE may cause rapid collapse. The blood may be confined retroperitoneally as a broad-ligament haematoma. Accidental haemorrhage must be considered in the diagnosis.

PAIN may be confused with the pain of contractions and the pain is said to be of a "tearing" nature. Rupture when complete produces a transient relief from pain and is followed by cessation of contractions.

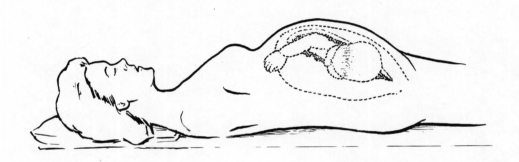

SHOCK depends on the rate of hae-morrhage: but a large tear will cause shock even without much blood loss. If the rupture is a dehiscence of a lower segment scar, there may be virtually no bleeding or shock. "Silent rupture" - completely symptomless - can occur and is only found on section for some other reason.

ALTERATION IN SHAPE OF ABDOMINAL SWELLING. The foetus is wholly or partly extruded into the abdominal cavity and quickly dies, whether or not the tear is complete (i.e. peritoneum also torn through) or incomplete. The uterus contracts and may be mistaken for a foetal head in the suprapubic region.

Vaginal examination reveals an empty pelvis.

RUPTURE OF THE UTERUS

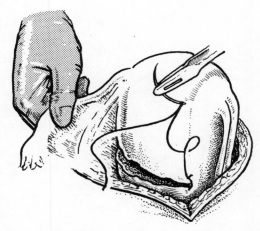

Once the diagnosis is reached laparotomy must be carried out with blood transfusion set up.

When the abdomen is opened the uterus is pulled out and inspected. Hysterectomy is usually the safest treatment, but if the tear is small without excessive bleeding or is easily accessible as in rupture of a previous classical scar, the simplest procedure might be repair and conservation of the uterus. In such cases the tear is closed with two continuous catgut sutures.

If hysterectomy is decided on, the tear will in most cases have half completed the operation. Subsequent steps in the operation are indicated below. If bleeding is severe this will be an operation in which speed is of importance.

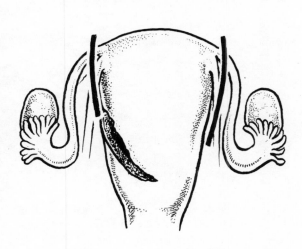

Division of the fallopian tubes and broad ligaments, leaving behind the ovaries and part of the tubes.

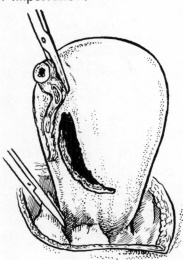

After incision of the peritoneum at the site of rupture the bladder is stripped from the uterine wall and a subtotal hysterectomy performed.

ACUTE INVERSION OF THE UTERUS

Acute inversion of the uterus is a very rare condition in modern practice but important because of its serious consequences.

First Degree (Incomplete)

The inverted fundus reaches the external os.   Diagnosis is made by vaginal examination.

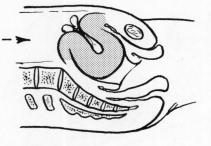

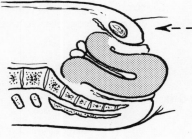

Second Degree (Complete)

The whole body of the uterus is inverted as far as the internal os and protrudes into the vagina.

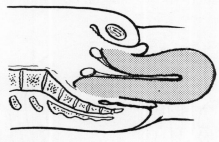

Third Degree

Prolapse of inverted uterus, cervix and vagina outside the vulva.

CAUSATION

1. Most commonly due to a too vigorous attempt at expression of placenta or to pulling on the cord.

2. It is favoured by laxity of the uterine muscles as in women of high parity, and by fundal attachment of the placenta. It can be brought on by any sudden bearing down effort.

CONSEQUENCES

1. Usually very severe shock and perhaps bleeding.   Death may follow.

2. The uterus may strangulate and slough off.

3. Inversion may become chronic.

4. Sepsis is common; and the shock may be followed by anuria and renal failure.

ACUTE INVERSION OF THE UTERUS

If the doctor is present when inversion occurs he should at once attempt to re-place the uterus by hand. He must not use too much force, and if not immediately successful, he should simply replace the inverted uterus in the vagina and institute treatment for shock. It is probably safer to leave the placenta if it is attached; removal might precipitate severe haemorrhage.

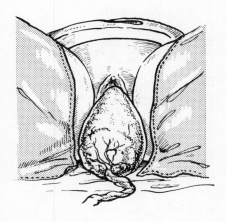

REDUCTION BY TAXIS

Under general anaesthesia an attempt is made to reduce the inversion by gradual replacement of the uterus, pressing first on that part of the corpus which was inverted last. The most difficult part to reduce is the retraction ring between upper and lower segments.

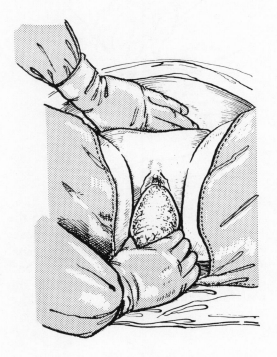

Once reduced, the hand is kept inside the uterus until ergometrine or oxytocin has produced a firm contraction.

ACUTE INVERSION OF THE UTERUS

REDUCTION BY HYDROSTATIC PRESSURE

If taxis fails, O'Sullivan's hydrostatic method should be attempted.

REDUCTION BY THE ABDOMINAL ROUTE

If other methods fail, the abdomen should be opened.

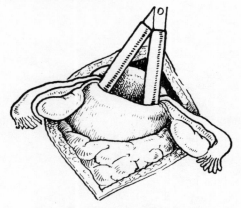

The constricting ring is stretched. Then the posterior part of the ring is divided and the fundus hooked up and resutured.

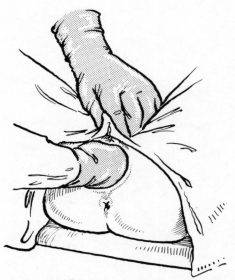

A douche nozzle is passed into the posterior fornice, and an assistant closes the vulva around the operator's wrist. Warm saline is run in (up to 2 gallons) until the pressure gradually restores the position of the uterus.

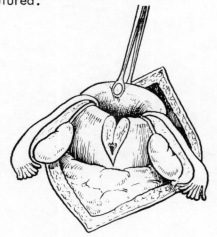

HAEMATOMA OF THE RECTUS SHEATH

A rare condition occurring mostly in multiparous woman as a result of coughing or sudden expulsive effort. Muscle fibres and branches of the deep epigastric veins are torn.

It is a condition most likely to be diagnosed on the history of sudden effort followed by pain.

If rupture occurs below the umbilicus, blood can track anywhere along transversalis fascia and is virtually retroperitoneal. If above the umbilicus the haematoma is more likely to be localised.

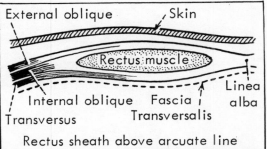

Rectus sheath above arcuate line

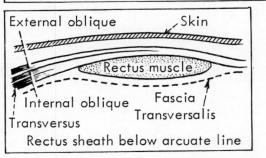

Rectus sheath below arcuate line

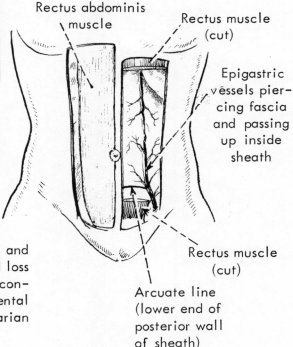

There is pain, possibly peritonism, and a vague abdominal swelling. If blood loss is large there may be collapse. The condition must be distinguished from accidental haemorrhage, rupture of uterus, ovarian cyst.

TREATMENT. If small and localised, the haematoma may be left to absorb. But usually operation is required, with evacuation of clot, ligation of any bleeding points, and closure with drainage.

TRAUMATIC NEURITIS (Syn. Obstetric Palsy)

Traumatic neuritis is a rare condition in which one or both legs show signs of motor and/or sensory nerve damage shortly after labour.

The lateral popliteal nerve which divides into the musculocutaneous and anterior tibial nerves is most commonly affected.

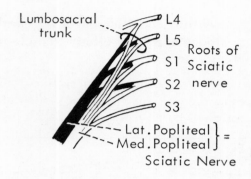

Theories of Causation

1. Prolapse of an intervertebral disc (L.4–5 or L.5–S.1). Disc prolapse is a flexion injury and may be caused by the exaggerated lithotomy position used for forceps delivery.

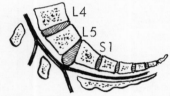

Disc being protruded by flexion

2. Foetal head may compress lumbosacral trunk as it crosses sacro-iliac joint (especially when pelvis is flat). The 5th lumbar nerve is the largest root of the sciatic nerve. Note how small is the foramen between L.5 and S.1 for the emergence of the 5th nerve.

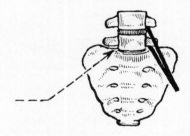

3. The sacrum may rotate back a little in labour, and put traction on the lumbosacral trunk.
Forceps delivery has a definite association with neuritis.

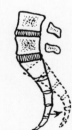

4. The popliteal nerve may be compressed between the head of the fibula and the lithotomy stanchion if no padding is used.

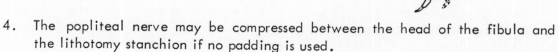

TRAUMATIC NEURITIS

PAIN is felt in the sciatic region (L.5 may contribute to the cutaneous supply to the back of the thigh) and there may be a tingling sensation in the lower leg.

MUSCULAR WASTING may be slight or extend so far as to involve the glutei (L.4,5 : S.1,2). Tension reflexes are variable but the ankle jerk is usually diminished and the knee jerk brisk.

FOOT DROP varies from weak dorsiflexion to complete paralysis of the peronei, tibialis anterior and extensor digitorum longus. The patient may be unable to flex her foot or extend her toes.

SENSORY IMPAIRMENT: Hyperalgesia (increased sensitivity to pinprick) and hypoaesthesia are demonstrated on the skin area over the dorsiflexors and peronei, usually to a minor degree.

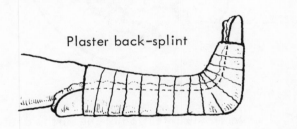

Plaster back-splint

Short leg-iron

TREATMENT: If disc prolapse is diagnosed or suspected, the patient is nursed with fracture boards under the mattress. Traction may be necessary to relieve the pain. The foot drop is protected by a blanket cage and a plaster back-splint. When walking begins a short leg iron may be required for several months until full function returns.

An episode of traumatic neuritis might be regarded as an indication for delivery by section in a subsequent pregnancy.

Backache associated with limping might result from sacro-iliac strain following parturition, or even from sacro-coccygeal strain (coxalgia); but in such cases there will be no evidence of a lower motor neurone lesion.

PUERPERAL INFECTION

Synonyms:- Puerperal Fever, Puerperal Sepsis, Childbed Fever.

Infection may enter through
one or more of these wounds :-

The PLACENTAL site is a raw
wound with gaping veins occluded
by thrombi - a good culture medium.

The CERVIX is nearly always torn
even in normal parturition.

The VAGINA is often torn, or
involved in an episiotomy.

The term PUERPERAL INFECTION covers only infection of the birth canal and spread therefrom.   Puerperal pyrexia may be due to an infection, genital or extra-genital.

NOTIFICATION of puerperal infection or pyrexia following childbirth or abortion is a legal obligation of the medical attendant. In England any temperature of $100.4^{\circ}F$ ($38^{\circ}C$) occurring in the first 14 days must be notified whatever the cause. In Scotland a distinction is still made between puerperal (i.e. genital) infection and infection in other organs, and the temperature of $100.4^{\circ}F$ must be sustained for, or recur in 24 hours within 21 days of childbirth or abortion.

In domiciliary practice the midwife must visit her patient twice daily during the first 3 days, and daily for a week thereafter. She must record the pulse and temperature (and the baby's temperature) at each visit; and if there is a rise in temperature after the first 24 hours, or any other condition requiring close supervision, a doctor must be summoned and the midwife's Supervising Authority informed.

316

PUERPERAL INFECTION

Sources of infection are:-

ENDOGENOUS – from organisms already in the genital tract;

AUTOGENOUS – from organisms elsewhere in the patient's body;

EXOGENOUS   – from attendants (hand, droplet infection), instruments, linen, lavatories, baths.

Overcrowding of puerperal wards and overworking of the attendants may lead to carelessness and oversight which can cause infection.

The vulva and perineum should be swabbed twice daily and after using a bedpan.   Ambulant patients may do this for themselves, or better still take 2 baths daily or use a bidet.   The patient sits astride the bidet and bathes her whole perineum.

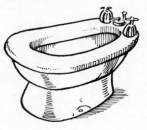

All pads, dressings and other waste must be disposed of rapidly, preferably in an incinerator. A central incinerator can be a fairly heavy furnace type of installation but individual ward incinerators allow immediate disposal of infective material and reduce the risk of cross-infection.

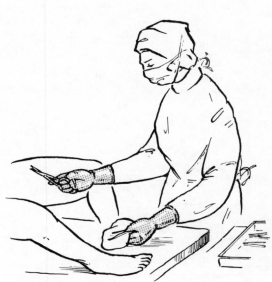

Treatment of the perineal area (swabbing, removing sutures) must be as aseptic a procedure as possible.   The nurse is gowned and masked, wears gloves and has a sterile tray of instruments.   The patient may also be masked if she has a respiratory infection; boils, paronychias, etc. must be covered with dressings.

PUERPERAL INFECTION—ENDOMETRITIS

The most common and usually mildest form of puerperal infection is ENDOMETRITIS.

4 Classical Signs:–

1. Pyrexia 100° – 102°F.
2. Pulse 100 – 120.
3. Fundal height not falling – poor involution.
4. Lochia remain red and have characteristic offensive smell.

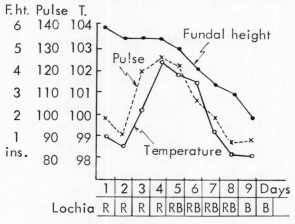

F.ht.	Pulse	T.										
6	140	104										
5	130	103										
4	120	102										
3	110	101										
2	100	100										
1	90	99										
ins.	80	98										

	1	2	3	4	5	6	7	8	9	Days
Lochia	R	R	R	R	RB	RB	RB	RB	B	B

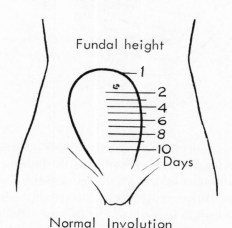

Fundal height

Normal Involution

Investigations. Because of the uncertainty in diagnosis and the need for expedition, a throat swab and MSSU are sent to the bacteriologist as well as vaginal and cervical smears. Intra-uterine smears which are more difficult to obtain are not in general use. (The uterine cavity may be normally colonised from the vagina by the 4th or 5th day.)

Treatment. A broad spectrum antibiotic is exhibited and changed to the drugs suggested by bacteriological sensitivity tests only if clinically unsuccessful. It should be maintained for at least 5 days.

Bacteriological evidence from the vagina and cervix is difficult to interpret unless there is a marked predominance of one organism.

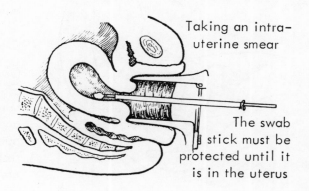

Taking an intra-uterine smear

The swab stick must be protected until it is in the uterus

PUERPERAL INFECTION—PARAMETRITIS
(syn. cellulitis)

Infection may spread from the uterus, from a cervical laceration, or even from thrombophlebitis or peritonitis into the loose areolar connective tissue, setting up a PARAMETRITIS. The infection may extend retroperitoneally in any direction, commonly between the leaves of the broad ligament, round the vagina or rectum, or even up to the loin. Sometimes infection spreads along the round ligament and might then point above the inguinal ligament, near the inguinal ring.

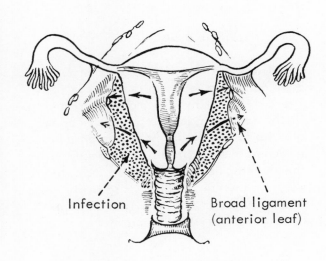

Infection   Broad ligament
                   (anterior leaf)

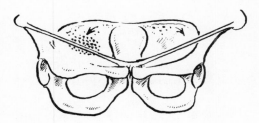

The condition occurs later than endometritis, usually in the second week and presents with fever and malaise. Pelvic examination reveals a large, often very hard mass and the lochia are red and heavy. Pain is less than might be expected.

Treatment: The appropriate antibiotic is given usually for 2 or more weeks, until the pelvis feels normal. If collections of pus appear they must be drained. A poor response to treatment calls for a search for spread: and the possibility of subphrenic abscess must be remembered.

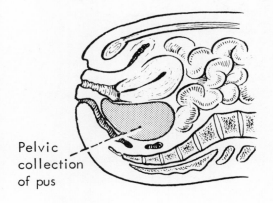

Pelvic
collection
of pus

319

PUERPERAL INFECTION—PERITONITIS AND SALPINGITIS

PERITONITIS and SALPINGITIS

These two conditions are almost indistinguishable and neither is common. The pelvic peritoneum may be involved in the same way as the parametrium and also be spread along the fallopian tubes. A generalised peritonitis may occur with the development of paralytic ileus; and very rarely the infection is so acute and fulminating that the condition of 'septic' or 'irreversible' shock is met with.

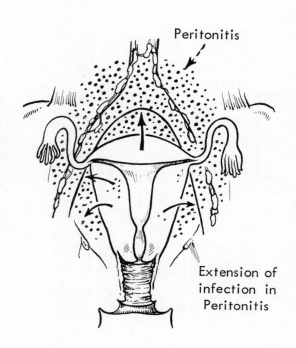

Peritonitis

Extension of infection in Peritonitis

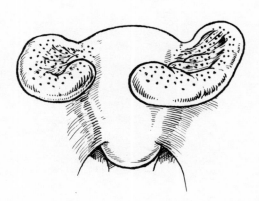

Acute Salpingitis.

Permanent blockage is unusual.

DIAGNOSIS and TREATMENT

In some cases it may be impossible to exclude acute appendicitis without an exploratory laparotomy; but otherwise treatment is along the same lines as described for parametritis. If laparotomy is carried out and only acute salpingitis found, the abdomen should be closed without drainage.

PUERPERAL INFECTION—THROMBOSIS

The anaerobic strepto-coccus has a predilection for veins and is the commonest infecting organism.

Common femoral vein

Deep femoral vein

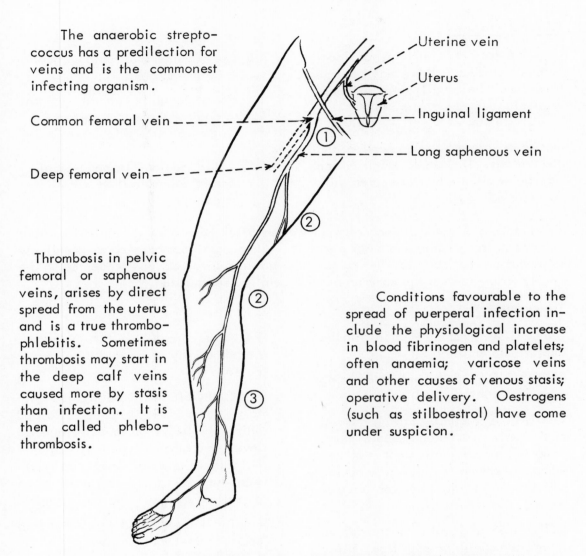

Uterine vein

Uterus

Inguinal ligament

Long saphenous vein

Thrombosis in pelvic femoral or saphenous veins, arises by direct spread from the uterus and is a true thrombo-phlebitis. Sometimes thrombosis may start in the deep calf veins caused more by stasis than infection. It is then called phlebo-thrombosis.

Conditions favourable to the spread of puerperal infection in-clude the physiological increase in blood fibrinogen and platelets; often anaemia; varicose veins and other causes of venous stasis; operative delivery. Oestrogens (such as stilboestrol) have come under suspicion.

In its mildest form thrombophlebitis is little more than inflammation of a super-ficial varix. At the other extreme is phlegmasia alba dolens, the classical 'white leg'. The leg is swollen, tender and cold, due to venous occlusion, lymphatic congestion and arterial spasm.

THROMBOPHLEBITIS

Clinical Features

The patient complains of local pain and stiffness. There may be some fever and the usual puerperal bacteriological smears must be taken.

There will be an area of tenderness over a vein, red, swollen and oedematous. The whole thigh or leg may be swollen when compared with its neighbour.

The examiner must palpate gently in the following areas:-

1. Femoral vein in femoral triangle.
2. Along the saphenous vein.
3. In the calf (for phlebothrombosis).

Ankle flexion (Homan's Sign) causes calf pain if thrombosis is present.

Phlebothrombosis is uncommon in women of childbearing age but is important because of the greater chance of embolism. Saphenous thrombophlebitis is unlikely to produce embolism unless the pelvic veins are also involved, and tenderness in the femoral triangle over the common femoral vein is a serious sign.

Treatment

INFECTION must be treated with the appropriate antibiotic.

TENDERNESS can be helped by using a cage to hold off the blankets.

OEDEMA is treated by raising the end of the bed to encourage venous return. After it has gone the patient is allowed up, wearing an elastic stocking which she should use for several months.

COLDNESS and PALLOR are due to interference with arterial flow, either because of congestion, or because of reflex arterial spasm. The leg should be allowed to remain cold at first to guard against gangrene.

PAIN is treated with analgesics. Morphine may be needed in the acute phase.

THROMBOSIS must be treated with large doses of heparin (up to 20,000 units, 8-hourly) while a therapeutic level of coumarin-type anticoagulant is building up. Anticoagulant treatment may have to be continued (as an outpatient) for as long as 6 months.

Physiotherapy should begin when pain and tenderness are abolished.

The practice of paravertebral sympathetic block is needed only if there is anxiety about distal blood supply.

THROMBOPHLEBITIS

Mild cases may respond to rest and an antibiotic: but usually a course of anticoagulant treatment is required. It should be maintained for at least 10 days at thrombotest level of 20% and heparin is used for the first few days to relieve discomfort and prevent further clot formation until a therapeutic anticoagulant effect is achieved.

Estimation of clotting factors should be carried out before treatment is begun.

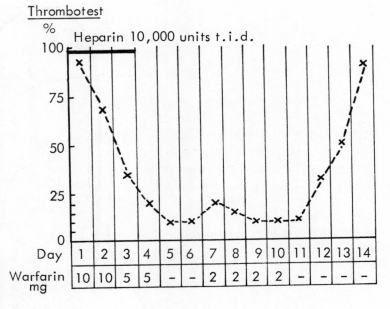

Thrombotest

Day	1	2	3	4	5	6	7	8	9	10	11	12	13	14
Warfarin mg	10	10	5	5	–	–	2	2	2	2	–	–	–	–

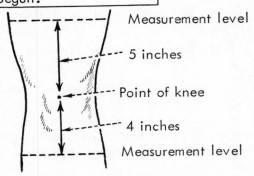

Measurement level

5 inches

Point of knee

4 inches

Measurement level

Reduction in swelling can be recorded by daily measuring at the same levels in thigh and calf. The levels at which measurements are made can be marked with indelible ink.

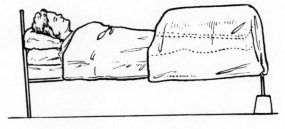

Venous flow should be assisted by raising the end of the bed. The patient should move her leg freely if it is not painful to do so and a leg cage should be used to encourage this. Local treatment should be restricted to kaolin poultices during the acute phase.

323

SYSTEMIC SPREAD OF THROMBOSIS

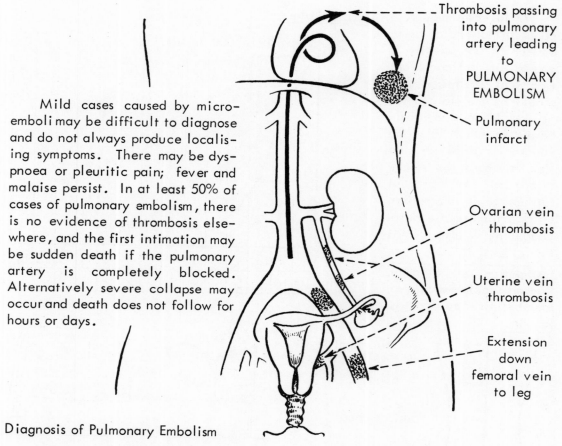

Thrombosis passing into pulmonary artery leading to **PULMONARY EMBOLISM**

Pulmonary infarct

Ovarian vein thrombosis

Uterine vein thrombosis

Extension down femoral vein to leg

Mild cases caused by micro-emboli may be difficult to diagnose and do not always produce localising symptoms. There may be dyspnoea or pleuritic pain; fever and malaise persist. In at least 50% of cases of pulmonary embolism, there is no evidence of thrombosis elsewhere, and the first intimation may be sudden death if the pulmonary artery is completely blocked. Alternatively severe collapse may occur and death does not follow for hours or days.

Diagnosis of Pulmonary Embolism

There is extreme dyspnoea, cyanosis and neck vein distension, passing into coma and death or severe shock. The differential diagnosis includes cardiac infarction and septic shock (page 330). If the patient is fit enough, some investigations may be carried out. X-rays may show dilated hilar arteries and dilatation of the right side of the heart, and the ECG may give information. Other diagnostic procedures include catheterisation of both sides of the heart to check the difference in pressure, scanning of the lungs after the injection of radio-active albumin to detect areas of ischaemia, and pulmonary angiography; but these would be undertaken in a special surgical unit.

PULMONARY EMBOLISM

Treatment of Pulmonary Embolism

This is still not clearly understood. Severe shock is treated along the lines suggested for septic shock (page 330) and heparinisation is started at once. Some patients will recover without further treatment but, in cases of massive embolism, the thrombus must be surgically removed or possibly broken down by streptokinase. The advice of a surgeon experienced in cardiovascular work must be obtained and the patient may be transferred to a special centre where modern techniques such as hypothermia and cardiopulmonary by-pass have improved the results of surgical intervention. Ligation of the inferior vena cava to prevent further embolism is only carried out if thrombotic emboli continue to form in spite of anticoagulants. It is a simple operation but has much morbidity in the form of oedema, ulcers, varices, and arteriospasm.

STREPTOKINASE INFUSION. This is dangerous but can be effective. Streptokinase is an enzyme cultivated from a strain of haemolytic streptococcus which activates plasma plasminogen to form the fibrinolytic enzyme plasmin. Antibodies to streptokinase are always present in human blood and must be neutralised before an effect is achieved.

If laboratory control is not at once available, and the patient's condition is serious, an initial dose of 1,250,000 units may be given, followed by 100,000 units four-hourly for 3 days. The services of a coagulation expert should be obtained as soon as possible. Anticoagulants are not given during streptokinase treatment, but must be started as soon as the streptokinase is stopped. (Fibrin must be allowed to develop when the plasmin level is being increased).

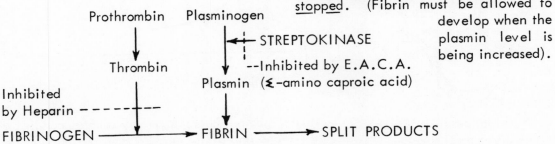

Side effects include fever (for which steroids should be given) and the risk of a serious coagulation defect. Streptokinase has a limited life and is very expensive; nevertheless it can achieve the breaking up of thrombotic emboli and its use may be justifiable.

ENGORGEMENT OF THE BREASTS

As the circulating oestrogens fall the anterior pituitary output of prolactin rises. If milk secretion outstrips milk removal (as with a weak or lethargic baby) the breasts become overfull, the venous and lymphatic drainage is obstructed and the breasts become oedematous, swollen, painful and too tender even to allow expression of milk. Engorgement may also be due to blocking of the ducts with inspissated colostrum or sebaceous matter during the antenatal period.   The treatment is to REST the breasts, SUPPORT them with a brassière or binding, give STILBOESTROL 15 mg thrice daily for at least 24 hours, and EXPRESS the milk as soon as tenderness is relieved.

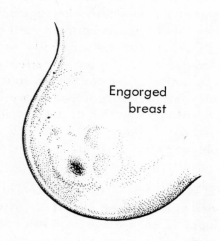

Engorged breast

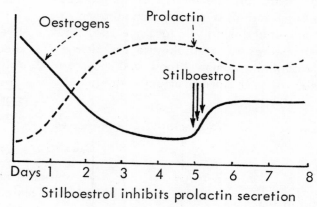

Stilboestrol inhibits prolactin secretion

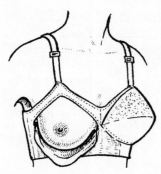

Nursing brassière which gives good support.

Engorgement is an extremely painful condition and analgesics may be required. Reduction in fluid intake, or the administration of diuretics may have a marginal effect but the depression of lactation by stilboestrol is the most important step.

BREAST INFECTION

Mastitis is a disease of lactation.

Infection (nearly always staph. aureus) enters through a cracked and abraded nipple, and sets up a local inflammation of parenchyma and interstitial tissue, which proceeds to abscess formation.

The presenting symptom is usually pyrexia. Then a painful area is felt and a 'flush' appears on the breast, usually radial in outline, red and tender but not fluctuant or swollen. At this stage an antibiotic should be given empirically (cloxacillin is a good choice as the organism is probably a penicillin-resistant staphylococcus), the breast is supported and stilboestrol given to suppress lactation temporarily or permanently. In many cases the infection will now subside.

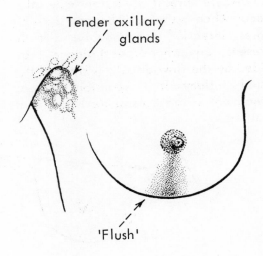

Tender axillary glands

'Flush'

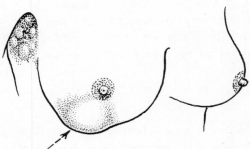

Painful, swollen area

The next stage is overt inflammation – a brawny swollen, painful breast which probably contains pus although not yet fluctuant. If deffinitely not ready for incision, a kaolin poultice or other source of heat may be applied for a day; but it is better to incise early than late. Lactation must be suppressed at this stage.

BREAST INFECTION

Under general anaethesia, a radial incision is made and all pockets of pus broken down. A drain must be left in for 3 days, stilboestrol is continued, and pus sent for culture and antibiotic sensitivity.

Acute breast infection may also occur when weaning is begun. In such cases infection is probably already present, and when the drainage provided by the flow of milk is stopped the usual inflammatory reaction occurs. Treatment is the same as for lactational mastitis.

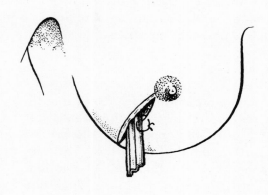

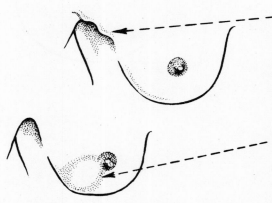

There is occasionally an extension of mammary tissue into the axillary tail, which becomes swollen and painful during lactation. It should soon regress but sometimes discomfort is so great that lactation has to be suppressed.

Galactocoele. This is an accumulation in a lobe of the breast whose duct is blocked by inspissated secretions. It is usually absorbed and should be left alone unless discomfort is severe.

(These two conditions must be distinguished from inflammation).

The lactating woman's chance of developing a breast infection is much reduced if she is properly instructed in the care of the breasts and nipples during the pregnancy and if engorgement is avoided in the early puerperium. If the patient has decided against breast feeding, lactation should be suppressed from the start.

PUERPERAL URINARY INFECTION

The puerperal woman is able to hold large amounts of urine in her bladder without feeling the need to empty it. The bladder tends to be atonic at this stage and particularly after a long labour.

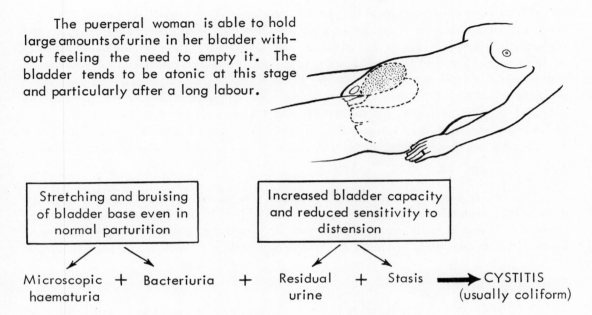

Stretching and bruising of bladder base even in normal parturition	Increased bladder capacity and reduced sensitivity to distension

Microscopic haematuria + Bacteriuria + Residual urine + Stasis ➡ CYSTITIS (usually coliform)

CLINICAL FEATURES

Low grade pyrexia. Dysuria (not always). Urine may have an offensive smell. Frequency of micturition. Loin pain and lower abdominal pain.

If there has been a urinary tract infection during the pregnancy, there is often an early recurrence post partum.

TREATMENT

Mid-stream specimen of urine (MSSU); also cervical and vaginal smears. A 'holding' antibiotic, e.g. nitrofurantoin 100 mg four times per day. Change later to the antibiotic indicated by the bacteriologist.

Encourage the patient to drink.

Micturition should be encouraged in the early puerperium. The kidney is not usually affected, unless there is an underlying pyelonephritis acquired earlier in the pregnancy.

SEPTIC SHOCK (Irreversible, Stagnant Shock)

This is due to the endotoxins of Gram-negative bacteria or to the exotoxins of Gram-positive bacteria. An anaphylactic basis has been postulated in which the pregnancy itself is assumed to 'prepare' the woman for the 'provocative' dose of toxin; but an identical type of shock may follow prolonged haemorrhage, pulmonary or coronary embolism, and also severe burns. The toxin produces by its sympatho-mimetic effect an intense vasoconstriction of the skin and viscera but not the cerebral or coronary vessels, an action which is of course temporarily effective in maintaining central venous pressure. However unless the vasoconstriction is relaxed the circulation becomes stagnant and septic shock appears, terminating in death.

Clinical Appearances

The patient is conscious, pale, anxious and sweating, with cold extremities, generalised abdominal pain and rigidity (peritonitis). There may be diarrhoea and vomiting. Pulse is rapid and thready, and blood pressure unrecordable. There may be a high temperature. Urinary excretion is scanty and likely to be blood stained.

Treatment

1. An intravenous catheter should be inserted into the saphenous vein in the leg, as a route for treatment. The bacteriologist must be given blood cultures and urine, and smears from throat, vagina and cervix.
2. Massive doses of broad spectrum antibiotics should be given at once: say, ampicillin 500 mg four-hourly supported by cephaloridine 500 mg eight-hourly.
3. The blood gases and pH must be monitored and metabolic acidosis corrected. Oxygen should be given continuously by face mask.
4. Prophylactic digitalisation with intravenous digoxin is advisable.

Suggested Mechanism of Shock

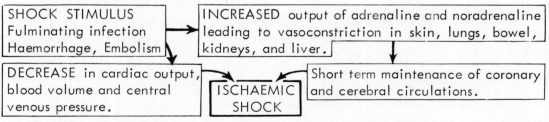

This may be reversible if blood volume is promptly expanded.

SEPTIC SHOCK

If the ischaemic shock is not reversed the patient passes on to the state of irreversible shock.

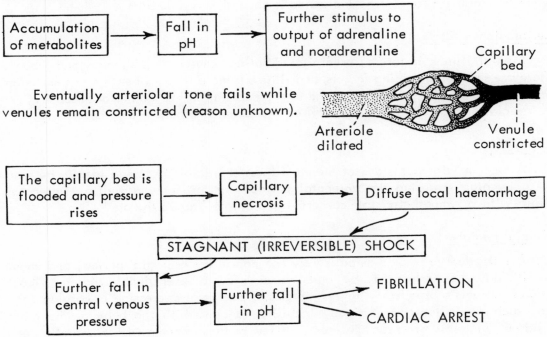

Accumulation of metabolites → Fall in pH → Further stimulus to output of adrenaline and noradrenaline

Eventually arteriolar tone fails while venules remain constricted (reason unknown).

Capillary bed

Arteriole dilated

Venule constricted

The capillary bed is flooded and pressure rises → Capillary necrosis → Diffuse local haemorrhage

STAGNANT (IRREVERSIBLE) SHOCK

Further fall in central venous pressure → Further fall in pH → FIBRILLATION / CARDIAC ARREST

The patient is now plainly moribund, passing into a state of mental confusion and eventually to coma. Because of the capillary haemorrhage the face and other parts of the body may become a dusky purplish colour, and epigastric pain may be complained of as the liver becomes oedematous and swollen.

The vasoconstriction must be overcome and the blood volume restored to a normal amount by transfusion of blood or plasma or plasma substitutes. Steroids have a vasodilating effect and probably protect the tissues against the toxin. A large dose, say 2 g of hydrocortisone should be given intravenously and repeated in 2 hours. If this is ineffective, a specific vasodilator such as phenoxybenzamine 5 mg or methyldopa 250 mg or guanethidine 10 mg should be given. It follows from this, that vasoconstrictor drugs such as noradrenaline and metaraminol should not be given to patients suffering from shock.

MENTAL ILLNESS IN THE PUERPERIUM

Depression is the commonest disturbance followed by schizophrenia. Mania is rare, and delirious states due to toxic exhaustion have almost disappeared as obtetric standards improve. The incidence is about 1 in 1,000 births.

Aetiological Factors

Mental illness is latent, precipitated but not caused by pregnancy and labour. There are some predisposing factors, and illness is more likely when the patient is an obsessional neurotic, or immature and overdependent on her mother or husband.

Social or marital stress - poverty, an inadequate husband - may contribute.

Prophylaxis

A woman with a history of mental illness or instability should ideally be seen by a psychiatrist during the antenatal period. In addition, a well run antenatal clinic with a sympathetic staff can provide a helpful 'group therapy'.

Clincial Features

A mild degree of depression is very common in the postnatal period, and about the 4th day the mother may be found weeping for no ascertainable reason. About 10% of patients subsequently have symptoms of puerperal depression in varying degrees such as irritability, fatigue, inability to cope with the baby or the other children, and loss of sexual interest. A few of these women will eventually need psychiatric treatment.

Acute Mental Illness

There is usually a latent period of about 2 days following confinement, and the first divergence from normal behaviour will be observed by the nursing staff. There may be confusion and disorientation in time and place: delusions ('The nurses are trying to poison me'); or an aversion to the baby.

Unless the patient is unmanageable (abusive, dirty, offensive to the other patients) she is better nursed in a single room in the obstetric unit in the first instance, in charge of a psychiatrist. Severe depression and attempts at suicide or infanticide must be guarded against, and the room should be on the ground floor. She should be given the baby, unless she is incapable of being trusted with it.

Sedatives and tranquillizing drugs will be prescribed, but if there is no improvement within a week, the patient is better transferred to a psychiatric unit.

CHAPTER 15

THE NEWBORN BABY

THE NEWBORN BABY

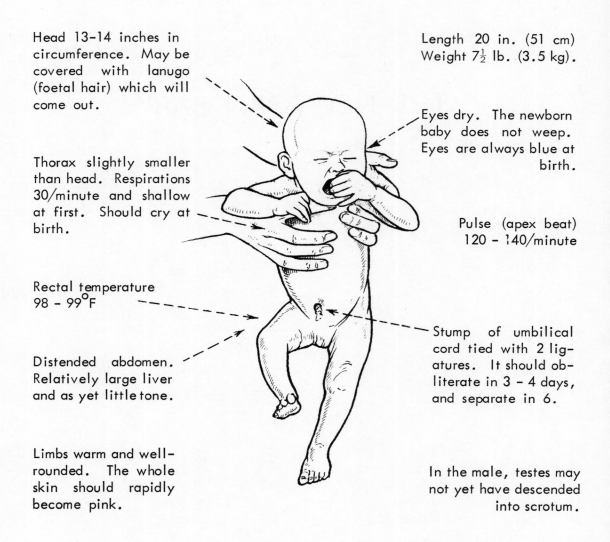

Head 13-14 inches in circumference. May be covered with lanugo (foetal hair) which will come out.

Thorax slightly smaller than head. Respirations 30/minute and shallow at first. Should cry at birth.

Rectal temperature 98 - 99°F

Distended abdomen. Relatively large liver and as yet little tone.

Limbs warm and well-rounded. The whole skin should rapidly become pink.

Length 20 in. (51 cm)
Weight 7½ lb. (3.5 kg).

Eyes dry. The newborn baby does not weep. Eyes are always blue at birth.

Pulse (apex beat) 120 - 140/minute

Stump of umbilical cord tied with 2 ligatures. It should obliterate in 3 - 4 days, and separate in 6.

In the male, testes may not yet have descended into scrotum.

The baby is covered in utero with a sebaceous secretion called 'vernix caseosa' (L., a cheese-like coating). This protects the skin against maceration while in the liquor amnii.

MANAGEMENT OF THE NEWBORN BABY

WIPING the EYES

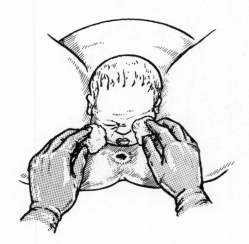

The eyes are swabbed with sterile cotton wool to remove any infective secretion (such as the gonococcus). The baby's lacrimal glands do not function and there is no antiseptic protection from tears. In some countries there may be a legal obligation to instil an antibiotic such as sulphacetamide or an antiseptic such as silver protein eye drops.

The cord is clamped and divided as soon as pulsations have ceased.

CLAMPING and LIGATING the CORD

No cord dressing is necessary. If ligation is done carelessly the baby may lose a great deal of blood in a very short time.

All clamps or ligatures should be at least 2 inches away from the umbilicus. This excludes the chance of clamping extruded bowel (e.g. Meckel's diverticulum) and keeps foreign bodies away from direct contact with the umbilicus.

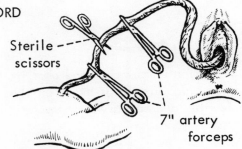

Sterile scissors

7" artery forceps

It is then ligated with 2 linen ligatures or a special clamp.

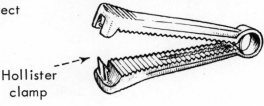

Hollister clamp

MANAGEMENT OF THE NEWBORN BABY

All mucus, blood and meconium must be sucked out before the infant has a chance to inhale it. Simple mouth suction can be used as shown here. A more effective method is the use of a hand sucker.

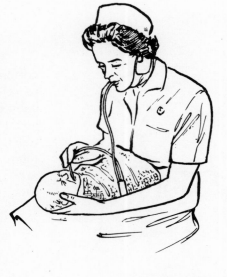

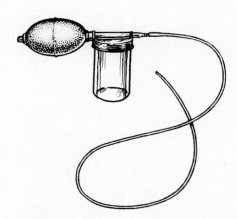

Suction is for mouth and pharynx only. No attempt is made by the midwife to clear larynx or trachea.

In hospitals a Venturi suction pump (connected to the oxygen supply) may be available and is the most convenient to use.

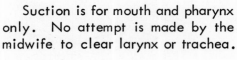

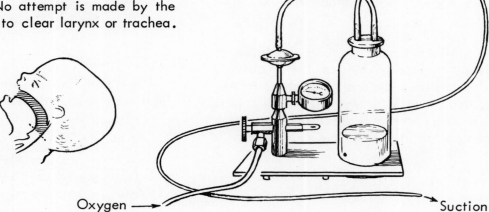

Oxygen →   → Suction

INSPECTION FOR CONGENITAL DEFECTS

Certain of the commoner defects should be noted at birth.

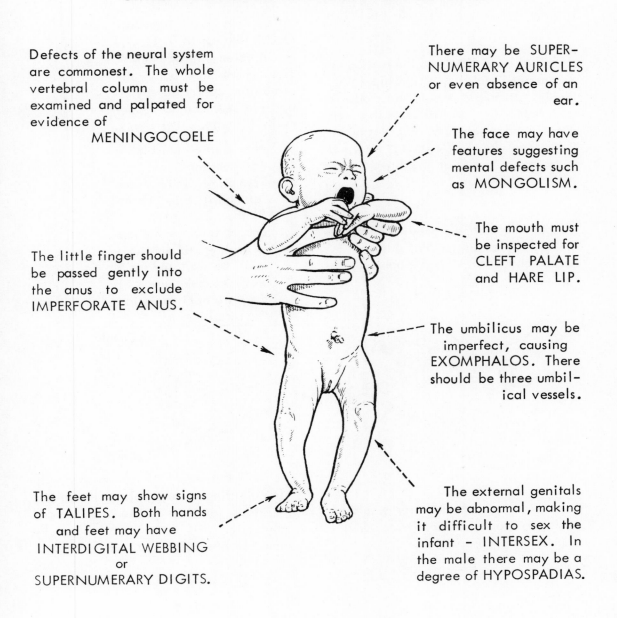

Defects of the neural system are commonest. The whole vertebral column must be examined and palpated for evidence of MENINGOCOELE

There may be SUPER-NUMERARY AURICLES or even absence of an ear.

The face may have features suggesting mental defects such as MONGOLISM.

The mouth must be inspected for CLEFT PALATE and HARE LIP.

The little finger should be passed gently into the anus to exclude IMPERFORATE ANUS.

The umbilicus may be imperfect, causing EXOMPHALOS. There should be three umbilical vessels.

The feet may show signs of TALIPES. Both hands and feet may have INTERDIGITAL WEBBING or SUPERNUMERARY DIGITS.

The external genitals may be abnormal, making it difficult to sex the infant - INTERSEX. In the male there may be a degree of HYPOSPADIAS.

ROUTINE PROTECTIVE TESTS

Tests for detecting CONGENITAL DISLOCATION of the HIP (CDH)

The term CDH includes various degrees of instability of the hip-joint. Ideally diagnosis should be made in the first week of life for the best outcome of treatment; but X-rays at this stage are difficult to interpret because so much of the hip-joint is still cartilaginous.

In the normal baby the flexed hip-joints should be capable of 90 degree abduction with the baby supine.

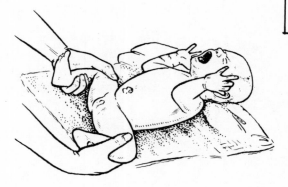

Limitation of abduction would be an indication for continued investigation and observation.

B.C.G. VACCINATION

0.1 ml. of Bacillus-Calmette-Guerin (B.C.G.) is injected intradermally. This gives the baby the immunity conferred by a positive reaction to tuberculin ('Mantoux Positive').

1. The mother must give her consent.
2. Premature babies are left until they reach $5\frac{1}{2}$ lb. (2.5 kg).
3. Babies born to mothers with open tuberculosis must be isolated for 6 weeks to make sure that they are not incubating the disease.

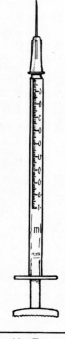

Ortolani's Test

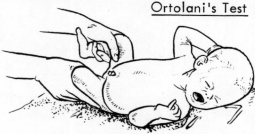

The flexed legs are grasped with the forefingers lying along the thigh. If the joint is dislocated forced abduction will cause a 'click' as the femoral head slips into articulation.

338

ROUTINE PROTECTIVE TESTS

Inborn Errors of Metabolism

This covers a group of rare diseases in which the basis is congenital deficiency of an enzyme controlling a metabolic step. Metabolism of proteins, carbohydrates, fats, purines can be affected.

The one at present most susceptible to early diagnosis is PHENYLKETONURIA (PKU) in which there is deficiency of phenylalanine hydroxylase, which converts phenylalanine to tyrosine. Progressive failure of mental development is the most important feature, and diagnosis is made by finding high blood phenylalanine levels (Guthrie Test) or phenylpyruvic acid in urine.

The GUTHRIE Test will demonstrate abnormal blood levels of phenylalanine.

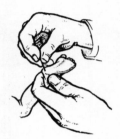

| Patient's Name .... |
| Ward .... |
| Date........................ |
| Date first feeding.............. |
| Bottle ☐   Breast ☐   Both ☐ |
| FILL ALL CIRCLES WITH BLOOD |
| ◯ ◯ ◯ ◯ |

The discs of filter paper are impregnated with blood taken from a heel stab.

The disc is placed on a culture of B. subtilis in which there is a special growth inhibitor. If phenylalanine is present in abnormal concentration the inhibitor is neutralised and growth of B. subtilis occurs.

URINE Test for PKU
('Phenistix' reagent strips)

The strip is impregnated with chemicals including ferric ammonium sulphate. Ferric ions at correct pH react with phenylketones to produce a greyish green colour.

The test end of the strip is pressed against a freshly wet napkin. A reading is taken after 30 seconds.

Phenylalanine levels are normal at birth and any rise depends on protein intake. Both these tests are useless before milk feeding is established.

NURSING CARE

The ideal cot for the newborn should be draughtproof and easily cleaned. It should be possible to raise and lower the head and there should be a box for the toilet materials provided separately for each baby.

The baby is wiped down and dried, dressed in nightgown and napkin, and placed in a cot in a room temperature between 65 – 70 degrees F.

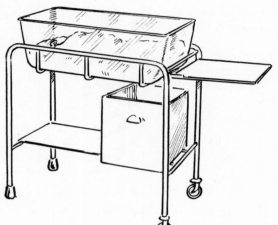

Rigid cots of metal or plastic are easily cleaned, but expensive. Canvas cots are cheap, but must be laundered.

The principal underlying all methods of nursing of the newborn is the avoidance of infection. A baby needs as much space as an adult, and overcrowding is bad. In the 'rooming-in' system, all changing and cleaning is done beside the mother and usually by the mother, the baby lives with her and is colonised by her organisms to which it should have some degree of immunity. Alternatively she sees the baby only for feeding and all nursing is undertaken away from the mother in circumstances allowing maximum precautions against infection.

Single rooms for mother and baby avoid the risks of mixed bacterial flora and cross-infection. They are also more restful – one crying baby does not disturb the others – but single room hospitals are expensive and require bigger staffs. The patients also need a day-room if loneliness is to be avoided. Many women like the company afforded by three and four bedded wards.

BREAST FEEDING

The first feed is usually sterile water. This makes certain of the baby's capacity to feed normally; and if regurgitation or inhalation occurs water is less damaging than milk or glucose.

The baby should be put to the breast within 12 hours of birth. The mother must be comfortable and be able to hold the baby in such a way that both are relaxed and at ease.

These preparations help to establish the milk ejection response.

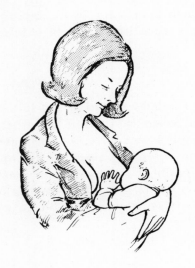

The baby may have to be taught to 'fix', i.e. to take a good grip of the nipple.

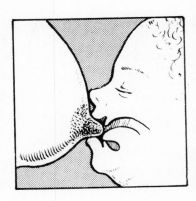

The baby feels the nipple at its lips.

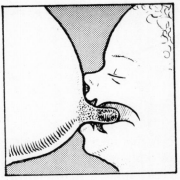

The nipple is 'fixed' – sucked into the mouth.

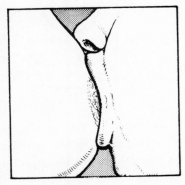

The baby's lips are in contact with the areola.

BREAST FEEDING

Once established on the breast, the baby requires about 20 oz. of milk a day and should get this in 6 feeds, taking 10 minutes at each breast, with a short rest in between to bring up swallowed air.   After the initial loss (before lactation is completely established) weight gain should be about 1 oz. (30 g) per day.

The baby should be put to the breast when it wants it and when the mother has milk, but complete 'demand' feeding is neither natural nor feasible: the ewe sometimes refuses the lamb.   An attempt at a 4-hourly schedule should be made.

Baby's Weight Chart in first 10 days

Days

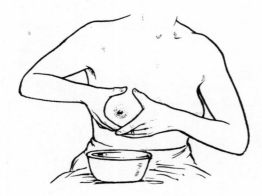
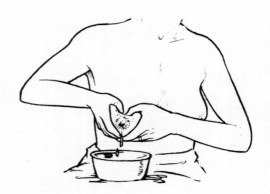

The fluctuating oestrogen levels also affect the supply of milk. The 'first flush' in the 4th to 5th days produces a plentiful supply which may then go away for a day or two before returning in abundance.   This variation (and variation in baby's appetite) may leave the breast still with milk at the end of a feed and it is important to empty it by hand or with a pump if lactation is to be maintained and engorgement avoided.

342

BREAST FEEDING

Another method of expressing milk is by means of the manual breast pump or 'breast reliever'. This is simple and easy to use but, if the breast is at all tender, its sustained suction can cause pain.

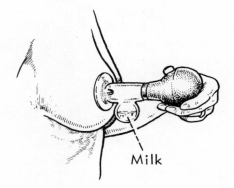

Milk

The Humalactor is a mechanical breast milker, driven by an electric motor, which produces a gentle, interrupted suction simulating closely the sensation of normal suckling.

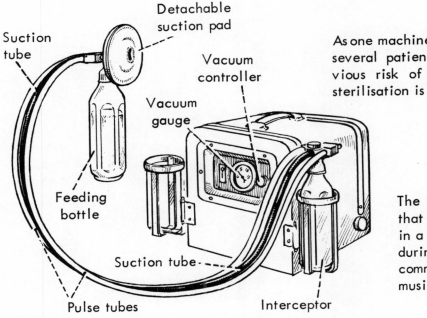

As one machine would be used by several patients there is an obvious risk of cross-infection if sterilisation is imperfect.

The makers emphasize that the mother must be in a state of relaxation during use. They recommend the use of soft music to achieve this.

ARTIFICIAL FEEDING

Artificial feeding is by cow's milk, usually made up from dried or evaporated concentrates. Cow's milk has three times as much protein as breast milk, but much less carbohydrate. Because of this, sugar is often added.

	Human milk	Cow's milk
Protein	1.0%	3.5%
Fat	3.5	3.5
CHO	7.0	4.5

Feeds are given every 4 hours, thus:-
  10 a.m. (10.00 hours)
  2 p.m. (14.00 hours)
  6 p.m. (18.00 hours)
  10 p.m. (22.00 hours)
  2 a.m. (02.00 hours)
  6 a.m. (06.00 hours)
(To allow the mother an undisturbed night, the 2 a.m. feed is omitted if the baby will 'allow' it).

Amounts are calculated on a basis of $2\frac{1}{2}$ oz. per lb. bodyweight (140 g per kilo) in 24 hours. Thus a 7 lb. baby will get 5 feeds of $3\frac{1}{2}$ oz. (90 g).

If the baby is hungry a teaspoonful of sugar may be added to the feed. A drink of boiled water may be given between feeds: or the feed may be increased. A fractious baby may be fed more or less on demand.

HOW TO MAKE UP A FEED
(This is a STERILE procedure)

1. Count out the required number of measures of dried milk into a sterile jug.

2. Add an equivalent number of ounces of boiling water.

3. Add sugar as required, pour into sterile bottle and fix on sterile teat.

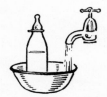

Cool the milk in cold water and ...

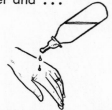

... test its temperature on the back of the hand. It should be at body heat.

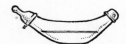

The old fashioned 2-teat bottle had the merit of allowing air to enter or escape as the feed was taken: but contamination was more likely to occur.

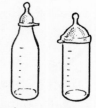

Bottles used to-day

ARTIFICIAL FEEDING

After each feed all utensils must be cleaned and sterilized either by boiling or storing in antiseptic.

CLEANING

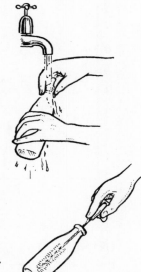

1. Rinse bottle and teat under cold tap, inside and out.

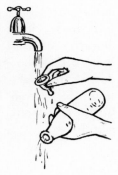

2. Clean teat inside and out, rub with salt to remove slime and rinse well.

3. Clean bottle with hot water and detergent. Use a brush, which must be boiled daily.

BOILING METHOD
Boil bottle and teat for 5 minutes in a pan big enough to cover them with water. Leave in pan, with lid on.

STERILIZATION

ANTISEPTIC METHOD (after cleaning)

(Hypochlorite is tasteless and harmless to the baby, e.g. 'Milton', 'Nobactin', 'Nursery Hysan').

1. Make up, every day, a supply of the antiseptic as instructed. Immerse bottle and teat, making sure bottle is full, and leave for at least 3 hours.

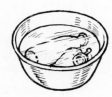

2. When feed is due, remove bottle and teat and pour in feed WITHOUT RINSING. Place cap on teat until ready to feed.

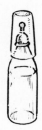

PHYSIOLOGY OF THE NEWBORN BABY

PHYSIOLOGICAL JAUNDICE occurs in about one third of normal babies between the 2nd and 5th days. It is due to the immaturity of the liver cells and the hyperbilirubinaemia caused by destruction of red cells. (Hb. level falls from 20 g per cent at birth to about 11 g by third month).

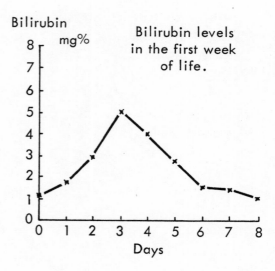

Bilirubin mg%

Bilirubin levels in the first week of life.

Days

STOOLS. Meconium – mainly cast-off cells, mucus, and bile pigment – is passed for the first 2 – 3 days. The bowel is sterile at birth but is colonised by bacteria within a few hours. Formed stools appear on the 5th day, usually light yellow in colour, with the odour of faeces. Breast-fed babies pass less faeces than bottle-fed ones.

URINE   The foetus drinks liquor and the kidneys excrete in utero.   Urine should be passed within a few hours of birth.

The passage of urine and faeces must be recorded – they are evidence of normal function.

RESPIRATORY SYSTEM. Complete expansion of the lungs is not achieved until about a week, and is helped by crying. The rate is about 30/minute; and there may be much irregularity.

The foetal lungs are airless and filled with blood, which becomes fully oxygenated with the first few cries.

GENITAL SYSTEM. Manifestations of oestrogen withdrawal may occur, known as the 'genital crisis' (consequent on cessation of placental circulation). There is sometimes swelling of the breasts and even a little colostrum secretion ("witches' milk"). The female may bleed a little from the vagina and the male may develop a transient hydrocele.   No treatment is required.

PHYSIOLOGY OF THE NEWBORN BABY

With the first breath the lungs expand and the pulmonary vessels increase in size. The DUCTUS ARTERIOSUS, which has a very muscular coat, actively contracts and diverts all the blood from the right ventricle to the pulmonary arteries. This will increase the left atrial pressure while the right atrial pressure is reduced by cessation of placental flow. Blood now tends to flow from left to right through the FORAMEN OVALE and this will cause its closure.

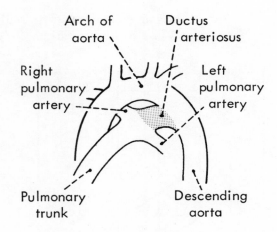

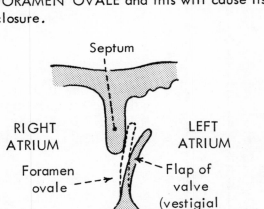

The DUCTUS ARTERIOSUS closes functionally almost at once and is obliterated by the 6th week. The FORAMEN OVALE closes gradually and may take months, but is functionally closed once the left atrial pressure is greater than the right.

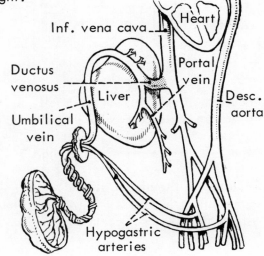

With the clamping of the cord the UMBILICAL ARTERIES are thrombosed and persist as the obliterated hypogastric arteries. The UMBILICAL VEIN obliterates by the 4 – 6th day and persists as the ligamentum teres of the liver. The DUCTUS VENOSUS obliterates a little later and persists as the ligamentum venosum.

CHARTED OBSERVATIONS

Baby charts must be kept in meticulous detail. An ill baby usually shows signs at once, always by failure to gain weight. A baby's condition can deteriorate very quickly.

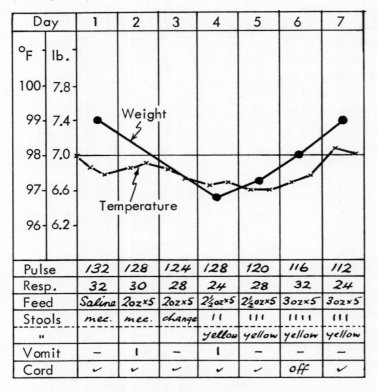

Day	1	2	3	4	5	6	7
Pulse	132	128	124	128	120	116	112
Resp.	32	30	28	24	28	32	24
Feed	Saline	2oz×5	2oz×5	2½oz×5	2½oz×5	3oz×5	3oz×5
Stools	mec.	mec.	change	ΙΙ	ΙΙΙ	ΙΙΙΙ	ΙΙΙ
"				yellow	yellow	yellow	yellow
Vomit	—	Ι	—	Ι	—	—	—
Cord	✓	✓	✓	✓	✓	off	✓

WEIGHT usually falls in first 3 – 4 days, even with artificial feeding. Birthweight should be regained in a week.

TEMPERATURE about 98 degrees F. but some instability is usual in the first week.

PULSE is taken by auscultating the apex beat. It is much faster than in the adult but should be regular.

RESPIRATION about 30 per minute at first and becoming slower. Irregularity is common in the first week.

VOMIT. Regurgitation should be noted if it occurs. It may cause respiratory infection, or be a sign of congenital abnormality, or of infection already present.

FEEDS. The first feed is usually boiled water or saline, in case the baby should inhale some fluid because of a congenital defect. (See Breast Feeding, page 341; Artificial Feeding, page 344.)

STOOLS. Meconium should give way to normal, formed stools by the 4th day. They should be yellow with a faecal odour, and are less frequent in breast fed babies.

348

ASPHYXIA

ASPHYXIA NEONATORUM

By this is meant failure of the newborn to establish spontaneous respiration. (Gr. Asphyxia = pulselessness: apnoea is a more accurate term.)

The initiation of respiration in the newborn depends on many stimuli including those received by the cutaneous nerves; and the high blood pCO_2 and low pO_2. A relatively high negative pressure is required to overcome the lung resistance to expansion, but lung compliance increases thereafter and progressively less effort is needed. The first breath is all important, and if respiration does not occur within one minute of delivery, a state of asphyxia may be said to exist.

CAUSES of Asphyxia

Antenatal: Any condition leading to placental insufficiency and foetal anoxia such as pre-eclamptic toxaemia, and accidental haemorrhage.

Natal: Foetal shock due to difficult delivery. Haemorrhage. Intracranial trauma. Cord accidents. Drugs and difficult anaesthesia.

Postnatal: Prematurity. (Immature respiratory centre. Immature alveolar system.)

Inhalation of blood, mucus or other foreign material.
Congenital abnormalities such as diaphragmatic hernia.

Two kinds of asphyxia are described:-

ASPHYXIA LIVIDA

General dusky cyanosis. Good muscle tone, strong but slow heart beat. Efforts at respiration are made and gasping occurs which should clear the cyanosis.

ASPHYXIA PALLIDA (foetal shock)

Skin is pallid and cold, lips cyanotic, no peripheral circulation, no muscle tone, heart beat weak and slow. Occasional shallow gasps which become less and less frequent.

Asphyxia livida may pass into pallida, or the baby may be born in a state of asphyxia pallida. A more flexible method of evaluating the condition of the newborn is the Apgar scoring system (see page 365).

ASPHYXIA

TREATMENT of Asphyxia Neonatorum

Every baby should have its mouth, pharynx and nostrils cleared by suction. (Page 336)

Every baby must be kept warm and handled gently. Babies should never be slapped or squeezed in an effort to stimulate respiration.

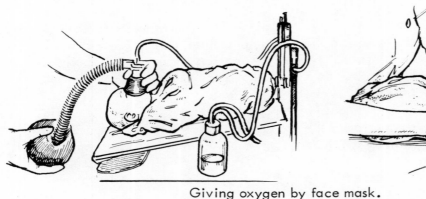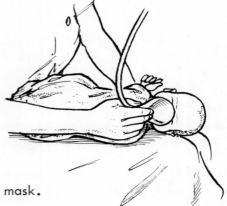

Giving oxygen by face mask.

TREATMENT of Asphyxia Livida

If no respiration has begun by one minute, oxygen should be given by face mask. The baby's head is kept lower than its heart either on a nurse's knee or on a resuscitation table. Note a warm towel to keep the baby from chilling. The oxygen pressure should be atmospheric and the mask must not be held so tightly on the baby's face as to exclude air.

DRUGS

Analeptic drugs are used much less than in former days. Lobeline, nikethamide (Coramine) and vanillic acid diethylamide (Vandid) all stimulate respiration, but have a narrow safety margin, and overdosage causes convulsions. They are useless in severe asphyxia.

If the respiratory depression is thought to be due to morphine or pethidine recently given to the mother, there is a specific antidote in nalorphine hydrobromide (Lethidrone) given in doses of 0.5 mg by injection into the umbilical vein.

ASPHYXIA

TREATMENT of Asphyxia Pallida

If this develops (or if the baby is born in this condition) oxygen must be given by positive pressure. Every obstetrician should know how to pass an endotracheal catheter in a newborn baby.

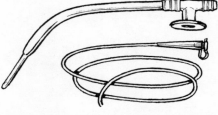

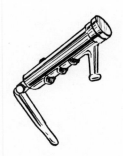

A straight-bladed laryngoscope is the most convenient.

A special endotracheal catheter is used, with shoulders near the tip to prevent its being inserted too far. The mucus aspirator also shown is small enough to pass through the catheter.

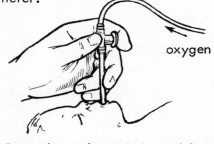

oxygen

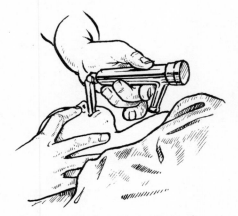

The neonatal larynx lies opposite C.3 and 4. The tip of the laryngoscope catches the epiglottis and pulls it forward to allow clear view of the vocal cords.

Once the catheter is in position and connected to the oxygen supply, the pressure is regulated by the finger on the escape hole of the catheter. It must not exceed 30 cm of water; and on modern resuscitation tables a water manometer is incorporated in the oxygen circuit, and 'blows off' above this pressure.

ASPHYXIA

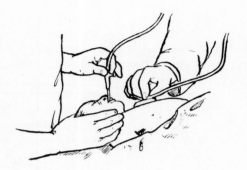

The first sign of recovery is a quickening and strengthing of the foetal heart, then colour improves and attempts at respiration are made. The baby is then placed in a warm, oxygen-filled cot and transferred to the nursery.

It may be necessary to employ positive pressure oxygen for up to an hour before spontaneous respiration begins, or death is recognised as inevitable. Even though some cause such as severe intra-cranial haemorrhage is suspected, attempts at resuscitation must be maintained as long as there are signs of life.

The insertion of an endotracheal catheter is a rather difficult technique to master, and it is customary to practise on stillborn babies.

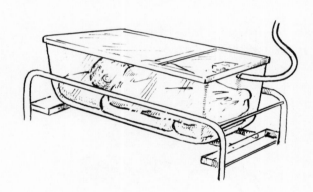

There are many other methods of resuscitating the newborn, ranging from mouth-to-mouth breathing, to the use of the most refined and expensive equipment such as the patient-actuated respirator, and the infant pressure chamber which makes use of four atmospheres of oxygen.

The technique described here is the one most generally practised and the apparatus required should be in every labour room.

MOULDING OF THE HEAD

The base of the skull and face are rigid with firm sutures. The vault of the skull is flexible and jointed by open sutures. This allows a certain amount of malleability to the skull vault. The bones may override each other and alter their contour.

This moulding is often characteristic for a presentation. In the normal vertex presentation the anterior parietal overlaps the posterior parietal bone and both overlap the occipital and frontal bones.

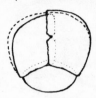 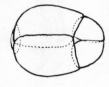 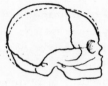

The skull is now asymmetrical and the occipito-frontal diameter is diminished but the mento-vertical diameter is increased. The shape is altered and the volume is slightly diminished.

Other presentations give different mouldings and contours:-

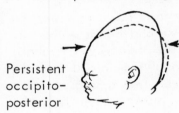 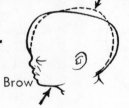 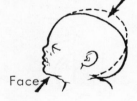

Persistent occipito-posterior

Brow

Face

Arrows indicate compression forces

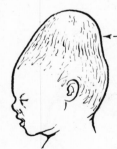 At birth the head looks elongated which is partly due to moulding but is also due to the formation of caput succedaneum. This is an oedematous, ecchymosed swelling of the tissues overlying the cervical os and lower uterine pole. It is greatest with prolonged and strenuous labour.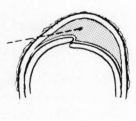

After birth reduction in the moulding occurs in 48 hours but most of it has gone within a few hours. The caput takes several days to disappear though the main oedema is gone in 36 hours.

BIRTH INJURIES

INTRA-CRANIAL HAEMORRHAGE. This means injury due to mechanical trauma rather than primarily to anoxia. It is seldom met with in present day practice.

The foetal brain is protected against damage in labour by:-

1. Softness and moulding of membranous bones.
2. Ability of fontanelles to 'give' slightly on pressure.
3. Cushioning effect of cerebro-spinal fluid.
4. Anatomical arrangement of dural septa with their free edges.
5. Plasticity of brain tissue.

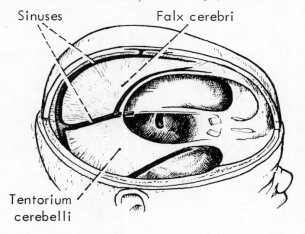

Sinuses   Falx cerebri

Tentorium cerebelli

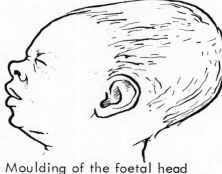

Moulding of the foetal head

Sometimes however distortion is excessive and a tear of the free edge of the tentorium cerebelli occurs involving blood vessels. Death occurs from increased intra-cranial pressure, especially on the brain stem and medulla.

This lesion is associated with difficult deliveries, such as high forceps, breech etc., but does occur after spontaneous vertex delivery. The signs and symptoms are those of asphyxia neonatorum and definite diagnosis is only made at post mortem examination.

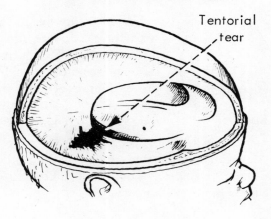

Tentorial tear

BIRTH INJURIES

The bones most commonly broken are the clavicle, humerus and femur as a result of too forcible delivery. In the case of the clavicle there may be no signs at all and callus is felt 2 weeks later. In the case of the long bones the Moro reflex will be absent in that limb and X-ray will be required. In healthy infants callus formation is rapid and splinting is only needed for 2 or 3 weeks.

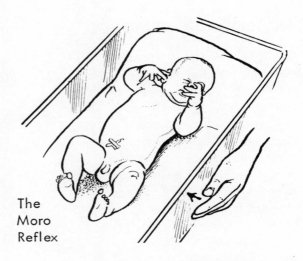

The Moro Reflex

In response to a sudden noise or vibration, the arms and legs are extended and then approach each other with slight shaking movements.

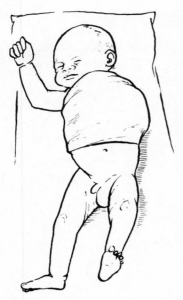

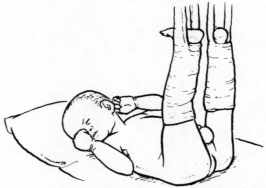

This splinting serves for clavicle and humerus. A pad must be placed between the arm and the chest wall: and as there is always some radial nerve paresis, the wrist should be in dorsiflexion.

The gallows splint is the most convenient method of treating fracture of the femur, and allows the baby to be kept clean easily. Feeding requires care and babies in this position must always be under observation.

BIRTH INJURIES

BRACHIAL PLEXUS DAMAGE

The commonest lesion is damage to the upper trunk at Erb's point caused by hyperextension of the neck in breech delivery and also in cases of shoulder dystocia. The abductors of the shoulder and the flexors of the arm are paralysed and the arm rotates forward and hangs in the characteristic 'waiter's tip' position.

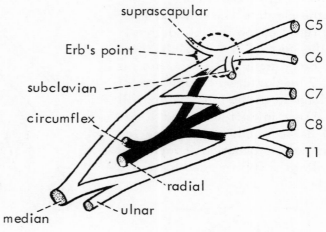

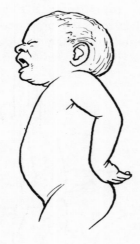

Erb's palsy

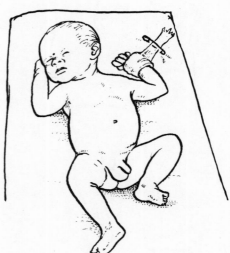

The arm must be kept in the position of maximum relaxation for the affected muscles and at first this is achieved by pinning the baby's arm to the pillow, in a position of flexion and abduction. If further treatment is required, a splint must be made.

BIRTH INJURIES

FACIAL PALSY

Paralysis of the facial nerve caused by pressure from the forceps made on the nerve as it emerges from the stylomastoid foramen. Recovery occurs in a matter of days, and any delay is an indication for further investigation.

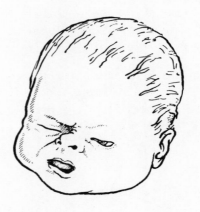

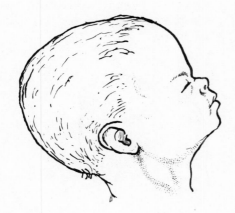

STERNOMASTOID TUMOUR

A painless lump in the sterno-mastoid muscle, appearing in the first week of life. It has tradition-ally been attributed to trauma, but its aetiology is unknown. Torticollis is an occasional sequel; and the mother should be instructed to put the muscle on the stretch for 3 or 4 periods a day. (This exercise is at first painful to the baby.)

357

BIRTH INJURIES

SUPERFICIAL HEAD INJURIES

Minor abrasions may be sustained during forceps delivery or from the use of the vacuum extractor. They need only local treatment as a rule, but:

1. Infection may pass into the skull via the emissary veins.
2. Dense connective tissue prevents vessel retraction, and scalp wounds bleed freely.

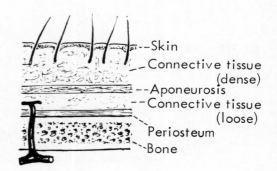

CAPUT SUCCEDANEUM

('Substitute Head'). This is a normal occurrence caused by pressure of the cervix interrupting venous and lymphatic scalp drainage during labour. A serous effusion collects between aponeurosis and periosteum disappearing a few hours after birth.

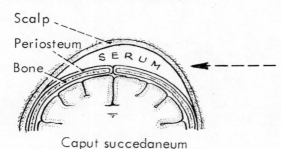

Caput succedaneum

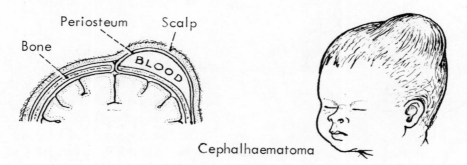

Cephalhaematoma

CEPHALHAEMATOMA is a collection of blood between periosteum and skull bone which is limited by the periosteal attachments at the suture lines. It is due to trauma and may not appear until several hours after birth. It should not be aspirated or drained and will normally be absorbed within a few weeks.

BIRTH INJURIES

SUBDURAL HAEMORRHAGE
(A rare condition)

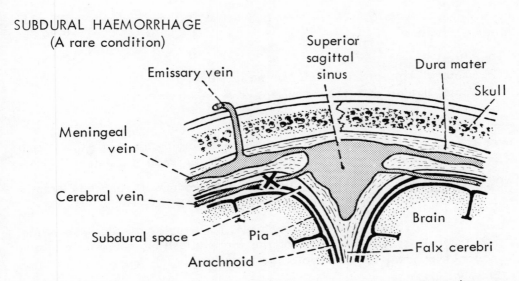

Bleeding arises from rupture of cerebral veins in the subdural space; a collection of blood extends over the frontal lobes; and the clinical picture is usually chronic failure to thrive along with cerebral irritation. In acute cases there will be a bulging fontanelle, convulsions and often retinal haemorrhages. Decompression by bilateral subdural tap is essential. The needle is introduced through the fronto-parietal sinus, just lateral to the anterior fontanelle.

DEPRESSION FRACTURE OF THE SKULL

This may be caused by the tip of the forceps blade in difficult delivery. If cerebral irritation or paresis is observed, elevation of the depressed area is done by passing an elevator through an adjacent burr hole – but usually no treatment is necessary.

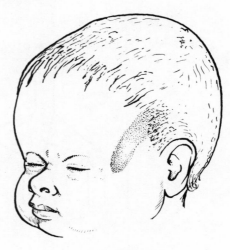

CONGENITAL DEFECTS

Many common defects are of unknown aetiology. Others can be explained by one of three mechanisms.

    A. Hereditary genetic defects.
    B. Chromosomal aberrations which may be familial.
    C. Incidental defects due to environment or of unknown aetiology.

A. Hereditary Genetic Defects

In each defect of this type the cause is usually a single abnormal gene. Such genes are, broadly speaking, of two types in their ability to produce a defect:-

    1. <u>Dominant Genes</u>. In this case the gene can produce the anomaly even if its opposite number in the gene pair is normal.

    Examples:- Achondroplasia, osteogenesis imperfecta, acholuric jaundice, sickle-cell anaemia, polyposis of the large intestine, neurofibromatosis, myotonia congenita, paramyotonia, polydactyly, syndactyly, arachno-dactyly.

Some of these such as the abnormalities of digits (see page 367) will be apparent at birth; others may be expected from family history.

    2. <u>Recessive Genes</u>. These genes can only express themselves when coupled with a similar gene. The incidence of the resulting defect will depend on the genetic make-up of the parents.

    Alkaptonuria may be taken as an example.

Where both parents are homozygous for the abnormal gene all offspring will be affected.

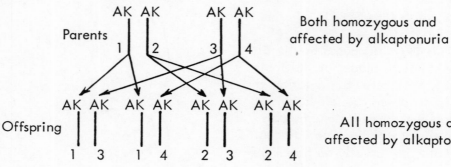

360

CONGENITAL DEFECTS

If one parent is homozygous for the gene and the other heterozygous 50% of the offspring will be affected. The other 50% will carry the gene but will be phenotypically normal.

With both parents heterozygous only 25% of the offspring will be affected, 50% will be phenotypically normal but carry the abnormal gene, and 25% will be completely normal.

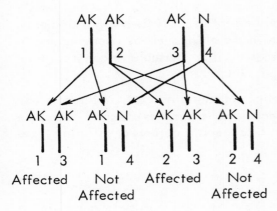

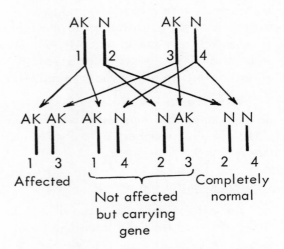

Examples of Recessive Gene Anomalies

Progessive infantile muscular atrophy, haemophilia, Christmas disease, para-haemophilia, congenital afibrinogenaemia, agammaglobulineamia, haemoglobin-opathies, inborn errors of metabolism. The last are numerous and affect various metabolic pathways. Their importance lies in the fact that if the defect is diagnosed early, the subsequent disease process may be prevented in some but not all by dietary means. This applies particularly to those genetic defects affecting carbohydrate and amino acid metabolism.

Defects of Carbohydrate Metabolism

Fructosuria, galactosuria, glycogen storage diseases, pentosuria.

Defects of Amino Acid Metabolism

Alkaptonuria, phenylketonuria, cystinuria, oxaluria, albinism.

Defects of Lipid Metabolism

Gaucher's disease, Niemann-Pick disease, Tay-Sach's disease, Hand-Schüller-Christian disease, Xanthomatosis.

CONGENITAL DEFECTS

Diagnosis

In the case of dominant gene anomalies the diagnosis is easy since one or other of the parents is bound to show signs of the defect. The only exception is where a new mutation arises in a family.

Recessive gene anomalies are much more difficult to discover since the parents are commonly heterozygotes and show no evidence of the disease. A careful family history extending to siblings of the foetus, siblings of the parents and grandparents, is essential. In the case of inborn errors of metabolism such as phenylketonuria which may lead to mental deficiency if untreated, it is advisable to carry out bio-chemical tests in all newborn infants (see page 339).

A further difficulty may arise in recognising genetic defects. With some abnormal genes the manifestation of their effects is not always expressed in the same way. Several members of a family may have congenital defects of differing types but due to the same gene.

Genetic Counselling

As with diagnosis, counselling in the case of dominant gene anomalies is straightforward from the scientific point of view.

Recessive gene anomalies require more detailed investigation and explanation. To a great extent the likelihood of a genetic defect manifesting itself depends on the genotype of the parents. As explained previously, if the parents are both homozygous for the abnormal gene all offspring are affected. If one is homozygous and the other heterozygous, 50% of the children will be affected, and with both parents heterozygous only 25% of offspring will be affected.

With some diseases the affected homozygous person is incapable of reproduction e.g. in progressive infantile muscular atrophy, and the disease is always transmitted by heterozygotes.

Another variation occurs in sex-linked genetic diseases. The abnormal recessive gene is carried on the X chromosome, as in haemophilia. In the case of females the abnormal recessive gene is usually repressed by its normal counterpart on the other X chromosome and female patients only rarely exhibit any signs of the disease. Manifestation of the disease occurs in males where the abnormal gene has no counterpart on the Y chromosome.

CONGENITAL DEFECTS

Mutations

Mutations of genes are possibly always occurring but harmful genes are constantly being eliminated and therefore effective spontaneous mutations are rare. This is shown by the following incidence figures:-

New cases of:-

Achondroplasia arise in 1 in 10,000 births.

Haemophilia arise in 1 in 10,000 male and 1 in 100,000 female births.

Tuberosclerosis arise in 1 in 60,000 male and 1 in 120,000 female births.

B.   Congenital Defects Due to Chromosomal Aberrations

These defects arise as a result of either an abnormal number of chromosomes or an abnormality in one chromosome, produced during cell division.

These abnormalities in chromosomes are produced during maturation of the ova and sperm. Abnormalities in number are due to failure of the chromosomes to separate in equal numbers when the germ cell divides.

Normal cells contain 44 somatic chromosomes plus 2 sex chromosomes, X and Y in the male, and 2 X chromosomes in the female, 46 in all. In the germ cells the number is reduced to 23 so that on fertilisation the zygote will contain the normal 46. The main chromosomal defects so far recognised are in association with the sex chromosomes. They arise by disjunction of chromosomes during meiosis. The following diagrams illustrate the variations which may occur in the mature ovum and sperm.

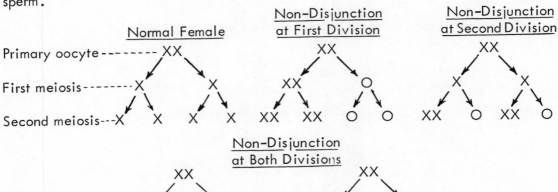

CONGENITAL DEFECTS

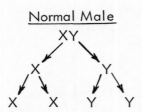

Normal Male

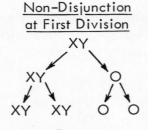

Non-Disjunction at First Division

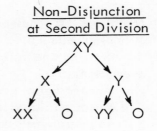

Non-Disjunction at Second Division

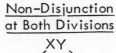
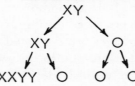

Non-Disjunction at Both Divisions

Many of these chromosomal aberrations result in the formation of cells incapable of taking part in fertilisation. With others however fertilisation can take place and the child produced will have an abnormal number of chromosomes. In some cases there may even be a mosaic chromosome structure, differing numbers of chromosomes being found in different cells of the body. This is probably due to non-disjunction of chromosomes during cell division in the embryo.

Several clinical syndromes are recognised as due to this kind of abnormality e.g.:-

	Chromosome Pattern	
Turner's Syndrome	44 XO	i.e. 45 chromosomes
	44 XO/XX	45 – 46 mosaic
	44 XO/XY	45 – 46 mosaic
	44 XO/XXX	45 – 47 mosaic
	44 XO/XYY	45 – 47 mosaic
Klinefelter's Syndrome	44 XXY	47 chromosomes

Few of these changes can be recognised at birth. Sometimes however extra autosomal chromosomes occur. This is found in one form of mongolism.

CONGENITAL DEFECTS

Another abnormality which may arise during meiosis is the formation of an abnormally long or short chromosome. Most chromosomes consist of a long arm and a short arm. When seen in pairs they almost form the outline of a St. Andrews cross.

When the two separate the short arm of one may pass to the other thus forming a very long chromosome. This will reduplicate itself and be passed on to the next generation. A chromosomal deformity of this kind may also be found in mongolism.

C. Defects Due to Environment

These defects arise during the first few weeks of pregnancy when foetal cells are differentiating to form various structures. The earlier the noxious agent acts the greater the disorganisation of the foetus and in many cases abortion probably results. Isolated defects are of later origin and are related to the time-table of organ development (see page 13).

Until recently environmental agents known to cause congenital defects in man were viruses, such as rubella, but now following the thalidomide tragedy it is realised that quite simple chemical substances may have disastrous results. Many congenital abnormalities are thought to be due to change in foetal environment but direct proof is lacking and at the present moment the majority of these lesions are of unknown aetiology.

Sign	0 points	1 point	2 points
Skin colour	Cyanosis Pallor	Periph. Cyanosis	Pink
Muscle tone	Flaccid	Moves Limbs	Good
Resp. effort	None	Gasps	Good
Heart rate	None	<100	>100
Response to stimulus	None	Slight	Good

The Apgar Scoring System (see page 349).

Evaluation is made 60 sec after delivery and the maximum score is 10 points. A score below 6 suggests that the baby may develop respiratory distress and perhaps hyaline membrane disease.

CONGENITAL DEFECTS

The obstetrician and the midwife should have some knowledge of the prognosis for the commoner abnormalities seen at birth, so that they can answer the mother's questions and initiate treatment when necessary.

MENINGOCOELE and MENINGOMYELOCOELE

Herniations of meninges and spinal cord through a bony gap due to a meso-dermal defect causing failure of fusion of vertebral arches (spina bifida) and failure of development of posterior dura mater. It occurs usually in the lumbo-sacral region.

MENINGOCOELE

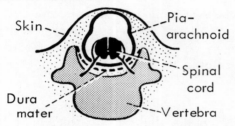

Herniation of pia-arachnoid is covered by skin (sometimes attenuated). There is no paralysis and surgical closure can be delayed for 6 months. Prognosis should be guarded until it is known for certain that nervous tissue is not involved. Otherwise the child will develop normally.

MYELOCOELE

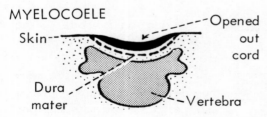

The internal surface of the cord is exposed. This defect is not compatible with life.

MENINGOMYELOCOELE

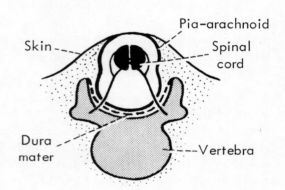

The cord is displaced as well as the membranes and neural epithelium forms the fundus of the sac. Skin cover is incomplete and infection inevitable unless closure is done within 24 hours. Paralysis of legs, bowel and bladder, and hydrocephaly, are normally present. Where immediate closure is practised, $\frac{1}{3}$ of the survivors will have little or no neurological deficit; the other $\frac{2}{3}$ will require many years of treatment for their multiple defects and may pass their whole lives paralysed and incontinent.

CONGENITAL DEFECTS

CLEFT LIP and PALATE

Lip or palate may be affected separately, but usually both are involved. The mother should be told that a good cosmetic result will be obtained when the lip is repaired at about 4 months and that after the palate is repaired at about a year the child will be taught to speak normally. Spoon feeding may be necessary if sucking is weak, and the cleft should be kept clean.

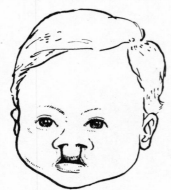

Bilateral cleft lip
('Hare lip')

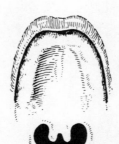

Cleft of soft
palate
(Bifid uvula)

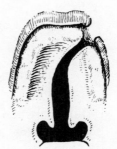

Unilateral cleft
palate

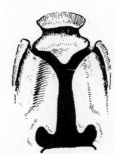

Bilateral cleft
palate

ACCESSORY DIGITS

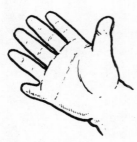

Small tags of flesh are common and can be removed with scissors. Fully developed extra digits must be surgically amputated at any time when the baby is big enough to withstand the operation.

CONGENITAL DEFECTS

OESOPHAGEAL ATRESIA with TRACHEO-BRONCHIAL FISTULA

The upper segment ends blindly at the level of the vena azygos arch and the distance of the blind end to the anterior alveolar margin is 10 cm.

It must be suspected antenatally in cases of unexplained hydramnios. In the neonate attempts at feeding lead to choking and cyanosis and there may be 'frothing' – excess of unswallowed mucus. If a sterile lubricated rubber catheter is arrested 10 - 12 cm from the alveolar margin, the diagnosis is almost certain. Antibiotic cover should be started and the paediatrician notified.

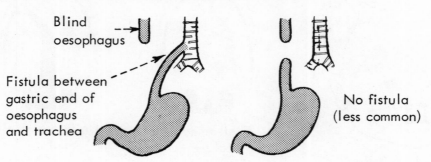

Blind oesophagus

Fistula between gastric end of oesophagus and trachea

No fistula (less common)

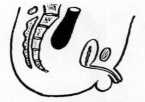

Failure of development of rectum

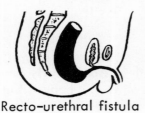

Recto-urethral fistula

IMPERFORATE ANUS

There is a wide variety of congenital ano-rectal abnormalities and a relieving colostomy may be an emergency measure. The passage of faeces must be noted: but fistula is often present and the observer may be confused by small amounts of faeces passed per urethram or per vaginam.

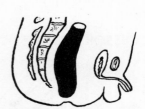

Cloacal membrane has failed to rupture

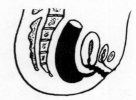

Recto-vaginal fistula

CONGENITAL DEFECTS

EXOMPHALOS

Some of the abdominal viscera lie within the umbilical cord and there is incomplete development of the abdominal wall. (It is a persistence of the normal situation in the 10 week foetus). The sac is a thin jelly-like membrane (the root of the cord) and the vessels of the cord run over the sac. The chances of repair depend on the size of the defect: but prior to operation the sac must be kept moist with saline swabs to prevent drying and cracking.

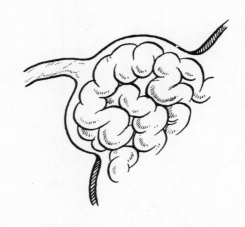

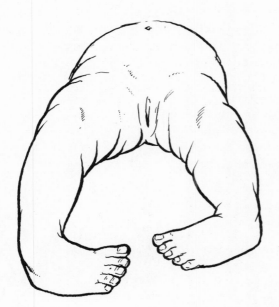

CLUB FOOT
(L. talipes = walking on the talus or ankle).

In true club foot there is always some resistance to complete passive correction. Treatment begins at birth in order to minimise the adaptive distortion of soft tissues and tarsal bones. The mother is taught to stretch and correct the deformity regularly and the baby must be referred at once to a paediatric surgeon. Operation is now seldom required.

CONGENITAL DEFECTS

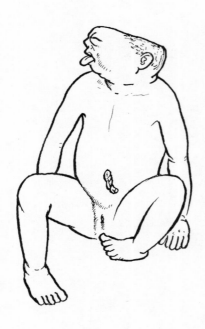

ANENCEPHALY is the failure of proper development of the cranium and scalp. The face and base of the skull are present. The head is frequently mistaken for a breech on palpation.

There is usually hydramnios – this is attributed to the inability of the foetus to swallow, the absence of foetal anti-diuretic hormone, and to the secretions of the exposed choroid plexus and meninges. The cause is obscure. X-ray shows the absence of a cranial vault.

Oestriol is practically absent from the maternal urine because the foetus has very little suprarenal tissue.

Anencephaly is about seven times more frequent in the female foetus than in the male.

Labour should be induced surgically after 34 weeks, but premature labour will tend to occur spontaneously when hydramnios is present. Sudden release of the liquor amnii may cause premature separation of the placenta and therefore bleeding.

The face is often the presenting part.

INIENCEPHALY is a condition giving a defect in the occipital bone in the region of the foramen magnum and fusing of the occiput to the ununited neural arches of an accompanying cervical spina bifida. This gives fixed extension of head and cervical spine.

Dystocia is rare because there is usually an associated hydramnios and premature labour.

However if the pregnancy goes to term there may be gross disproportion as the sterno-bregmatic diameter tries to negotiate the pelvis. A destructive operation or Caesarean section will deliver the foetus. The condition is incompatible with life.

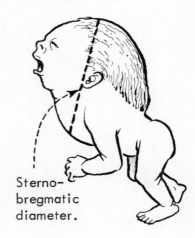

Sterno-bregmatic diameter.

CONGENITAL DEFECTS

HYDROCEPHALUS (water in the head) causes the head to enlarge. Some develop after birth but the antenatal development is of importance obstetrically.

A hydrocephalic head may fill the lower segment and give disproportion, obstructed labour, and uterine rupture. The lower segment seems unduly liable to rupture in these cases.

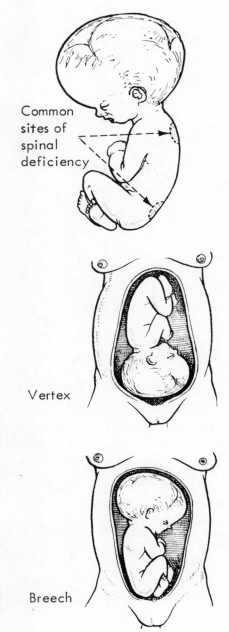

Common sites of spinal deficiency

Vertex

Breech

The diagnosis of hydrocephaly may be difficult because the head is not so hard as a normal head (two thirds of these cases present by the head) and fills the lower segment and paradoxically may not be recognised on vaginal examination. The head is not engaged and does not feel as rigid as normal. The bones may give on pressure ('egg shell' crackle). The sutures and fontanelles are wide.

If the foetus presents by the breech the head fills the fundus and may be difficult to define.

X-ray shows the large head with wide sutures and fontanelles. The bones of the cranium are not as distinct as usual and areas of thinning may show (craniolacunae - 'paw marks'). Ultrasound will measure the biparietal diameter and its growth.

Hydramnios is associated with hydrocephaly but, in this case, there is usually an accompanying meningocoele. A breech birth showing a meningocoele always suggests a co-existing hydrocephalus. A breech birth with extended arms may wrongly simulate hydrocephaly.

CONGENITAL DEFECTS

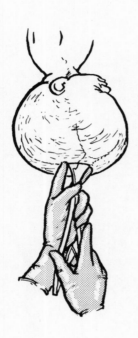

A hydrocephalic head presenting can be reduced by perforation of the cranium through a fontanelle or suture and draining off the cerebrospinal fluid. It may be difficult to stabilise the head at the brim. A Drew-Smythe cannula, a rigid spinal needle or a cranial perforator is used per vaginam.

A needle may be introduced through the abdominal wall to collapse the head. The bladder should be empty and there is a risk of perforating a uterine sinus.

The collapsed head allows delivery to proceed readily. It may be stimulated by traction of vulsellum forceps on the head.

If the presentation is breech the collapse of the head is usually easier as the head is fixed by the presence of the foetal body in the vagina.

The decompression can be accomplished by inserting a straightened male metal catheter through a meningocoele into the cranium, or by transection of the spine to gain access to the canal if there is no meningocoele. Other methods are by perforators through the mastoid region, or roof of the mouth.

Labour may be induced but marked degrees of hydrocephalus usually lead to premature labour.

Minor degrees of hydrocephaly may be delivered normally, or lead to section.

Some cases with hydrocephalus are compatible with life.

Future development in treatment may be so successful that Caesarean section becomes the method of choice.

CHAPTER 16

VAGINAL BLEEDING IN PREGNANCY

VAGINAL BLEEDING IN PREGNANCY

ECTOPIC PREGNANCY

6 – 8 weeks
Decidual bleeding

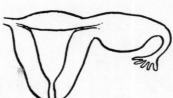

ABORTION

Up to 13 weeks
Chorio-decidual
bleeding

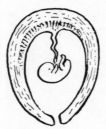

After 13 weeks

Normally or
abnormally
situated placenta

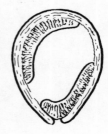

ANTE-PARTUM HAEMORRHAGE

After 28 weeks

Abruptio

Placenta
praevia

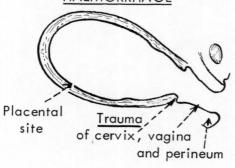

INTRA-PARTUM HAEMORRHAGE

Abruptio

Placenta
praevia

Excess
show

Vasa
praevia

Obscure causes

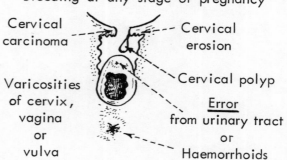

THIRD STAGE OR POST-PARTUM HAEMORRHAGE

Placental
site

Trauma
of cervix, vagina
and perineum

OTHER CAUSES of Staining or
Bleeding at any stage of pregnancy

Cervical
carcinoma

Cervical
erosion

Cervical polyp

Varicosities
of cervix,
vagina
or
vulva

Error
from urinary tract
or
Haemorrhoids

ECTOPIC PREGNANCY

Ectopic pregnancy is one in which the products of conception are developing outside the uterus. By far the commonest site is the fallopian tube.

The fallopian tube is about 12 cm long. Its diameter varies from 1 mm in the interstitial portion to about 5 mm at the fimbriated end.

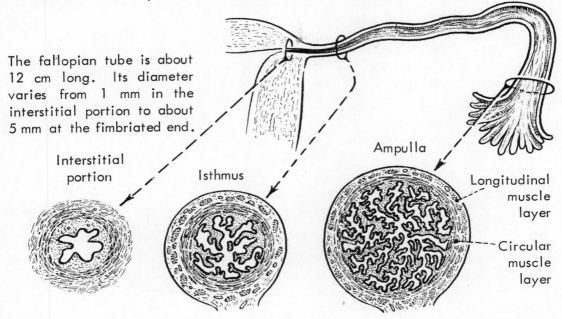

Interstitial portion

Isthmus

Ampulla

Longitudinal muscle layer

Circular muscle layer

The musculature is of two layers, an inner circular and an outer longitudinal, and peristaltic movements are particularly strong during and after ovulation. The mucosa is arranged in plications or folds which become much more complete and plentiful as the infundibulum is approached.

The mucosa consists of a single layer of ciliated and secretory cells, resting on a thin basement membrane. There is no submucosa and the epithelium is in direct contact with the muscle; and there is no decidual reaction, so muscle is easily invaded by the trophoblast.

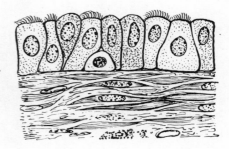

TUBAL PREGNANCY—AETIOLOGY

Ectopic implantation must be regarded as fortuitous: but there are some recognised predisposing factors.

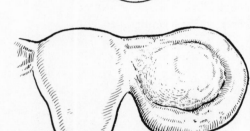

Zona pellucida

The zona pellucida is said to protect the ovum against premature implantation, and if owing to some delay, it has disappeared before the fertilised ovum reaches the uterus, tubal implantation will occur.

Delay might be due to:-

1. Preceding tubal or pelvic inflammation with residual chronic infection and distortion by adhesions.

Chronic salpingitis

2. Migration of ovum across the pelvic cavity to the fallopian tube on the side opposite to the follicle from which ovulation occurred.

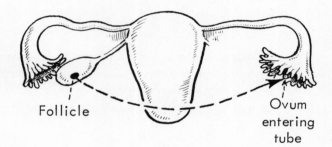

Follicle

Ovum entering tube

3. Congenital abnormality of the tube such as hypoplasia, elongation, diverticulae.
   Diverticulae are occasionally seen and, in theory, present a cul-de-sac in which the ovum may lodge.

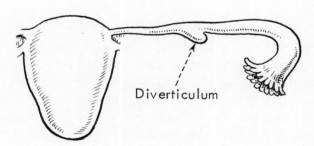

Diverticulum

TUBAL PREGNANCY—IMPLANTATION

Because there is no decidual membrane in tubal mucosa, and no submucosa, the ovum rapidly burrows through the mucosa and embeds in the muscular wall of the tube, opening up maternal blood vessels and causing necrosis of muscle and connective tissue cells.

Wall of tube

Pseudo-capsularis of muscle tissue in which ovum is embedded

Compressed lumen of tube

Villi eroding maternal vessels

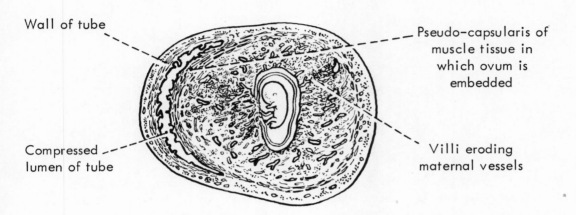

The ampulla is the commonest site of implantation, followed by the isthmus.

Interstitial implantation is rare (but very dangerous because it ends in severe haemorrhage).

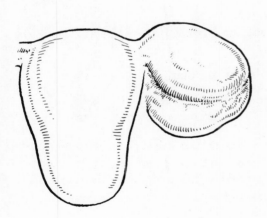

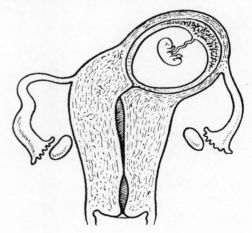

TUBAL PREGNANCY—TERMINATION

The muscle wall of the tube has not the capacity of uterine muscle for hypertrophy and distension and tubal pregnancy nearly always ends in rupture and the death of the ovum.

RUPTURE INTO LUMEN OF TUBE (TUBAL ABORTION)

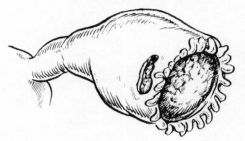

This is usual in ampullary pregnancy at about 8 weeks. The conceptus is extruded, complete or incomplete, towards the fimbriated end of the tube, probably by the pressure of accumulated blood. There is a trickle of bleeding into the peritoneal cavity, and this may collect as a clot in the pouch of Douglas. It is then called a pelvic haematocoele.

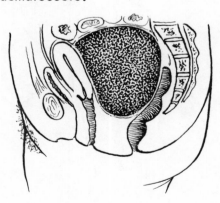

RUPTURE INTO THE PERITONEAL CAVITY

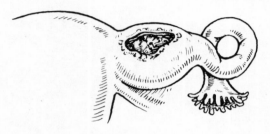

This may occur spontaneously, or from pressure (such as straining at stool, coitus or pelvic examination) and occurs mainly from the narrow isthmus before 8 weeks, or from the interstitial portion at 12 weeks. Haemorrhage is likely to be severe.

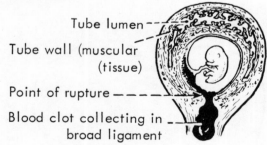

Tube lumen

Tube wall (muscular (tissue)

Point of rupture

Blood clot collecting in broad ligament

Sometimes rupture is retroperitoneal between the leaves of the broad ligament – broad ligament haematoma. Haemorrhage in this site is more likely to be controlled.

TUBAL PREGNANCY—EFFECT ON UTERUS

The uterus enlarges in the first three months almost as if the implantation were normal, and may reach the size of a gravid uterus of the same maturity. This is a source of confusion in diagnosis.

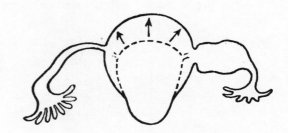

The uterine decidua grows abundantly, and when the ovum or embryo dies, bleeding occurs as the decidua degenerates. Rarely it is expelled entire as a decidual cast; and is replaced within a few weeks (perhaps before clinical diagnosis) by normal endometrium.

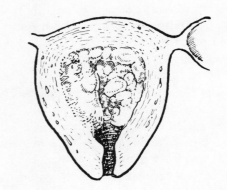

Enlargement of Non-Gravid Uterus

The picture shows a non-gravid uterus enlarged to the size of a 16 weeks' pregnancy. It was seen at laparotomy carried out in the 34th week of an abdominal pregnancy in which the placenta was attached to the pelvic floor and the broad ligament.

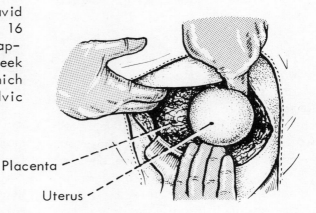

Placenta

Uterus

TUBAL PREGNANCY—SYMPTOMS AND SIGNS

Tubal pregnancy can present in many ways and misdiagnosis is common.

PAIN in the lower abdomen is always present and may be either stabbing or cramp-like - 'uterine colic'. It may be referred to the shoulder if blood tracks to the diaphragm and stimulates the phrenic nerve, and it may be so severe as to cause fainting. The pain is caused by distension of the gravid tube, by its efforts to contract and expel the ovum, and by irritation of the peritoneum by leakage of blood.

VAGINAL BLEEDING occurs usually after the death of the ovum and is an effect of oestrogen withdrawal. It is dark brown and scanty ('vaginal spotting') and its irregularity may lead the patient to confuse it with the menstrual flow. In about 25% of cases tubal pregnancy presents without any vaginal bleeding.

INTERNAL BLOOD LOSS will, if gradual, lead to anaemia. If haemorrhage is severe and rapid (as when a large vessel is eroded) the usual signs of collapse and shock will appear. Acute internal bleeding is the most dramatic and dangerous consequence of tubal pregnancy but it is less common than the condition presented by a slow trickle of blood into the pelvic cavity.

PELVIC EXAMINATION in the conscious patient will demonstrate extreme tenderness over the gravid tube or in the pouch of Douglas if a haematocoele has collected. If the pregnancy is sufficiently advanced and rupture has not occurred, a cystic (and very tender) mass may be felt in the fornix; but often tenderness is the only sign elicited.

PERITONEAL IRRITATION may produce muscle guarding, frequency of micturition, and later a degree of fever, all leading towards a misdiagnosis of appendicitis.

SIGNS AND SYMPTOMS OF EARLY PREGNANCY must be expected, all of which can confuse the clinical picture. When implantation occurs in the isthmus, tubal rupture may occur before the patient has missed a period, and pregnancy tests may be negative until the 40th day.

ABDOMINAL EXAMINATION will demonstrate tenderness in one or other fossa. If there has been much intraperitoneal bleeding there will be general tenderness and resistance to palpation over the whole abdomen.

TUBAL PREGNANCY—DIFFERENTIAL DIAGNOSIS

1. Salpingitis.
2. Abortion.
3. Appendicitis
4. Torsion of pedicle of ovarian cyst.
5. Rupture of corpus luteum or follicular cyst.
6. Lateral displacement of gravid uterus (page 266).

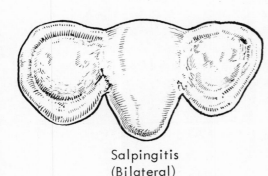

Salpingitis
(Bilateral)

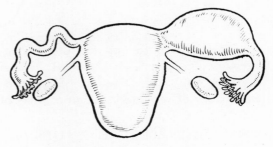

Tubal pregnancy

1. SALPINGITIS

Swelling and pain are bilateral, fever is higher, and a positive pregnancy test is unusual.

2. ABORTION, threatened or incomplete.

Bleeding is more profuse and the blood is red rather than dark brown. The pain is milder and more like a small labour. The uterus is larger and softer and the cervix patulous or dilated. Curettage may help but naked eye appearances cannot be relied on.

3. APPENDICITIS

The area of tenderness is higher and localised at McBurney's point. There may be a swelling if an appendix abscess has formed but it is not so deep in the pelvis as a tubal swelling. Fever is greater and a positive pregnancy test and amenorrhoea unlikely.

TUBAL PREGNANCY—DIFFERENTIAL DIAGNOSIS

4. TORSION of PEDICLE of OVARIAN CYST.

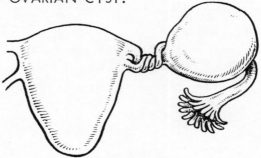

The mass so formed can usually be felt separate from the uterus, while a tubal pregnancy usually feels attached.   Tenderness may be marked, and intraperitoneal bleeding may produce fever.   Signs and symptoms of pregnancy are absent but there is a history of repeated sudden attacks of pain which pass off.

5. RUPTURE of CORPUS LUTEUM.

It is virtually impossible to distinguish this by examination from a tubal pregnancy, but such a severe reaction is rare.

ALWAYS TAKE A CAREFUL HISTORY

ALWAYS <u>THINK</u> OF TUBAL PREGNANCY

AIDS TO DIAGNOSIS

<u>Culdocentesis</u> (passing a needle through the posterior fornix into the pouch of Douglas).   Intraperitoneal blood does not readily clot: and if such blood is obtained it is an indication for laparotomy.   However, an unruptured tubal pregnancy will not be revealed by this procedure;   nor will endometriosis; and if inflammatory adhesions fix the pelvic organs, the intestine may be perforated.

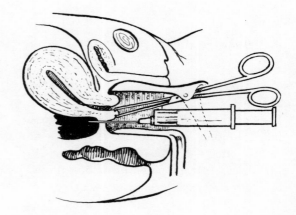

LAPAROSCOPY

Laparoscopy

The pelvic cavity can be inspected by means of an endoscope, passed either through the posterior fornix of the vagina (culdoscopy) or through the abdominal wall (laparoscopy). This method of investigation has become much more effective with the development of the Cold Light System, whereby a light source from outside the body is transmitted to the endoscope along a flexible fibreglass cable, illuminating the cavity with a brilliant light, which gives off no heat.

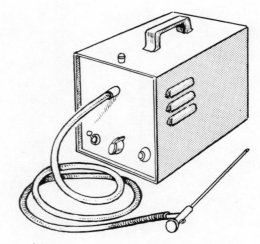

Laparoscopy is obviously of use in diagnosing the case with equivocal signs and symptoms, and especially so when an unruptured tubal pregnancy is suspected. The abdominal approach avoids the risk of injuring structures fixed in the pelvis, and unnecessary laparotomy is avoided. (A per-abdominal cautery instrument has also been devised so that sterilisation by cautery of the fallopian tubes can be carried out under direct vision.)

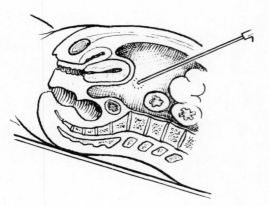

But:-

1. Even laparoscopy may not reveal an early undisturbed tubal pregnancy.
2. A general anaesthetic is required, the procedure must be carried out in theatre, and the woman's abdomen must be distended with gas (carbon dioxide or helium) which may subsequently cause discomfort.
3. The perforation made by the modern laparoscope amounts to a laparotomy scar an inch long.
4. The equipment is expensive, and the technique requires experience.

TUBAL PREGNANCY—TREATMENT

1. Once the diagnosis is made the next step is laparotomy which should not be delayed.

2. If haemorrhage and shock are present, blood transfusion should be given at once. If there is delay in obtaining blood, plasma should be given and operation proceeded with. The patient's condition will improve as soon as the bleeding is controlled.

3. In the less acute case pelvic examination under anaesthesia may be undertaken, although it is unlikely to yield more information than examination of the conscious patient. Such an examination must be made in circumstances which allow immediate laparotomy if the palpating fingers should rupture the gravid tube. The best place to do it is in the theatre.

4. If a tubal pregnancy is found the blood should be sucked and mopped out and salpingectomy performed. Conservation and repair of the tube even if possible is unwise because of the danger of recurrence, unless there is a compelling reason such as a previous salpingectomy in a patient who very much wants more children.

5. At operation all the pelvic organs should be inspected. If the diagnosis turns out to be a tubal or appendix abscess, it is best simply to remove all pus and close the abdomen with drainage unless the operator is experienced in pelvic surgery.

ABDOMINAL PREGNANCY

Abdominal pregnancy is very rare. The ovum is expelled from the tube and re-implants elsewhere in the pelvis; or implantation occurs primarily in the peritoneum.

CLINICAL FEATURES
1. There is a history of 'threatened abortion' with irregular bleeding.
2. Continual abdominal discomfort is felt, and foetal movements are painful.
3. Foetal abnormality is common and foetal mortality is high. Foetal death may be followed by suppuration with abscess pointing into bowel or bladder; or by calcification and lithopaedion formation.

The ovum may be expelled intra- or retro-peritoneally. The trophoblast develops its connection with the nearest blood supply (usually on the broad ligament and back of uterus); and in the retroperitoneal situation the proximity of great vessels will increase the risk of haemorrhage.

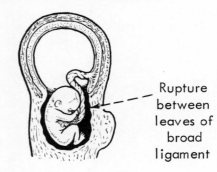

Rupture between leaves of broad ligament

DIAGNOSIS is difficult
1. Palpation is unreliable even when foetal limbs are easily felt.
2. X-rays should show a foetus in an abnormal position in the abdominal cavity.
3. Small doses of oxytocin may help by causing the uterus to contract so that it can be palpated separately from other masses.

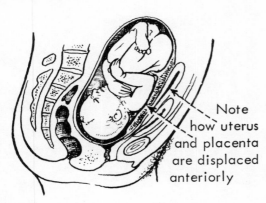

Note how uterus and placenta are displaced anteriorly

Recovery is apt to be slow while the placenta is being absorbed, and the pregnancy test will remain positive for about four weeks.

TREATMENT. Once diagnosed or strongly suspected, it is better to perform laparotomy in the interests of the mother. The foetus is removed, the cord tied, and the abdomen closed. NO ATTEMPT IS MADE TO DETACH THE PLACENTA. The absence of a contractile uterus leaves no means of controlling haemorrhage.

ABORTION

The termination of a pregnancy before the 28th week.

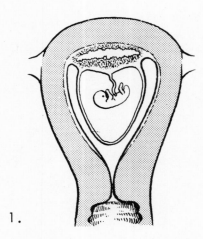

1.

Haemorrhage occurs in the decidua basalis leading to local necrosis and inflammation.

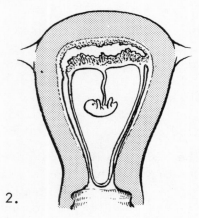

2.

The ovum, partly or wholly detached, acts as a foreign body and initiates ·uterine contractions. The cervix begins to dilate.

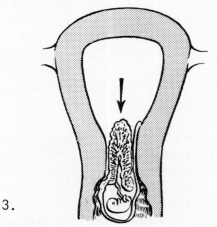

3.

Expulsion complete. The decidua is shed during the next few days in the lochial flow.

Up to 12 weeks before the placenta is fully developed, abortion is likely to be complete, as shown.

From the 12th to the 24th week the gestation sac is likely to rupture expelling the foetus, while the placenta is retained.

From the 24th week onward the mechanism resembles normal labour although the placenta is more often retained.

ABORTION

Once an abortion is declared inevitable, because of the amount of blood loss or dilatation of the cervix, it becomes either:-

COMPLETE or INCOMPLETE

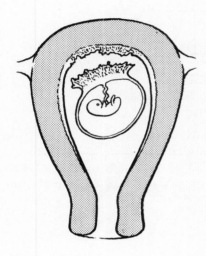 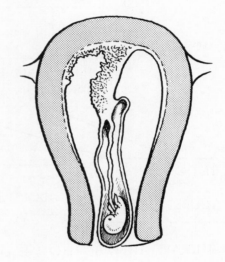

Uterine contractions are felt 'like a small labour', the cervix dilates and blood loss continues. The foetus and placenta (often with membranes intact) are expelled complete.

The uterus contracts and no further treatment is needed except perhaps for a haemorrhagic anaemia.

In spite of uterine contractions and cervical dilatation, only the foetus and some membranes are expelled. The placenta remains partly attached and bleeding continues.

This abortion must be completed by surgical methods.

ABORTION

Classification is based on a mixture of clinical, pathological and moral concepts, and is sufficiently flexible to suit a condition in which diagnosis must often be a matter of supposition. Sepsis can complicate any type of abortion and is commonly due to criminal interference.

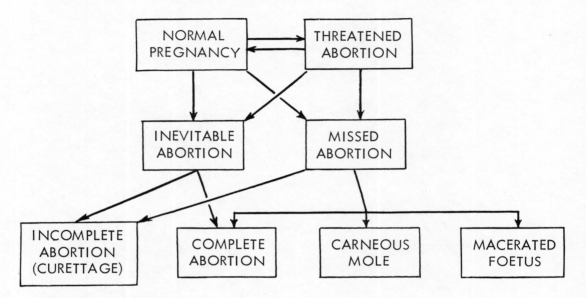

A THERAPEUTIC ABORTION is one performed electively by a qualified medical practitioner for medico-legal indications.

Under the Abortion Act of 1967 this may be done if two registered medical practitioners are of the opinion that:-

1. Continuance of the pregnancy would involve risk to the life of the pregnant woman, or of injury to the physical or mental health of the pregnant woman, or any existing children of her family, greater than if the pregnancy were terminated; or

2. there is a substantial risk that if the child were born it would suffer from such physical or mental abnormalities as to be seriously handicapped.

In (1) above, account may be taken of the pregnant woman's actual or reasonable forseeable environment.

ABORTION

AETIOLOGY.   In most cases the cause is unknown.

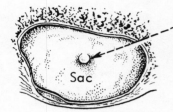

Abnormal Development of the Ovum

Of those embryos recovered from abortion about half are said to be abnormal.

Sac

Maternal Conditions

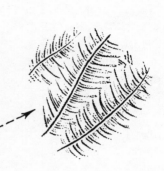

High fever, congestive cardiac failure, severe Rh iso-immunisation, chronic renal disease are all associated conditions. 'Hormonal Imbalance' – not a well defined condition – usually refers to progesterone deficiency as indicated by pregnanediol excretion rate (see page 397) and by 'ferning' of cervical mucus when dried on a slide. This peculiar pattern is evidence of unopposed oestrogen activity.

Mechanical causes are rare but recognised:

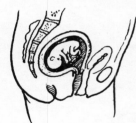

Incarceration of Gravid Uterus
The growing uterus cannot escape from the pelvis because of retroversion.

Cervical Incompetence
Severe lacerations may make it impossible for the uterus to contain a gestation beyond the 4th month.

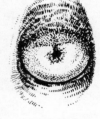

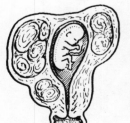

Fibroids
A uterus distorted by fibroids may be unable to accommodate the growing foetus.

Congenital Abnormality of the Uterus
may interfere with the development of the growing foetus.

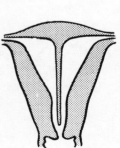

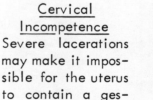

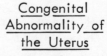

389

ABORTION

CLINICAL FEATURES

Haemorrhage is usually the first sign and may be very heavy if placental separation is incomplete.

Pain is usually intermittent, 'like a small labour'. It ceases when the abortion is complete.

Cervical Dilatation means that abortion is inevitable.

THREATENED ABORTION. Abortion is said to threaten when any bleeding occurs before the 28th week. It may even be accompanied by pain, yet the abortion process may not have begun in utero and the pregnancy may continue.

Some women have a tendency to bleed in the early months for no known reason. There may be incidental causes such as cervicitis, cervical polyp, rarely carcinoma.

Treatment of threatened abortion.

The patient is confined to bed and given a sedative drug such as promazine 50 mg three times per day. Urine is sent for a pregnancy test; and after 48 hours the cervix is inspected. If all is normal the patient gradually becomes ambulant and is sent home.

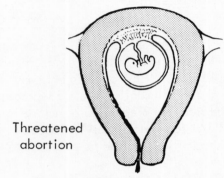

Threatened abortion

Bleeding is slight, not retroplacental, and cervix is closed. Pregnancy is likely to continue.

INEVITABLE ABORTION. Here bleeding is also slight and cervix still closed. Clinically the woman has a threatened abortion: but bleeding is retroplacental and the ovum already dead. The condition is really one of <u>inevitable abortion</u>.

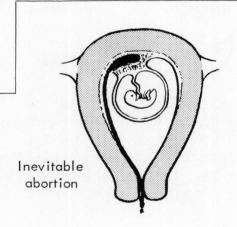

Inevitable abortion

ABORTION—DIFFERENTIAL DIAGNOSIS

TUBAL PREGNANCY

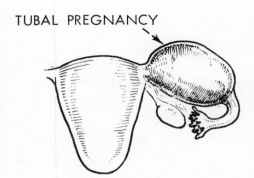

The swollen tube may not be felt separate from the enlarged uterus. There is usually a history of severe pain and slight bleeding; but exploratory laparotomy may eventually be resorted to.

FIBROIDS

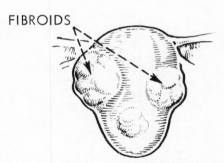

The irregularity of the mass should be felt unless the patient is very fat. Bleeding may be heavy but there will be no history of amenorrhoea. Abortion and fibroids may co-exist.

METROPATHIA HAEMORRHAGICA
may simulate abortion so closely that the distinction can be made only on the histological appearances.

PYOSALPINX

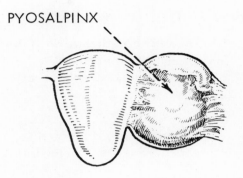

The uterus may be involved in adhesions and there is often irregular bleeding. There will be no evidence of pregnancy however, and there may be systemic signs of infection.

OVARIAN CYST

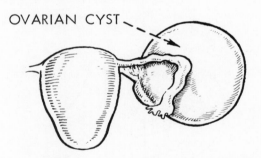

There may have been a period of amenorrhoea followed by heavy bleeding. But ovarian cysts usually have pedicles and the non-gravid uterus should be felt separately.

Much uterine bleeding has no organic explanation and the patient accepts or supplies a diagnosis of abortion for want of anything better.

ABORTION—TREATMENT

SURGICAL TREATMENT of INCOMPLETE ABORTION

1. It must be done in theatre with the patient anaesthetised.
2. The patient may bleed:
   (a) before admission to hospital
   (b) while in hospital
   (c) during the operation

   } Blood loss may be large and facilities for blood transfusion must be to hand.

3. The operator must, all the time, remember the ease with which a gravid uterus can be perforated by a metal instrument.

'Digital Curettage' is tried first.

Removal of Placental tissue with ovum forceps.

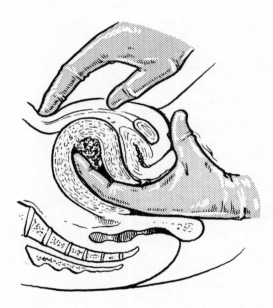

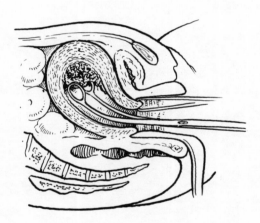

The surgeon presses on the fundus with the external hand and clears out as much of the cavity as he can reach with the internal finger.

The open blades are rotated to grasp tissue and then gently withdrawn. Before using any instrument inside the uterus oxytocin, 5 units, should be given intravenously to cause contraction and thickening of the uterine wall.

ABORTION—TREATMENT

CURETTAGE. A blunt curette is used first but if this is ineffective the operation is completed with a sharp curette.

PACKING the UTERUS. This is only necessary if bleeding continues from an empty uterus and oxytocin is not effective; or if the uterus still has products of conception but curettage is considered too dangerous.

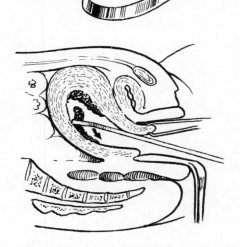

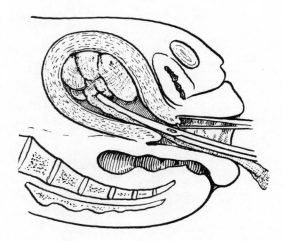

The concave side of the curette loop is pressed against the wall and pulled down. It is then reapplied on another part of the wall. Do not push the curette up the uterine wall.

It is important to pack the whole cavity, not just the lower part.
Dry sterile gauze is used and the pack should be withdrawn in 12 hours.

EVACUATION BY SUCTION. This is becoming the method of choice for therapeutic abortion up to 12 weeks, but is regarded as a gynaecological procedure. Suction is applied by inserting a tube of glass, plastic or steel through the dilated cervix, using a pressure of about 0.6 kg/cm^2 from an ordinary theatre suction machine. The operation is speedy and blood loss rather less than with the curette.

Suction tubes

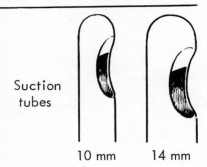

10 mm   14 mm

MISSED ABORTION

The retention of an ovum, after its death, for a period of several weeks.

Death of the ovum occurs unnoticed; or is marked by some vaginal bleeding which ceases after treatment for threatened abortion. However enlargement of the breasts ceases and the uterus shrinks as liquor is absorbed. Pregnancy tests will be negative about a week after death, and at least two negative results should be obtained.

If retained for long enough, the gestation may end up as a

CARNEOUS MOLE   or   MACERATED FOETUS

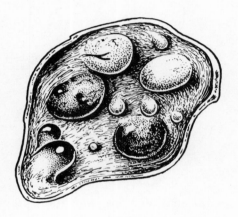
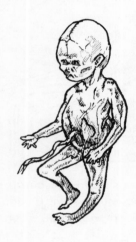

A carneous mole is a lobulated mass of laminated blood clot. The projections into the shrunken cavity are caused by repeated haemorrhages in the chorio-decidual space. In very early pregnancies (up to 12 weeks) complete absorption of the dead ovum may occur.

The skull bones collapse and override and the spine is flexed (changes known as 'Spalding's sign' when seen on X-ray). The internal organs degenerate and the abdomen is filled with bloodstained fluid. The skin peels very easily.

Pathological changes in the foetus such as mummification (foetus papyraceous) and calcification (lithopaedion) are exceedingly rare.

MISSED ABORTION

MISSED ABORTION

Treatment

If left alone most missed abortions will be spontaneously expelled, but during the waiting period there is a slight risk of hypofibrinogaemia (see page 407).

If the uterus is not larger than the size of an eight to ten week pregnancy it may be emptied by curettage. This operation requires experience and as bleeding is free until the uterus is emptied, transfusion facilities must be available.

If the uterus is too large for the curette attempts at inducing abortion may be made by giving a three day course of stilboestrol, 10 mg three times per day, to 'sensitise' the uterus, following with intravenous oxytocin. If no abortion follows the patient should be left alone; and while waiting for spontaneous expulsion, the blood fibrinogen level should be checked at weekly intervals and a watch kept for signs of purpura.

SEPTIC ABORTION

This is an incomplete abortion complicated by infection of the uterine contents, usually as a result of criminal interference. The clinical features are those of abortion complicated by a varying degree of fever; and while severe septicaemia can occur with any organism, it is best exemplified by describing the effects of Cl. Welchii infection (page 398).

Treatment

When sepsis is suspected, cervical and high vaginal smears, a specimen of urine and blood culture are sent to the bacteriologist and a broad spectrum antibiotic exhibited pending his report. Unless bleeding is heavy it is better to wait 24 hours before evacuating the uterus. This allows the antibiotic to produce its effect and reduces the risk of dissemination.

Perforation of a septic uterus is particularly easy and if the sepsis is due to criminal interference, a perforation may already exist. In a few cases necrosis of such extent may be found that hysterectomy must be carried out.

HABITUAL ABORTION

Habitual abortion indicates the occurrence of at least 3 consecutive spontaneous abortions.

Aetiology

A recurring factor must be suspected but is seldom identified although search is made for any of the various conditions mentioned on page 389.

Treatment

Treatment is usually empirical and when success is obtained the psychological effects of close medical supervision cannot be discounted.

CERVICAL INCOMPETENCE

In gross cases, repair is undertaken electively in the non-pregnant state, but where there is only functional evidence of suspected incompetence (repeated abortions at 12 weeks or over) the insertion of a cervical suture as early as possible is sometimes practised, again on empirical grounds.

A non-absorbable, inert suture such as tantalum wire is used. Under anaesthesia the cervix is grasped with a vulsellum and the suture inserted as shown. It is removed at about 36 weeks when all risk of abortion or prematurity has passed.

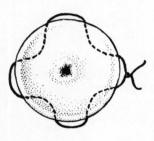

Four 'bites' are taken as high up the cervix as possible and the suture tied tight.

This treatment does no harm and its use is associated with a success rate of 75% after three abortions. Difficulties may arise when abortion threatens in spite of the suture which must be removed if the conceptus is definitely going to be expelled.

HABITUAL ABORTION

HORMONE TREATMENT

A progesterone (such as hydroxyprogesterone caproate 250 mg twice weekly) is given either empirically or after demonstration of suspected hormonal deficiency by urinary assay or by inspection of cytological appearances of the vagina.

URINARY PREGNANEDIOL EXCRETION

This estimation is performed in most laboratories, but wide variations reduce its practical value. Repeated low values are taken as a sign of progesterone deficiency.

8 weeks	3 mg/24 hours
12 "	4 "
16 "	6 "
20 "	9 "
24 "	11 "

URINARY OESTRIOL EXCRETION

Up to 20 weeks the amounts excreted are too variable to be of any guidance, but thereafter, when the foetal adrenal gland begins to make a significant contribution to oestrogen production, a more or less constant increase should occur. In the pre-viable stage of pregnancy, a level below 3 mg oestriol in 24 hours suggests hormone deficiency; but the technique is time-consuming and repeated serial observations are required.

VAGINAL CYTOLOGY

In pregnancy there is a proliferation of cells from the intermediate layers of the vaginal epithelium, the most abundant being the 'navicular' cell – an oval or boat-shaped cell with thickened borders, clear basophil cytoplasm and a vesicular nucleus.

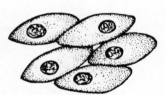

Navicular cells

When progesterone is deficient there is a change in the pattern and the number of cornified and pyknotic cells increases. These are cells of a more angular outline with small pyknotic nuclei, often oesinophil in reaction. When these cells surpass 20% of a cell count ('a high karyo-pyknotic index') a state of progesterone deficiency is diagnosed.

The 'ferning' of cervical mucus due to the same cause is described on page 389.

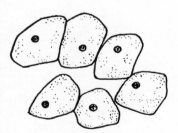

Pyknotic cells

CLOSTRIDIUM WELCHII SEPTICAEMIA

This bacillus can, in adverse conditions, form spores as a defence. These are very resistant and destruction requires high temperatures (over 120°C for up to 50 minutes).

Clostridium welchii may be found in the vagina in some cases of uterine infection without being the cause of the patient's symptoms. It is an obligatory anaerobe and requires dead tissue such as torn muscle or blood clot for growth. The 'gas gangrene' with which it is associated is due to the fermentation of the carbohydrate of the destroyed tissue.

TOXINS are produced:- A lecithinase which breaks down cell protein
A haemolysin
A fibrinolysin ⎱———⎰ These allow
Hyaluronidase ⎰   ⎱ spread.

DIAGNOSIS is clinical and not bacteriological (which takes 36 hours). The signs are pain, high temperature, profound shock with peripheral collapse although consciousness is retained; and a severe haemolytic anaemia and jaundice. Any urine in the bladder will be heavily contaminated with blood ('port wine urine').

TREATMENT

ANTIBIOTICS AND ANTITOXINS. Besides the usual specimens the bacteriologist will require an anaerobic blood culture. Polyvalent antiserum is given and large doses of penicillin must also be given, of the order of 1 mega-unit 4-hourly.

HAEMOLYSIS and RENAL FAILURE. The haemolytic anaemia is so severe that large amounts of blood must be given (up to 9 or 10 pints) in spite of the near certainty of renal failure. Electrolytes and blood urea must be monitored and acidosis corrected by bicarbonate. A day or two after operation the patient is transferred to a renal dialysis unit.

SHOCK. Septic shock is severe in the presence of Cl. Welchii infection, and should be treated along the lines described on page 330.

SURGERY. Once the shock is overcome and the blood pressure stabilised over 100 systolic, the uterus should be emptied by curettage.

PLACENTA PRAEVIA (PP)

A low implantation of the placenta in the uterus, causing it to lie alongside or in front of the presenting part.

The cause is unknown. The incidence is greater in multigravidae and there is an association with other foetal abnormalities. Twin pregnancy with its large placental bed is prone to low implantation of at least a part of the placenta. PP is divided into four types or degrees, of which the first two are the commonest.

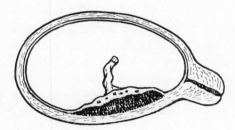

Type 1

The lower margin of the placenta dips into the lower segment. ('Low implantation').

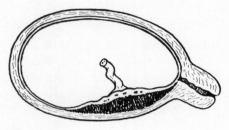

Type 2

The placenta reaches the internal os when closed but does not cover it. ('Marginal').

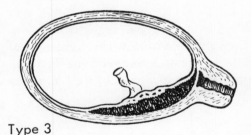

Type 3

The placenta covers the internal os when closed, but not when fully dilated. ('Partial' or 'Incomplete').

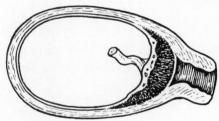

Type 4

The placenta covers the os even when the cervix is fully dilated. ('Central' or 'Complete').

Allocation to a particular type is usually made by palpation prior to delivery, or by observation at Caesarean section; so there is a subjective bias. In addition the dilating cervix may alter a classification; what was Type 1 at two fingers dilatation may become Type 2 at four fingers.

399

PLACENTA PRAEVIA

SIGNS and SYMPTOMS

Painless bleeding usually occurs about the 32nd week when the lower segment is beginning to form, although sometimes there is no bleeding until the onset of labour. The loss may be slight or considerable. Abdominal examination will reveal non-engagement usually with a high presenting part. Vaginal examination at this stage may cause uncontrollable haemorrhage and must never be done.

MANAGEMENT

If the pregnancy is at 37 weeks or more the best treatment is to carry out an Examination Under Anaesthesia (EUA) in theatre. However bleeding usually occurs early in the third trimester, and an expectant policy may be followed which will give the foetus a chance of reaching an acceptable weight and maturity.

After 3 days without fresh staining, speculum examination is made to exclude incidental causes of APH (page 374) and after the 34th week X-ray localisation of the placenta is carried out. If normal implantation is demonstrated the patient may go home, but if clinical signs such as bleeding and non-engagement of the head persist, then whatever the X-ray evidence the patient must be kept in hospital until the foetus is of a mature size – usually about 37 to 38 weeks, at which point EUA is carried out. If second heavy bleeding occurs after admission to hospital it is advisable to carry out EUA there and then.

EXAMINATION UNDER ANAESTHESIA

This is done in theatre set and staffed for Caesarean section. The treatment of PP to day may be summarised as being section for every degree except Type 1, when the membranes may be ruptured, and if no bleeding occurs spontaneous delivery may be awaited.

TYPE OF SECTION

As a rule the lower segment operation is done and the operator either cuts rapidly through the placenta or passes his hand above or below it. If the EUA has started torrential haemorrhage, classical section would have a slight advantage in speed.

BLEEDING AT OPERATION

Because of the poor retractile quality of the lower segment there is sometimes difficulty in obtaining control of bleeding after delivery of baby and placenta. Hysterectomy might ultimately be necessary.

PLACENTA PRAEVIA

If dangerous haemorrhage occurs in a situation in which rapid transfer to hospital is not possible, attempts might be made to control the bleeding by pressure of the presenting part on the placenta. The foetus is almost certain to die and the mother may sustain severe lacerations.

Willett's forceps

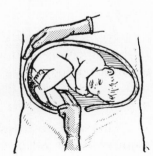

Willett's forceps in position

The membranes are ruptured and the placenta may have to be torn through as well. The forceps are applied to the foetal scalp and traction applied by a weight of up to 1 lb. The baby's scalp is certain to become torn and infected, and if it is dead the mother runs a risk of C. welchii infection.

Bringing down a Leg

Usually podalic version must first be done, and is easier by the external technique. Bipolar podalic version is only possible if at least two fingers can be passed through the cervix, and the manoeuvre is difficult unless the baby is small. Once the leg is down labour must be left to advance if section cannot be done in time. Never attempt accouchement forcé (forcible delivery through an incompletely dilated cervix).

Bipolar version

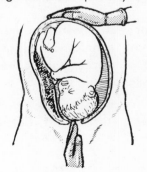
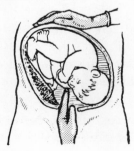

PLACENTAL LOCALIZATION BY X-RAYS

Soft Tissue Radiography (STR)

The uterus, placenta and liquor have the same radiodensity but can be clearly distinguished from the more opaque shadow of the foetal skin and subcutaneous fat, especially when the foetus is mature. This technique will display a normal implantation but not one in the pelvis where bone density intervenes.

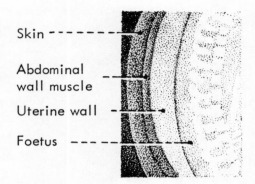

Skin

Abdominal wall muscle

Uterine wall

Foetus

Presenting Part Displacement

This technique is useful when STR does not show an upper segment implantation and the presentation is vertex. Postural X-rays are taken with the patient erect and semi-recumbent and gravity should cause the vertex to descend to within 2 cm of the symphysis and promontory, provided bladder and rectum are empty. A constant displacement of the vertex suggests placenta praevia. AP films will show lateral displacements.

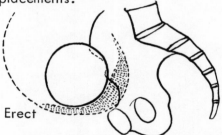

Erect

Anterior displacement in case of anterior PP.

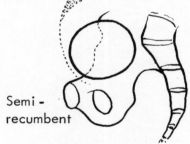

Semi-recumbent

The vertex is within 2 cm of promontory, excluding posterior PP.

Some radiologists will outline the bladder or rectum with air or contrast media if the diagnosis is in doubt, but other radiological techniques such as amniography or arteriography have proved too dangerous or too complex for routine use. In the best hands X-rays can produce an accurate diagnosis in 95% of cases but some experience is needed.

Placental localisation can also be carried out by ultrasound, but the equipment required is not yet generally available.

ABRUPTIO PLACENTAE (ACCIDENTAL HAEMORRHAGE)

This is bleeding due to complete or partial separation of a normally situated placenta from its site after 28 weeks gestation. It can on occasion occur earlier.

The amount of bleeding may vary from being all revealed with none retained (external accidental haemorrhage) to complete retention (concealed accidental haemorrhage). Part revealed and part concealed is the most common. All bleeding being concealed is uncommon. As a rule the greater the concealed element, the greater the shock.

Concealed Haemorrhage

This is a grave emergency. There is pain and collapse. The uterus is tender and 'wooden' to touch. The foetal heart is absent. A blood transfusion is organised and the patient's blood fibrinogen is checked (normal – at least 400 mg).

Rapid Tests

5 ml blood into 1 ml thrombin – normally should give rapid coagulation.

5 ml blood into dry tube – normally should give blood clot formation in 5 – 10 minutes.

Commercial testing outfits are available which can quickly demonstrate fibrinogen levels below 100 mg. It is postulated that the body fibrinogen is mobilised to deal with the bleeding and is thus depleted.

Concealed haemorrhage

Treatment

Morphine, 10 – 15 mg to combat shock.

Blood Transfusion beyond clinical estimate of need.

Fibrinogen. Up to 6 gm are given initially if required or concentrated plasma (1 bottle plasma contains 1.0 gm fibrinogen).

When shock is relieved patient tends to go into labour. If not, then the membranes are ruptured artificially and oxytocin may be given. The aim is to complete delivery in 4 – 6 hours from the incident.

Drew-Smythe cannula

Caesarean section may be the method of choice. There may be severe post-partum bleeding. The condition may be fatal.

When shock is passing off the blood pressure rises and albuminuria is present.

ABRUPTIO PLACENTAE

The shock phase may have been so severe as to cause ultimate renal failure with first haemoglobinuria, then oliguria or anuria.

This is due to renal cortical necrosis or lower nephron nephrosis.

The urinary output is checked carefully.

Afibrinogenaemia if untreated or inadequately treated leads to massive clotting failure and catastrophic bleeding. Epsilon aminocaproic acid is used to inhibit fibrinolysin (see page 410).

Heavy blood loss and shock can cause pituitary necrosis leading to Sheehan's disease.

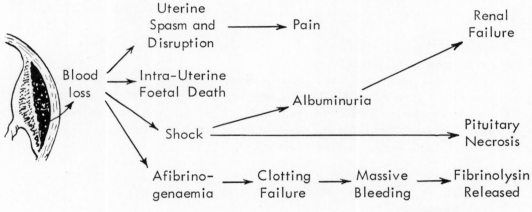

Couvelaire uterus (utero-placental apoplexy) is the term used to describe an extravasation of blood into the uterine wall especially at the borders and spreading into the broad ligament tissues. There may be splits of the uterine musculature and peritoneum with blood stained fluid in the abdomen.

Death is due to uncontrolled bleeding and shock or later by renal or pituitary failure.

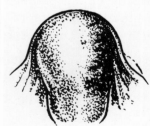

Couvelaire uterus

ABRUPTIO PLACENTAE

Minor retroplacental bleeding sometimes occurs. There is a tender spot on the uterus if the placenta is to the front. There is complaint of pain but little systemic upset.

Albuminuria and high blood pressure tend to follow. Treatment is bed rest, sedation and observation. Further episodes may occur, and induction of labour or Caesarean section may then be considered.

At delivery an old blood clot is found in a crater in the placenta.

Foetal growth tends to be retarded.

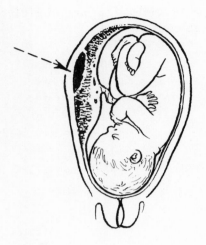

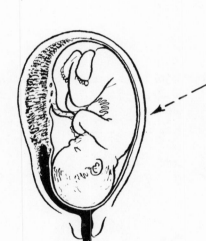

External bleeding alone causes little upset.

Treatment is by bed rest, sedation and observation. Haemoglobin and fibrinogen levels should be estimated.

The pregnancy is allowed to continue. Bleeding of this type could be due to placenta praevia or excessive show prior to labour.

The mixed bleedings (concealed and external) are dependent on the concealed element for the systemic upset and this will dictate the treatment.

In 100 cases of antepartum haemorrhage 36 – 40 will be due to abruptio of some degree, 34 – 38 to manifestations of placenta praevia, 16 will be of unknown origin and the rest 8 – 10 will be from incidental causes (e.g. cervical polyp).

ABRUPTIO PLACENTAE

The aetiology of abruptio is unknown but several factors have been postulated as linked causes.

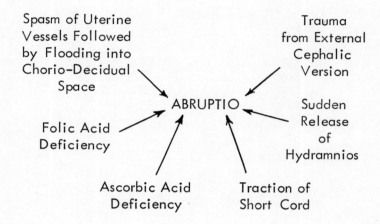

Spasm of Uterine Vessels Followed by Flooding into Chorio-Decidual Space

Trauma from External Cephalic Version

Folic Acid Deficiency

ABRUPTIO

Sudden Release of Hydramnios

Ascorbic Acid Deficiency

Traction of Short Cord

Certain patients seem susceptible to abruptio but again the reason is unknown.

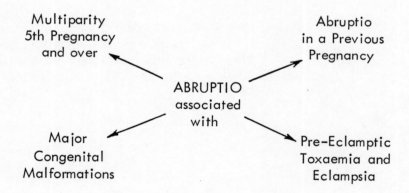

Multiparity 5th Pregnancy and over

Abruptio in a Previous Pregnancy

ABRUPTIO associated with

Major Congenital Malformations

Pre-Eclamptic Toxaemia and Eclampsia

Age irrespective of parity is not a factor.

COAGULATION FAILURE IN PREGNANCY

The coagulability of blood is controlled by two mechanisms:-

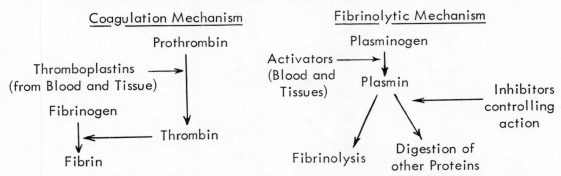

Coagulation Mechanism

Fibrinolytic Mechanism

These two mechanisms are normally in a state of dynamic equilibrium. The coagulation mechanism is activated whenever vascular endothelium is breached. Fibrinolysis prevents vascular occlusion as soon as endothelial integrity is restored and removes the fibrin scaffold when no longer required in areas of repair.

Deficiency or absence of blood clotting can be brought about in two ways:-

1. Depletion of fibrinogen and other factors due to the formation of either a large blood clot or multiple small intravascular thrombi. Frequently both lesions are present due to escape of tissue thromboplastins into the blood stream.

2. Excessive production of plasminogen activators resulting in lysis of any clot formed.

These usually form two phases of the coagulation defect syndrome. Phase 1 depletion of fibrinogen is always present and, by the nature of the lesion causing it, is apt to initiate the phase of fibrinolysis.

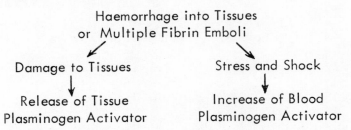

Phase 2 is particularly liable to occur in pregnancy since plasminogen activator is present in high concentration in the uterus, placenta and lungs.

COAGULATION FAILURE IN PREGNANCY

Once these two phases are in operation a further complication arises due to their interaction. Fibrin strand formation takes place in three steps.

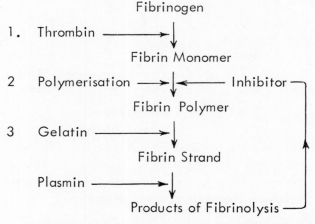

The products of fibrinolysis interfere with the second step and result in poor clot formation which is more susceptible to fibrinolysis. A vicious circle is therefore set up.

In addition to the coagulation defect the patient frequently exhibits symptoms of stress of a degree quite unrelated to the magnitude of the original causative condition. This is probably due to inadequate inhibition of the digestive action of plasmin.

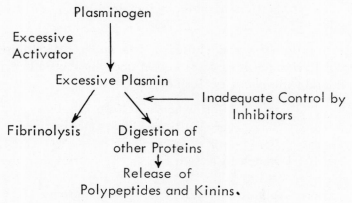

Kinins which are the result of digestion of α_2 globulins cause pain, increased permeability of capillaries, contraction of some smooth muscles and relaxation of others.

COAGULATION FAILURE IN PREGNANCY

The position may be summarised as follows:-

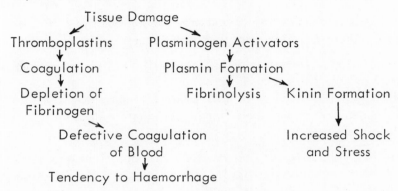

Tissue Damage

Thromboplastins   Plasminogen Activators

Coagulation   Plasmin Formation

Depletion of   Fibrinolysis   Kinin Formation
Fibrinogen

Defective Coagulation   Increased Shock
of Blood   and Stress

Tendency to Haemorrhage

AETIOLOGY

The coagulation failure syndrome is associated mainly with four conditions in pregnancy.

1 <u>Concealed Accidental Haemorrhage</u>

Clot ≡ depletes fibrinogen

Damage to uterus and placenta ≡ escape of thromboplastins and plasminogen activators into general circulation.

2. <u>Amniotic Fluid Embolism</u>. This is of sudden onset frequently preceded by violent uterine contractions. Multiple small emboli lodge in the lungs. Venous and pulmonary arterial pressures are increased.
Multiple small intravascular fibrin clots are formed as well as amniotic emboli. Fibrinolysins are probably released from the damaged lung.

3. <u>Retention of a Dead Foetus</u>. A coagulation defect may occur in this condition but only if the dead foetus is retained for at least one month. Thromboplastins causing intravascular thrombi, and plasminogen activators are liberated from the degenerating placenta and foetus.

4. <u>Septic Abortion</u>. The mechanism is similar in this condition, various factors being liberated by the necrotic tissues. The condition is complicated by the presence of infection which may cause a kind of Schwartzman reaction.

COAGULATION FAILURE IN PREGNANCY

DIAGNOSIS AND TREATMENT

Although a coagulation defect may be obvious the difficulty lies in diagnosing the phase. There are theoretically three phases.

1. Coagulation. Thromboplastins may still be circulating in the blood even after the available fibrinogen is consumed.
2. Fibrinogen Depletion. In this phase thromboplastins are no longer present but fibrinogen and other blood clotting factors are depleted.
3. Fibrinolysis.

The first phase is of extremely short duration and scarcely influences the approach to treatment. Difficulty lies mainly in differentiating phases 2 and 3 due to the fact that the patient's condition is usually critical and specific laboratory tests are too time-consuming.

Fibrinogen deficiency can be quickly demonstrated by the Fibrindex (Ortho) or other similar test. The occurrence of an episode of intravascular fibrinogen-fibrin conversion is suggested by a low platelet count.

Fibrinolysis is suspected when any clots which have formed disappear when the blood is left to stand. If no clots have formed the patient's plasma may be tested against normal whole blood or euglobulin clots. Lysis occurs if fibrinolysins are present. Nevertheless, difficulty is experienced in making a definite diagnosis in many cases.

It is wisest to treat these cases expectantly by concentrating on the circulatory condition. Whole blood, and if necessary fibrinogen, should be given. Specific fibrinolytic inhibitor, epsilon-amino-caproic acid (EACA) should be kept for those patients who do not respond to these measures and whose lives are endangered by continuing haemorrhage.

Concealed accidental haemorrhage is the commonest cause of coagulation failure. In such a case the following steps should be carried out.

1. Treat shock.
2. Determine blood group.
3. Replace blood lost.
4. Carry out fibrindex test.
5. Give fibrinogen, if necessary.
6. If patient continues to bleed, test for fibrinolysins.
7. Give EACA if required.

HYDATIDIFORM MOLE

A degenerative or neoplastic condition of the trophoblast.

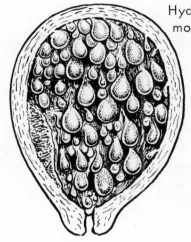

Hydatidiform
mole in situ

A part or the whole of the villous structure changes to a mass of hydropic vesicles of varying size. Some normal placental tissue may persist and nourish the embryo; but usually the whole trophoblast is involved and the embryo is absorbed.

Microscopic Characteristics

1. Trophoblastic proliferation.
2. Hydropic degeneration of vesicles.
3. Destruction of villous blood vessels.

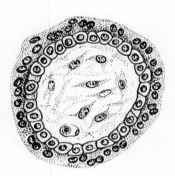

Normal chorionic
villus

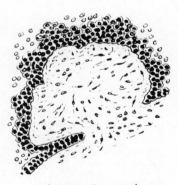

A hydatid vesicle
showing trophoblastic
proliferation

The trophoblastic cells retain the ability to invade maternal blood vessels by which they are nourished.

411

HYDATIDIFORM MOLE

HORMONAL EFFECTS

The proliferating cytotropho-blast continues to secrete HCG; and usually (but not always) large amounts of HCG are excreted in the urine. Serial dilutions of over 1 in 500 may be obtained in the so called 'quantitative' pregnancy tests.

Effects of increased HCG levels;

1. Ovaries are stimulated to develop multiple lutein cysts which regress when the mole is delivered. The ovaries may be as large as tangerines and are often easily palpable.

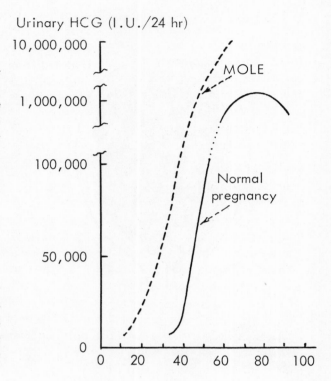

2. Hyperemesis may be very severe. This has been attributed to high HCG levels but may be due to the early increase in oestrogen level.

3. Pre-eclampsia early in the second trimester is associated with mole, and the high HCG level has been considered as a cause, but excessive uterine enlargement may contribute.

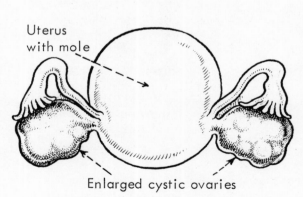

Uterus with mole

Enlarged cystic ovaries

HYDATIDIFORM MOLE

CLINICAL FEATURES   Haemorrhage occurs about the 12th week and may be slight
or heavy. If continued, sepsis often intervenes.

Anaemia may be a good deal more severe than the amount of blood loss seems to justify. There is often a large amount of blood clot retained in the uterus and this is sometimes a cause of pelvic cramp.

Normal symptoms of pregnancy are accentuated, such as breast discomfort, sickness. There may be early pre-eclampsia.

Uterine enlargement is usually beyond the expected degree, and quickening is not felt (although the patient may be confused about this).

DIAGNOSIS can be difficult
1. Sometimes a few vesicles are passed per vaginam, but often only blood comes and diagnosis is made at curettage for incomplete abortion.
2. A positive result from a pregnancy test on a 1 in 500 dilution of urine is strongly suggestive. But some moles do not secrete such amounts of HCG.
3. Absence of foetal parts on X-ray examination will exclude normal pregnancy if there is firm evidence of maturity; but dates can be wrong.
4. If ultrasonoscopy is available a definite diagnosis can be made.

TREATMENT   1. Because of the invasive nature of trophoblastic tissue, there are always risks of severe haemorrhage and uterine perforation.
2. If abortion has not begun spontaneously, medical induction with stilboestrol and oxytocin should be tried.
3. If unsuccessful, dilatation and curettage must be performed. This is done in theatre with facilities for laparotomy if necessary. Blood and oxytocin infusions should be in position and 4 pints of blood should be available.
4. The technique varies with the operator, but one method is to dilate the cervix with great care until an ovum forceps can be introduced. Molar tissue is removed with forceps and blunt curette until the cavity feels fairly empty and bleeding is slight. The uterus is packed and curettage repeated in 48 hours.

FOLLOW-UP. A hydatidiform mole may become malignant so the patient must be watched for at least a year.
1. The pregnancy test must be negative by 6 weeks after delivery of the mole. Tests should be repeated at 3 monthly intervals.
2. The patient should be warned not to start another pregnancy during this follow-up year so that the significance of positive tests is not obscured.

CHORIONEPITHELIOMA

Any malignant condition originating in chorionic epithelium.

It is uncommon and is usually a sequel to a mole but may follow abortion or normal pregnancy. Functioning trophoblast cells persist in the myometrium and after a varying period – sometimes several years – begin to proliferate. Histological appearances vary very much and are not well correlated with the degree of invasiveness: but there are two broad categories.

1. INVASIVE MOLE
(Syn: chorionadenoma destruens)

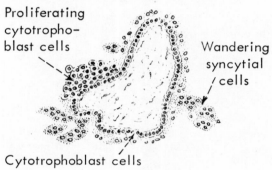

Proliferating cytotropho-blast cells

Wandering syncytial cells

Cytotrophoblast cells

Cyto- and syncytiotrophoblast proliferate, and there are signs of villus formation. The myometrium may be invaded by wandering syncytial cells.

2. CHORIONCARCINOMA

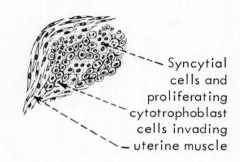

Syncytial cells and proliferating cytotrophoblast cells invading uterine muscle

Villous formation is absent. Masses of syncytial cells of irregular size mingle with a proliferation of cyto-trophoblast cells. There are no vessels, but many blood cells. Mitotic figures are common.

SYMPTOMS AND SIGNS

1. Irregular bleeding accompanied by a persistently positive pregnancy test, usually following a molar pregnancy. If tumour is found in the uterus it will be friable and haemorrhagic.
2. Because of the natural invasiveness of trophoblastic tumour, metastasis is common although the histological appearances may be almost benign. Common sites are the genital tract and lungs. Dyspnoea, haemoptysis, chest pain are serious signs.

CHORIONEPITHELIOMA

DIAGNOSIS

This is simple if the biopsy shows frank carcinoma, (and the pregnancy test is repeatedly positive often in high titre). But:-

1. Although all trophoblast cells secrete HCG, the concentration may be below that required to give a positive result with a conventional pregnancy test.
2. Trophoblast cells may be embedded in myometrium, out of reach of the curette.
3. Even when biopsy is obtained histological appearance is not by itself diagnostic.

The patient may exhibit 'clinical choriomatosis' – a positive pregnancy test, irregular bleeding, pulmonary shadows on X-ray, haemoptysis without any histological evidence of tumour being obtained; and the clinician may find himself obliged to advise radical treatment for cancer without being certain of the diagnosis. At the present day attempts are being made to refine assays of HCG, and to improve arteriographic techniques which would show up presence of persisting trophoblastic tissue.

TREATMENT

This is always aimed at cure, since metastases may regress after extirpation of the primary, and cytotoxic drugs exert a systemic effect. Successful treatment is indicated by a persistently negative pregnancy test.

Total hysterectomy must always be performed, with preservation of the ovaries in young women. When the diagnosis is definitely chorioncarcinoma, or when there is evidence of metastasis, or when there is still secretion of HCG a fortnight after operatiom, cytotoxic drugs should be used.

Cytotoxic Drugs are antimitotic substances which interfere with cell division.

Methotrexate prevents the formation of folinic acid from folic acid (essential to trophoblastic tissue) and is specific for chorionepithelioma. Cyclophosphamide is usually given as well, and is an all-purpose cytotoxic drug.

They have many serious side effects – stomatitis, diarrhoea and vomiting, intestinal ulceration, pancytopaenia, alopecia. Such conditions are usually reversible, but because of them cytotoxic drugs may not be used prophylactically.

Dosage is controlled by daily white cell counts, and is of the order of methotrexate 15 mg, cyclophosphamide 200 mg for 3 five-day courses with a rest in between.

CARCINOMA OF THE CERVIX IN PREGNANCY

The incidence is said to be about 1 in 6,000 pregnancies. The results of treatment should be as good as in the non-pregnant woman unless diagnosis has been delayed.

The presenting symptom is usually bleeding; and speculum appearances suggest the need for biopsy. Cervical cytology discovers some cases of malignancy before symptoms appear. Histological diagnosis is made difficult by the high steroid hormone levels of pregnancy and expert opinion must be taken. Diagnosis, including the use of cone biopsy where indicated, must be pursued with the same determination and urgency as in the non-pregnant patient.

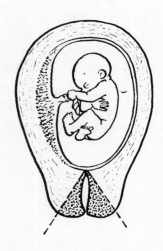

TREATMENT

1. If a definite diagnosis of non-invasive cancer is made (ie.e if the cone biopsy shows no sign of spread through the basement membrane) the pregnancy may be allowed to continue until the foetus is of a size to justify delivery.

2. If the cancer is invasive and considered curable, the pregnancy should be terminated forthwith by hysterotomy or classical section. (Any delay in the interests of the foetus increases the risk to the mother).

A cone biopsy must reach to the internal os and include all the epithelium of the canal and the portio vaginalis.

The operation causes severe bleeding and there is an obvious risk of abortion which must be accepted.

3. Thereafter treatment becomes a gynaecological problem. Radical Caesarean hysterectomy has been advocated, to avoid delay once the diagnosis is made: but the thorough clearance of pelvic connective tissue and lymph nodes must increase the risks of operation when done in the presence of the immense vascularity of the pelvis in pregnancy.

CHAPTER 17

OBSTETRICAL OPERATIONS

INDUCTION OF LABOUR—SURGICAL

Surgical Induction

This means bringing about the onset of labour by artificial means. It is achieved surgically by rupturing the membranes and withdrawing liquor, or medically by giving oxytocin.

Indications

1. Suspected Placental Insufficiency. It is known that foetal mortality increases as pregnancy passes the delivery date, especially in older women, so post-maturity is a frequent indication. Some maternal diseases such as pre-eclampsia, hypertension, diabetes also affect the placenta adversely, and it is usual to in-duce labour in such patients 2 or 3 weeks before term.
2. Maternal Disease. The pregnancy might have to be terminated in the mother's interests in cases of severe pre-eclampsia, eclampsia, chronic renal disease and cardio-respiratory failure.
3. Suspected or Potential Disproportion. Induction might be attempted in an effort to obtain a baby of deliverable size.
4. Foetal Disease. A foetus affected by Rh factor incompatibility may have to be delivered prematurely. Induction is usually carried out in the case of foetal monsters.

Surgical Induction (Artificial Rupture of Membranes: Amniotomy)

Either the hindwaters or the forewaters can be ruptured, and the instruments most commonly used are:-

The Drew-Smythe Cannula   or   Goodwin's Amniotomy Forceps
         (for hindwaters)   (for forewaters)

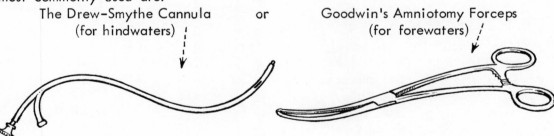

The cannula is shaped to pass behind the foetal head and puncture the amnion in the region of the neck.

The forceps are shaped to fit the cervico-vaginal angle. The teeth tear a hole in the amnion in front of the foetal head.

SURGICAL INDUCTION

Hindwaters Rupture

The patient is placed in the lithotomy position, cleaned and draped. No anaesthetic is necessary, but nervous patients will benefit from sedation, and a full explanation should be given of the proposed operation. The operator, gowned and gloved, inserts one or two fingers gently into the vagina and cervix, and if possible sweeps the membranes off the uterine wall. The cannula is passed up behind the foetal head, the stilette

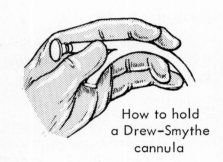

How to hold a Drew-Smythe cannula

pressed home, and with the assistance of gentle movements of the cannula, sideways and downwards, a free flow of liquor is produced. As much as can be obtained is drained off. In primigravidae, it is often easier to pass the cannula under direct vision.

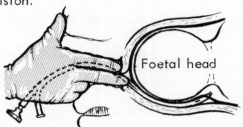

Passing the cannula by hand.

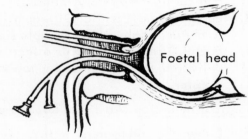

Passing the cannula under direct vision.

Forewaters Rupture

The preparation is the same, but amniotomy forceps are used to tear the amnion covering the internal os. Liquor should trickle out of the vagina, and if the presenting part is mobile, it should be gently pushed up to allow a free flow.

With both types of amniotomy as much liquor as possible should be removed, and it must of course be inspected for meconium. On completion the foetal heart should be listened to to make sure that the change in its environment has not harmed it.

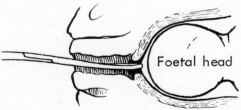

COMPLICATIONS OF SURGICAL INDUCTION

1. Failure to Bring about Labour.

'Failed induction' means failure of labour to ensue within an arbitrary time-limit, varying between 12 and 48 hours. About 80% of patients will go into labour within 24 hours, but all methods of induction are subject to this un-reliability and consequently lead to an increased incidence of Caesarean section.

2. Sepsis.
Delay in the onset of labour leads inevitably to infection of the uterine cavity from the vagina after about 48 hours. Both mother and child are involved, and the foetus may develop intra-uterine pneumonia. (There is an excessively rare condition called vagitus uterinus in which the foetus can be heard giving faint kitten-like cries while still in utero. It occurs when the membranes are ruptured and anoxia is stimulating foetal respiratory effort.)

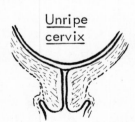

Unripe cervix

An unripe cervix is hard, long, closed and not effaced.

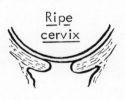

Ripe cervix

A ripe cervix is soft, effaced or becoming effaced and admits the finger.

Precautions

1. An attempt at selection of cases for induction should be made. Factors associated with successful surgical induction are:-

a) The state of the cervix - the riper the better.
b) the maturity - the later the better.
c) the level of the presenting part - the lower the better.
d) the parity of the patient - it is more difficult to induce labour in women of high parity.

2. The aseptic precautions described should be observed scrupulously; but of course the vagina cannot be sterilised.

3. The interval between induction and birth should be kept as short as possible by following amniotomy with oxytocin induction within 12 or 24 hours.

4. Antibiotic cover should be prescribed as a routine 24 hours after amniotomy unless the patient is well established in labour. Before doing this, vaginal swabs should be sent to the bacteriologist.

5. The presence of purulent discharge following amniotomy in a patient not in labour should be regarded as an indication for section.

COMPLICATIONS OF SURGICAL INDUCTION

3. <u>Bleeding</u>. The cannula may start bleeding, either foetal or maternal, which can be so severe that section is indicated. The best method of identifying the source of the blood is Kleihauer's test, a laboratory procedure. After treatment the foetal cells stand out dark in a field of 'ghost' maternal cells.

Precautions

When the presenting part is high, forewaters rupture will avoid this complication. Unfortunately forewaters amniotomy in such circumstances may be technically impossible, especially if the cervix is unripe.

---

4. <u>Prolapse of the Cord</u>. This occurs with an ill-fitting presenting part.

Rupture hindwaters rather than forewaters in such cases, examine the patient with the complication in mind, and watch for sudden foetal distress.

---

5. <u>Placental Separation</u> (abruptio). This may be caused by the sudden reduction in pressure as the liquor is drained off, and occurs in cases of hydramnios.

In such cases cross-matched blood should be to hand. Labour is usually quick and surgical intervention unnecessary.

---

6. <u>Pulmonary Embolism of Amniotic Fluid</u>. This very rare occurrence causes shock that is usually fatal. Symptoms of pulmonary embolism including intense dyspnoea may appear; and often death arrives so quickly that the diagnosis remains presumptive until histological demonstration of vernix and lanugo hairs in the lungs. Amniotic embolism may occur immediately after amniotomy but is usually preceded by strong uterine contractions. If the patient survives the initial shock a coagulation defect is inevitable.

There is no known way of preventing the occurrence of amniotic fluid embolism. The treatment of severe shock has been described on page 330.

> Surgical induction commits the obstetrician to delivering his patient within about 72 hours, if necessary by section. He must be sure that interference is justified.

INDUCTION BY OXYTOCIN

Medical Induction

Oxytocin is a hormone from the posterior pituitary gland, now prepared synthetically.

Oxytocin increases the intensity and frequency of uterine contractions when administered at or near term. Sensitivity to oxytocin varies very much, and to detect this and avoid overdosage administration is begun with very small doses which are gradually increased as indicated by the behaviour of the uterus.

Effects of Overdosage

Excessively strong and painful contractions may be produced, or the uterus may go into tetanic spasm – a continuous contraction causing great pain and killing the foetus. Rarely the contractions may be of such intensity as to cause rupture of the uterus.

Administration

1. By Intravenous Infusion. A typical scheme of administration would be to start with a concentration of 2 units/litre of 5% dextrose, then 4,8 and finally 16 units/litre. Infusion is begun at the rate of 12 drops/minute for 15 minutes, increasing to 24 and then 48 drops for the same period. When the concentration is changed the rate goes back to 24 drops. When good contractions are obtained at any one stage, the concentration and rate are maintained at that level. The infusion may be stopped once labour is fully established.

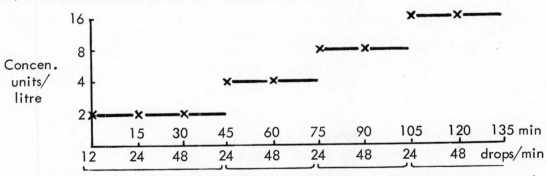

2. By Buccal Absorption. Tablets are placed in the buccal pouch adjacent to the upper molars and oxytocin is absorbed through the buccal mucosa. As with infusion the dosage is gradually increased and maintained at that level which first produces effective and regular contractions. The patient must not eat, drink or smoke during treatment, lest she alter her rate of buccal absorption.

COMPLICATIONS OF OXYTOCIN INDUCTION

1. Failure to bring about labour.
Oxytocin by itself and in the dosage described is not very effective and is usually combined with amniotomy. The 2 methods together are likely to have a 90% success rate (labour ensuing within 24 hours of the oxytocin induction).

<u>Precautions</u>

1. The factors influencing successful amniotomy are just as important with oxytocin and attemps should be made at selection.
2. It is probable that higher dosages than those described here can be given with safety but they are not yet generally in use because of the great need for caution.

---

2. Persistent rapidity or irregularity of the foetal heart.

The oxytocin administration must be stopped.

---

3. Strong contractions or tetanic spasm.

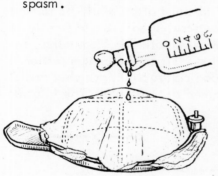

1. Patients receiving oxytocin must be under continuous observation and the drug is not suitable for domiciliary use.
2. Infusion must be stopped at once, and tablets spat out.
3. Chloroform should be given from a dropper bottle on to a Schimmelbusch mask to relieve pain and depress uterine contractions. This may have to be kept up for half-an-hour or more, and the patient may even then carry on with a painful and rapid labour. If contractions cannot be controlled in this manner, the patient may require section.

---

4. Rupture of the uterus

1. Oxytocin must never be given to patients who might be regarded as prone to this condition. These include women of high parity or who have had a previous section, and women suffering from disproportion (or suspected disproportion) or malpresentation.

2. Rupture is suspected because of the pain, the alteration in abdominal shape, the difficulty in palpation, the shock (see page 307). Treatment is immediate laparotomy.

OTHER METHODS OF INDUCTION

Castor Oil

This drug is absorbed from the small intestine and its action is therefore systemic. It is traditionally given in a 2 oz. dose (57 ml) followed by a soapsuds enema and then a hot bath, and will sometimes precipitate contractions in a patient who was about to go into labour spontaneously. Castor oil is probably retained in modern practice only because it satisfies the need of the midwife and her patient for a harmless treatment that has the name of action.

Quinine

This drug increases uterine irritability and will lower the threshold of response to other methods of induction. Nausea and tinnitus are unpleasant side-effects when quinine is given orally, and there is an association with foetal distress which has put the drug out of favour except in cases of intra-uterine death. Rectal administration is more pleasant for the mother, and 0.25 gm by suppository every 6 hours started at the time of amniotomy has no ill effect on the foetus.

Oestrogens

These hormones are of no use when the foetus is alive, but are occasionally used in an attempt to induce labour in cases of intra-uterine death. Large doses are given e.g. stilboestrol 10 mg 4-hourly (if the patient will tolerate it) for several days, followed by oxytocin; but their effectiveness is debatable.

Sparteine Sulphate

Sparteine is an alkaloid of the curare group which has an effect on the uterus similar to oxytocin. It has not been found to have any advantage over oxytocin, and as it is less safe and less reliable in its action it has not been extensively used.

Intra-Amniotic Injection of Hypertonic Saline

This method is of use in cases of intra-uterine death when oxytocin is contra-indicated. As much liquor as possible is withdrawn from the amniotic sac by paracentesis, and replaced with a slightly larger volume of 20% sodium chloride which would of course kill a live foetus. The average injection-delivery period is about 36 hours and a success rate of over 90% is claimed. However amniocentesis must carry a definite though slight risk of sepsis, and most women with an intra-uterine death can be left to go spontaneously into labour.

EPISIOTOMY

EPISIOTOMY   (Gr. A cutting of the pubic region)

Making an incision in the perineal body at the time of delivery.

INDICATIONS

1. To prevent a perineal tear or excessive stretching of the muscles. A tear is less controllable and may involve the anal sphincter, and overstretching will pre-dispose to prolapse in later years.

2. To protect the foetus if it is premature or is being forced repeatedly against an unyielding perineum which is obstructing delivery.

3. To prevent damage from an abnormal presenting part – occipitoposterior positions, face presentations, after-coming head in breech deliveries, all instrumental deliveries. In such cases it may be done before the perineum is distended. The obstetrician must himself put the tissues on the stretch before cutting.

TYPES OF INCISION

1. The median incision is easiest to make and to repair, but in the event of extension it does not give any protection to the anal sphincter.

2. The posterolateral incision is more difficult to repair as the edges retract unequally. Anatomical apposition is sometimes difficult to achieve and infection may appear. It gives the best protection against sphincter damage, and best answers the purpose of the operation.

3. The 'J-shaped' incision is a theoretical compromise which becomes a posterolateral incision in practice.

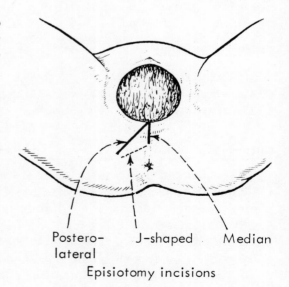

Postero-   J-shaped   Median
lateral

Episiotomy incisions

EPISIOTOMY

ANAESTHESIA

In the conscious patient the best method is to inject 10 ml of lignocaine 1%. Five minutes are required for this to be given and take effect; and if time is short deep breaths of Trilene or Entonox will serve.

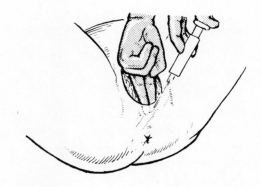

TECHNIQUE

Two fingers are placed as shown to protect the foetal head, and a long clean cut is made with scissors. It is important to start from the fourchette, otherwise anatomical apposition will be difficult when the repair is undertaken. Too long an incision will open up the ischiorectal fossa and fatty tissue will be seen, but provided there is no infection this does not affect healing.

The timing of an episiotomy must be learnt by experience. If done too soon, blood loss will increase, if delayed too long, a tear of the vagina or deep perineal muscles will occur.

The repair of an episiotomy is carried out in the same way as the repair of a perineal tear, described on page 300.

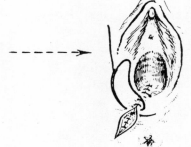

VERSION

Turning the foetus inside the uterus so as to obtain a more favourable presentation.

External Cephalic Version in which the foetus is turned from a breech or transverse lie to vertex presentation is the most common manoeuvre today. All manipulation is from outside the abdomen.

It should be attempted from the 32nd week onward and if unsuccessful it is customary after the 35th week to make an attempt with the patient anaesthetised. Good abdominal relaxation is necessary and chloroform or halothane will also reduce uterine tone. The mother's skin should be powdered to prevent excoriation by the operator's hands.

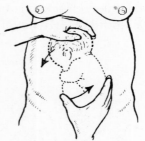

1. The breech must be eased out of the pelvis.

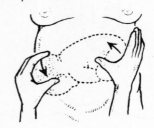

2. The left hand applies pressure to the head and the foetus is flexed between the two hands to allow it to slide round.

3. Once past the transverse the hands simply push the foetus into position.

Complications

1. The placenta may be partly separated. The foetal heart must be checked on completion and the vagina examined for bleeding.
2. Excessive force may rupture the uterus.
3. There may be unsuspected complications such as an abnormal uterus or short umbilical cord.

Contra-Indications

1. Toxaemia (as predisposing to placental bleeding).
2. Previous scar on the uterus.
3. Multiple pregnancy or foetal abnormality.

The commonest causes of failure are too large a foetus or too little liquor, or 'splinting' of the foetus by extended legs.

VERSION

Internal Podalic Version in which the operator has one hand inside the uterus to turn the foetus to breech presentation is the other type of version which has an occasional indication today.

It is attempted only at full or nearly full dilatation, with the membranes ruptured, either to correct a transverse lie or to turn a second twin which is not engaging, and in both cases the object is to achieve delivery by breech extraction.

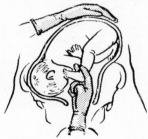

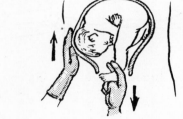

1. The anterior foot is grasped by the heel. (Pulling on the posterior limb tends to turn the baby's back to the back of the uterus: if possible both feet should be grasped.)

2. Downward traction is made on the leg and the outside hand presses the head upwards.

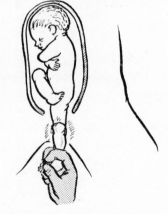

3. Gentle traction is made on the delivered leg until the breech is fixed, then the other leg is extracted and the foetus delivered by breech extraction.

Complications

There is a risk of uterine rupture, of injury to the foetus, and of infection.

Ideally this operation should only be undertaken when laparotomy can be resorted to in case of rupture. It should never be attempted when the uterus has contracted down on an impacted foetus and the lower segment is thin. In such circumstances even if the foetus is dead classical Caesarean section may be the method of choice unless embryotomy is preferred.

OBSTETRIC FORCEPS

The obstetric forceps are designed to grasp the foetal head when it is in the vagina and effect delivery by traction without causing injury.

A pair of forceps consist of two arms which can be articulated.

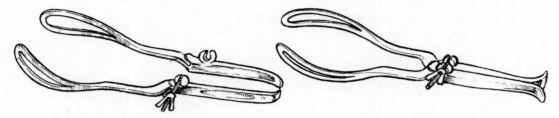

The blades have two curves:

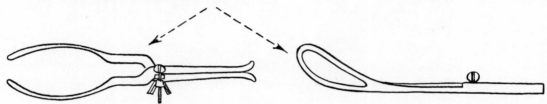

The cephalic curve is adapted to provide a good application to the foetal head.

The pelvic curve allows the blades to fit in with the curve of the birth canal.

There are several kinds of lock:

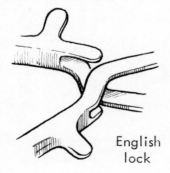

English
lock

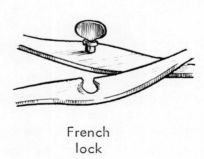

French
lock

OBSTETRIC FORCEPS

Because of the pelvic curve which would necessitate traction 'round a corner' some forceps have detachable rods which allow traction in the pelvic axis (axis traction).

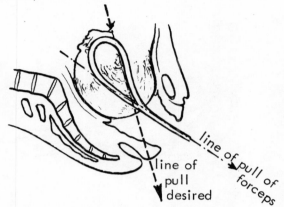

axis traction rod pulling in axis of pelvic curve

Forceps operations are of two kinds:

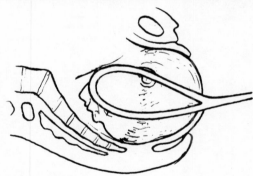

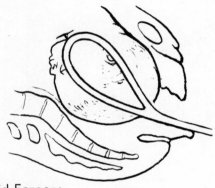

Low Forceps

The foetal head has reached the perineal floor and is visible at the vulva.

Mid Forceps

Engagement has taken place and the leading part of the head is at or below the level of the ischial spines.

Application of the forceps when the head has not engaged (i.e. when the greatest diameter has yet to pass through the brim) is known as a 'high forceps'. It is dangerous for both mother and child, and has been replaced by Caesarean section.

OBSTETRIC FORCEPS

There are very many different patterns. The forceps shown here are all well known and are identified with the **three** main operations – the low forceps, the mid forceps, and the rotation-extraction forceps delivery.

Wrigley's Forceps

Wrigley's Forceps are designed for use when the head is on the perineum and local anaesthesia is being used. It is a short light instrument with pelvic and cephalic curves and an English lock.

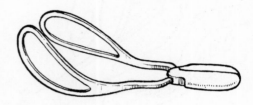

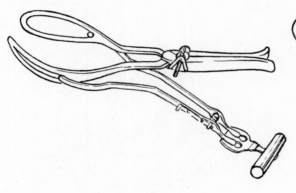

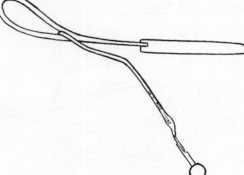

Milne Murray's Axis Traction Forceps

In theory the axis traction rods which were designed to apply traction to a head high in the pelvis are now obsolete; but in practice they are often of considerable help and the action of the rods allows the forceps blades to move more naturally along the pelvic curve without hindrance from the operator's hands. The forceps have an English lock and an additional screw lock to maintain a firm application, and the traction rods are connected in such a way as to give the best mechanical advantage. This instrument is a little awkward for the beginner, and the traction rods if used may damage the perineum unless a large episiotomy is made.

OBSTETRIC FORCEPS

Kielland's forceps were originally designed to deliver the foetal head at or above the pelvic brim. They are used today for rotation and extraction of the head which is arrested in the deep transverse or occipito-posterior positions.

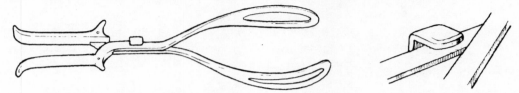

They have very little pelvic curve and are virtually an axis traction forceps so a large episiotomy is needed. The shallowness of this curve allows safe rotation inside the vagina.

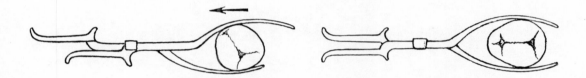

The claw lock allows the blades to slide up and down on each other and correct asynclitism of the foetal head.

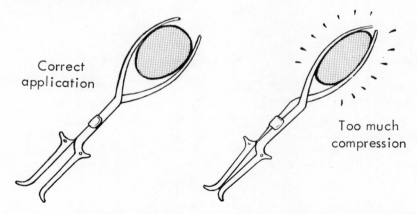

Correct application

Too much compression

This range of movement allowed by the claw lock makes it possible to apply lethal compression to the foetal head if the instrument is used improperly.

USE OF OBSTETRIC FORCEPS

INDICATIONS FOR THE USE OF FORCEPS

1. Second Stage Delay. When progress is absent or slow and the patient is tiring, whatever the position of the occiput. This covers a wide variety of attitudes to the second stage; but in general it may be said that the second stage should not last over an hour in a primigravida and half-an-hour in a multigravida.

2. Foetal Distress.

3. Maternal Distress. When the mother is exhausted by a long labour or is emotionally unequal to the demands of a second stage; or when some condition such as cardiac failure or hypertension makes the effort of the second stage undesirable.

CONDITIONS AND PREPARATIONS FOR FORCEPS DELIVERY

1. The cervix must be fully dilated. If the forceps are applied before this stage is reached the operator may produce severe lacerations and haemorrhage.

2. Except when the head is on the perineum the bladder should be emptied by catheter.

3. The patient should be in the lithotomy position, although some operators find delivery easier with the patient in the left lateral position. She must be cleaned and draped and aseptic precautions must be observed. Negligence in this respect will almost certainly lead to genital infection.

4. For low forceps operations local anaesthesia may be used provided it is acceptable to the mother. It avoids the risks of general anaesthesia and allows the mother to assist in the delivery by bearing down when asked.

5. If general anaesthesia is used, it should be given by an experienced anaesthetist. The stomach must be emptied by gastric suction, the patient should receive premedication, and endotracheal intubation is probably the safest technique.

6. Mechanical suction should be available for mother and child, and the head end of the bed or table used for the operation should be capable of being lowered rapidly if vomiting should occur when the patient is under the anaesthetic.

USE OF ANAESTHESIA FOR FORCEPS DELIVERY

Local anaesthesia for forceps delivery is usually a combination of local in-filtration and pudendal nerve block. Lignocaine 1% without adrenaline is satis-factory and up to 50 ml may be used with safety.

Local infiltration

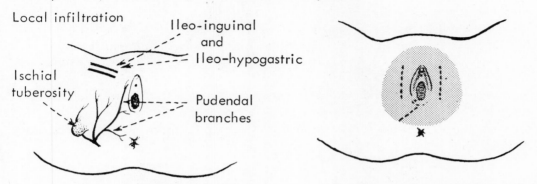

Principal nerves supplying vulva and perineum.

Area of vulva and perineum which should be infiltrated.

Local infiltration is usually all that is needed for low forceps operation.

Pudendal Nerve Block

The forefinger is placed on the ischial spine (behind which runs the pudendal nerve) and a long needle is passed via the ischiorectal fossa. When needle point, spine and finger are in conjunction, 5 ml of lignocaine are injected. It is advisable to withdraw the plunger before injecting to make sure that the needle is not in a blood vessel. The needle, preferably a guarded one can be passed per vaginam if the operator finds it easier.

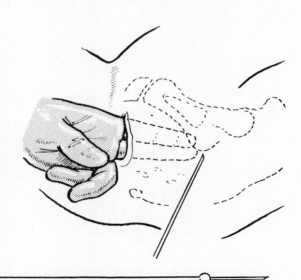

A transvaginal guarded needle.

LOW FORCEPS DELIVERY

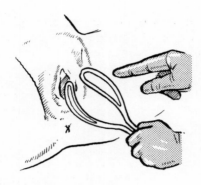

1.   Choosing the left blade.

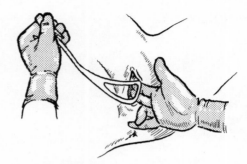

2.   Applying the left blade.

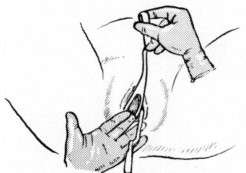

3.   Applying the right blade.

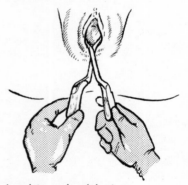

4.   Locking the blades.

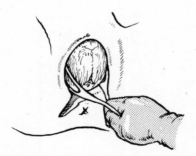

5.   Gentle traction with an episiotomy at crowning.

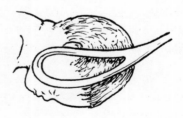

6.   The correct cephalic application (in the mento-vertical line).

MID FORCEPS DELIVERY

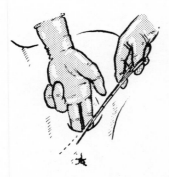

1. Making a large episiotomy before starting.

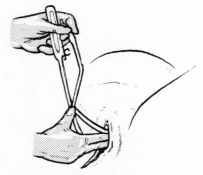

2. Applying the left blade.

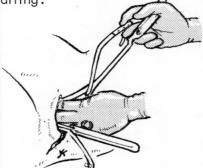

3. Applying the right blade.

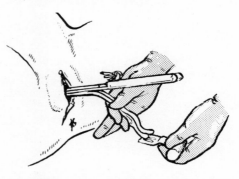

4. Locking the rods and applying the handle.

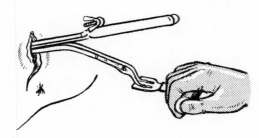

5. Traction, keeping traction rods parallel to the shank.

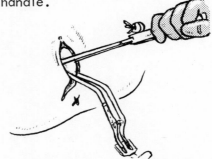

6. As the head crowns the forceps are held by handles and the head is lifted over the perineum.

TRANSVERSE AND O.P. POSITIONS OF VERTEX

It is usually necessary to rotate the head into the occipito-anterior position before effecting forceps delivery, unless the head is low in the pelvis. Rotation is done either with Kielland's forceps or manually.

The first step is to ascertain the exact position. This is not always easy especially if there has been much moulding or caput.

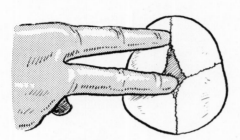 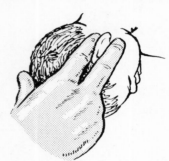

The four sutures and the diamond of the anterior fontanelle may be palpated. It must be distinguished from the other fontanelles.

An ear may be palpable. The root of the pinna must be identifed to distinguish left from right. Gentle traction on the ear may itself correct the position.

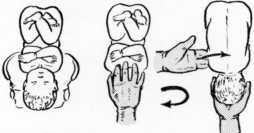

Manual Rotation

The right hand grasps the head anteriorly as shown, while the left hand, through the abdominal wall, pushes the shoulder forward. The head may have to be pushed up slightly to achieve this, and once round it must be held in position until the forceps blades have been applied.

Complications of Manual Rotation

1. Like all vaginal manipulations it increases the risk of infection.
2. The cord may prolapse during rotation, but delivery usually follows at once.
3. There is an increased risk to the foetus, and delivery without rotation is preferable from that aspect. However unless the head is low in the pelvis it is usually impossible to deliver it in the O.P. position without excessive and traumatic force.

DELIVERY WITH KIELLAND'S FORCEPS

The position of the occiput must be known. In this illustration it is lying R.O.L.

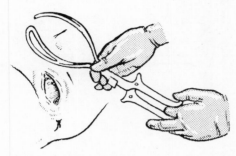

1. Holding forceps with the knobs directed towards foetal occiput.

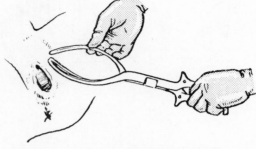

2. The anterior blade must be applied first.

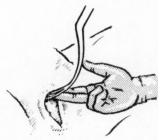

3. The blade is guided, concavity upwards, between head and cervix.

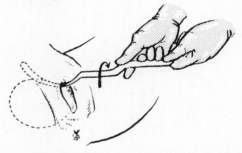

4. Once the blade is completely inside it is gently rotated away from occiput.

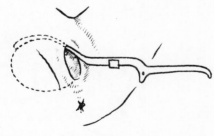

5. It now lies with the concavity of the blade applied to left (uppermost) side of the foetal head.

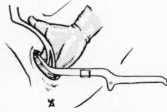

6. The posterior blade is applied directly in the usual manner. The guiding hand must be well inside the vagina.

DELIVERY WITH KIELLAND'S FORCEPS

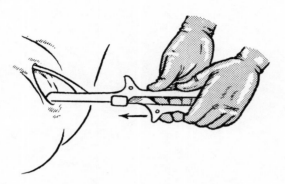

7. The forceps are locked. Note how their position shows asynclitism.

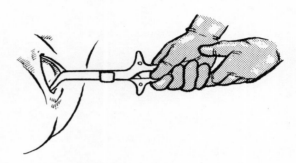

8. Asynclitism is corrected and the forceps blades are opposite each other.

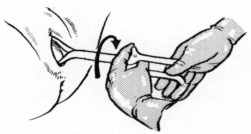

9. The head is gently rotated to the O.A. position.

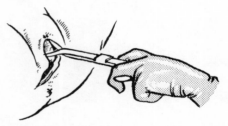

10. More or less at the same time traction is applied in the pelvic axis. A large episiotomy is needed.

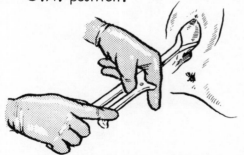

11. To prevent over compression of the baby's head, a thumb is kept between the handles.

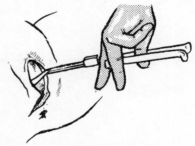

12. As the head extends, the direction of pull must be altered upwards.

DELIVERY WITH KIELLAND'S FORCEPS

Other methods of applying the Anterior Blade.

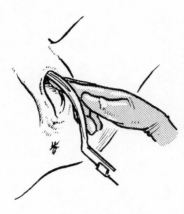

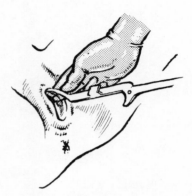

1. The Direct Method. The buttocks must be overhanging the edge of the delivery bed.

2. The 'Wandering' Method. The blade is applied laterally and then gently eased round to the front.

Delivery of the Head in the Occipito-Posterior Position

This is the easiest and often the best method of delivering a foetus with the head in the persistent O.P. position. It was once regarded as 'bad obstetrics'; but if the head is at or near the perineum, it is likely to be deliverable with very little traction, and the foetus is spared the risk inherent in any manipulation. It is important to remember that delivery in this position distends the perineum more than in the O.A. position, and a large episiotomy will be necessary.

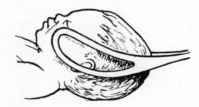

OTHER APPLICATIONS OF FORCEPS

Other Applications of the Forceps

The correct cephalic application is with the head O.A. as shown   - - - - →

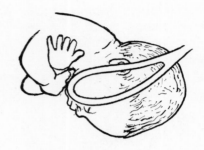

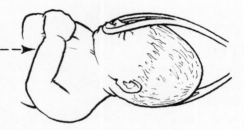

- - - - → Sometimes an oblique grip is obtained. This is undesirable as it may cause intracranial haemorrhage.

If the head is transverse it is permissable to apply the forceps laterally, obtaining an antero-posterior application. Manual rotation or by Kielland's forceps is better.   _ _ →

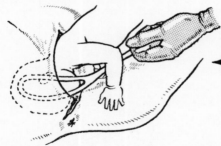

← - - - - In a breech presentation the safest method of delivering head is by applying the forceps once it has entered the pelvis.

In a face presentation (mento-   - - - - →
anterior) the forceps may be applied direct. (Mento-posterior positions must be rotated – see page 235.)

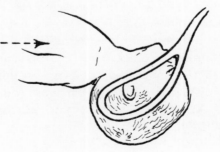

442

COMPLICATIONS OF FORCEPS DELIVERY

LACERATIONS
1. Perineal tears are inevitable unless episiotomy is done at the right time.
2. Vaginal wall may be split especially if compressed between ischial spine and foetal head.
3. Cervical tears may be caused during rotation with Kielland's forceps. After delivery the vagina and cervix should be carefully palpated and all damage repaired.

HAEMORRHAGE
Except from lacerations, haemorrhage is no more likely than after spontaneous delivery. If the uterus is 'atonic' (i.e. if contractions have ceased for some time before delivery) intravenous ergometrine or oxytocin should be given.

INJURIES TO BABY
If the blades have been properly applied, the foetal head should be protected by the rigid case of the forceps blades. Where excessive traction force has been applied, there may be bruising, facial nerve palsy or depression fracture of the skull (see page 359).

FAILED FORCEPS
This is an old term which means that an attempt to deliver with forceps has been unsuccessful. The causes are:-
1. Unsuspected disproportion.
2. Misdiagnosis of the position of the head.
3. Incomplete dilatation of the cervix.
4. Outlet contraction (very rare in an otherwise normal pelvis).

TREATMENT
1. If the patient is in good condition and the cause is undiagnosed malposition, an attempt at correction may be made by an experienced operator. Antibiotic cover should be started and general anaesthesia used.
2. If the cause is incomplete dilatation of the cervix and mother and child are in good condition, the patient should be sedated with morphine 15 mg and promazine 50 mg, given intravenous fluids and antibiotic cover, and observed for a while to see if labour advances.
3. If disproportion is present, or if the patient is exhausted and lacerated, Caesarean section should be carried out. In such circumstances there is a good argument for the classical operation which avoids the oedematous and easily torn lower segment.

VACUUM EXTRACTOR

The vacuum extractor is a traction instrument used as an alternative to the obstetric forceps. It adheres to the baby's scalp by suction and is used in the conscious patient to assist the maternal expulsive efforts.

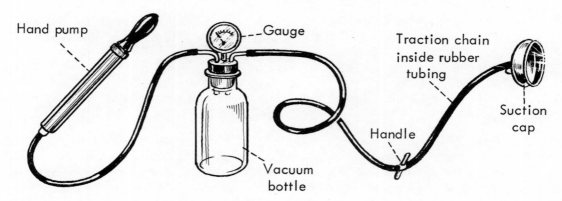

The suction cup obtains its grip by raising an artificial caput. Negative pressure is raised by 0.2 kg/cm^2 every two minutes to a maximum of 0.8. The patient is in the lithotomy position, using inhalation analgesia as required, and the same aseptic precautions are observed as for forceps operations. Probably the most convenient anaesthetic is a pudendal block.

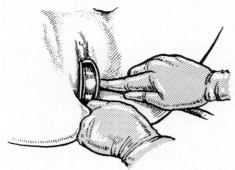

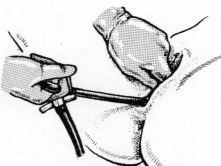

1. The cup is insinuated into the vagina. When applying it to the scalp, the fontanelles and sutures should be avoided.

2. Traction is made downwards with the right hand while the left hand presses against the cup and the foetal head, pressing them against the sacrum.

VACUUM EXTRACTOR

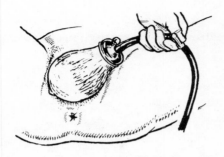 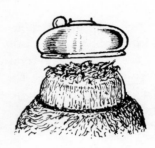

3. As the head is delivered an episiotomy may be necessary.

4. The artificial caput made by suction cup immediately after delivery.

The Place of the Vacuum Extractor

In inexperienced hands it is a simpler and safer instrument than the forceps and it is easier to learn how to use it. It is not however foolproof and serious injury can be done to the foetus by ill-judged and clumsy applications.

It finds its greatest use in second stage delay with the head low in the pelvis and can effectively take the place of the low forceps operation. When the head is in mid-cavity its relevance is not quite so clear although such deliveries are often feasible with the vacuum extractor. Sometimes there is delay in the first stage of labour for no obvious reason; the head is engaged and well flexed but the contractions are poor and the cervix remains three quarters dilated. In such circumstances the application of the forceps would be impossible, but the vacuum extractor may be applied as soon as enough foetal head is exposed to take the suction cup, and in this sort of case the instrument is worth a trial. The knob on the back of the cup allows the operator to feel when spontaneous rotation of the head is occurring as a result of traction and descent.

Precautions to be Observed:

1. The cup adheres to a caput succedaneum artificial or real. Application should take 10 minutes to allow caput to form.
2. The cup should not be kept applied for longer than 45 minutes. After this time there is an increased risk of necrosis.
3. Prolonged or excessive traction should not be used. There should be frequent pauses, and the maximum period during which traction is applied should not exceed 30 minutes.

SYMPHYSIOTOMY

The cutting of the symphyseal joint to allow vaginal delivery of a live child. With the increasing safety of Caesarean section this operation has become almost obsolete.

The anatomical advantage gained by separating the symphysis is mainly an enlargement of the outlet.

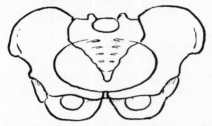

Pelvis with contracted outlet. Pubic angle 70°. Intertuberous diameter 3 in. (7.5 cm).

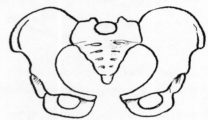

Separation of symphysis up to 5 cm increases intertuberous diameter by 4 cm and widens pubic angle. The true conjugate is increased by only 0.8 cm.

Symphysiotomy might very occasionally be indicated today in cases of labour obstructed in the second stage by outlet contraction, with the head engaged and the cervix fully dilated.

Complications

The greatest strain during the operation is taken by the soft tissues especially the vestibule, and if it tears the urethra and bladder will tear also. Also this area is full of erectile tissue and extremely vascular.

The complications met with are urinary fistula or incontinence; haemorrage which may be difficult to control; and sepsis. Although the sacro-iliac joints are put on the strain, there is not usually any subsequent backache or postural difficulty.

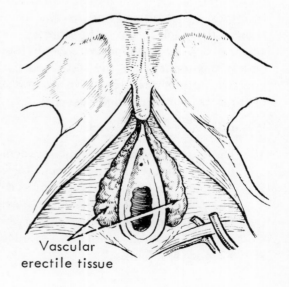

Vascular erectile tissue

SYMPHYSIOTOMY

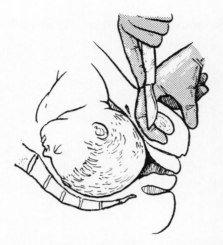

1. The patient is anaesthetised and placed in a semi-lithotomy position, with two assistants holding the legs and supporting the pelvis firmly to prevent the innominate bones springing suddenly apart when the symphysis is cut. A catheter is in the empty bladder and it is useful to have the obstetric forceps in position if they can be properly applied.

2. A transverse incision is made over the symphysis down to the rectus sheath which is opened longitudinally to give access to the vesico-pubic space. (Care must be taken to avoid damaging the urethra at this point.)

3. A finger is passed down behind the symphyseal joint, and the fibrocartilage divided with a strong knife down to but not including the sub-pubic ligament. It is very important at this point to get the assistants to allow slight separation so that the last fibres are cut on the stretch and the operator knows when to stop. The sub-pubic ligament if intact protects the vestibule.

4. Once about 4 cm of separation are achieved the baby is delivered with the assistance of a large episiotomy, again to protect the vestibule as much as possible.

5. The wound is then closed. A tight corset for a few days is advisable and bladder drainage should continue. The patient may get up in about ten days. The symphysis usually heals well but there will be a permanent separation of about 1.5 cm which may allow subsequent deliveries without interference.

CAESAREAN SECTION

Delivery of the foetus through incisions in the abdominal wall and uterus.

Classical section: – A longitudinal incision in the upper uterine segment.

This operation is quick and easy, but it is an abdominal operation rather than a pelvic one and more often followed by peritonitis and ileus. The involution of the uterus may not allow sound healing, and the scar may rupture in a subsequent pregnancy. Abnormal adhesions often develop.

Lower Segment section: A transverse incision in the lower uterine segment.

This operation takes rather longer, and may involve the operator in haemorrhage difficult to control. As a pelvic operation it is less prone to be followed by complications. The scar heals well and is very unlikely to rupture in a subsequent pregnancy.

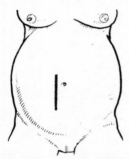

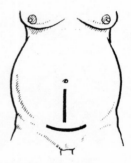

The incision for the Classical section is paramedian, one third above the umbilicus, two thirds below.

The incision for the lower segment section is midline subumbilical, or transverse suprapubic. The transverse incision heals very well, but access is reduced.

The lower segment section is today the operation of choice. Indications for classical section are:

1. Fibroids distorting the uterus.
2. Impacted transverse foetal lie.
3. An ill patient, when speed is important.
4. Following a failed trial of forceps. (The lower segment tends to be very oedematous and friable and the foetal head difficult to extricate from the pelvis).
5. When an inexperienced surgeon is operating in an emergency.

TECHNIQUE OF CLASSICAL SECTION

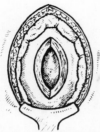

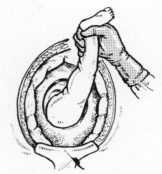

Abdominal contents are packed off and the uterus is opened in the midline. If the placenta is anterior (40% of cases) it is cut through or pushed aside at once. Bleeding is ignored.

The easiest way to remove the baby is to pull it out gently by the legs.

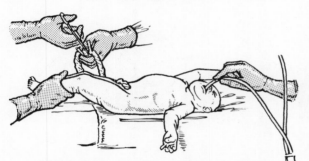

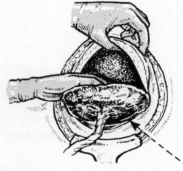

The baby's mouth and pharynx are sucked out, and the cord divided by the assistant.

Ergometrine is given and placenta and membranes separated. All membrane must be removed.

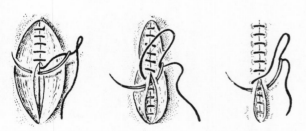

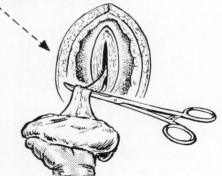

The wound is closed in 3 layers. Some haemostatic sutures may be required.

TECHNIQUE OF LOWER SEGMENT SECTION

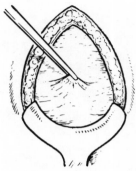

Pelvic contents are packed off, and the loose uterovesical peritoneum picked up.

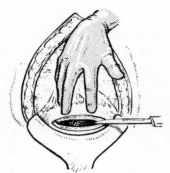

Peritoneum is cut to expose lower segment, and a small transverse incision is made.

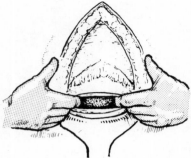

The incision is widened with the fingers.

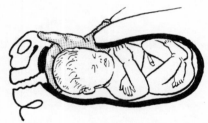

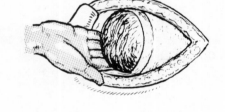

The operator's right hand is passed into the uterus to lift the baby's head, while the assistant presses on the fundus to push the baby out.

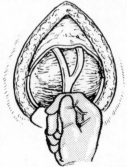

Sometimes it is necessary to extract the head with forceps.

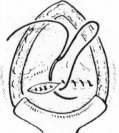

The placenta is delivered as before, and ergometrine given. The uterine wound is closed with 2 layers of No. 2 catgut.

COMPLICATIONS OF CAESAREAN SECTION

HAEMORRHAGE

If the lower segment incision tears at the angles during extraction of the foetus, the large uterine vessels may be entered and haemorrhage will be severe. The patient can very quickly pass into a state of collapse even to the extent of needing cardiac massage. If the operator cannot stop the blood loss with large artery forceps, or by suturing, temporary control may be obtained by compressing the aorta. If this does not allow a repair, subtotal hysterectomy must be carried out.

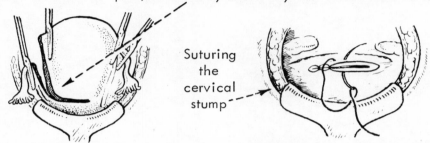

Suturing
the
cervical
stump

It is because of this ever-present risk of haemorrhage that the lower segment operation must never be done unless crossmatched blood is immediately available, and an intravenous drip of saline should always be set up.

POST-OPERATIVE DISTENSION

Gaseous distension of the bowel is almost the rule after section, but the lax condition of the abdominal muscles, although it accentuates the swelling, reduces the pain of distension.

WOUND DEHISCENCE and INFECTION

Owing to the distension the wound is under tension and dehiscence is much more common after section than after any other abdominal operation. Unless very small, resuture should be carried out in theatre. A remote sequel is ventral hernia.

PARALYTIC ILEUS

A condition of 'incipient ileus' – distension, reduced bowel sounds, no flatus – is the rule for the first 24 – 48 hours, but flatus should be passed by then. If not, gastric suction and parenteral fluids should be started forthwith until the condition has resolved.

PULMONARY EMBOLISM

Pulmonary embolism has an association with Caesarean section and is the commonest cause of the mortality arising from the operation.

ABDOMINAL HYSTEROTOMY

Termination of pregnancy by the abdominal route before the 28th week. This is the best method of performing abortion after the 10th week. Curettage may be attended by severe bleeding at this stage which would be difficult to control.

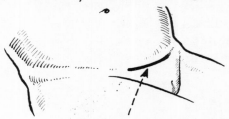

A transverse suprapubic incision is used. The scar will become almost invisible.

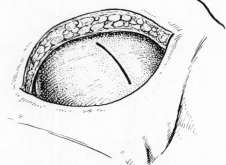

A midline incision is made in the body of the uterus.

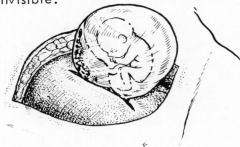

An attempt is made to squeeze out the gestation sac unruptured.

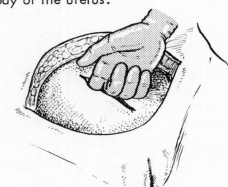

Ergometrine is injected intravenously and the cavity is gently curetted with the finger.

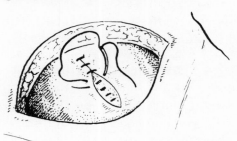

The uterus is then closed with 2 layers of catgut. Haemostatic sutures may be needed to control oozing.

VAGINAL HYSTEROTOMY

This operation is indicated only when termination is called for in a parous woman who also has a degree of prolapse. It is rarely performed at the present day.

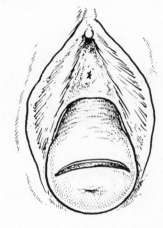

An incision is made across the front of the cervix.

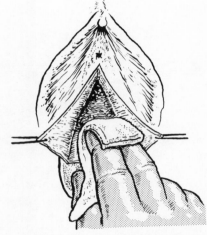

The vaginal wall has been separated and the bladder mobilised and pushed up out of the way.

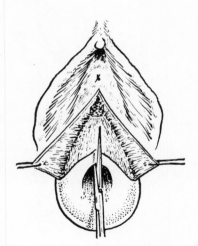

The cervix is divided up to the internal os, and the uterus evacuated with ovum forceps, and curette.

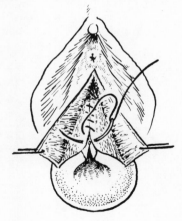

The cervical wound is closed with a continuous catgut suture.

DESTRUCTIVE OPERATIONS

Operations designed to reduce the bulk of the foetus and allow delivery per vaginam. Only dead or grossly abnormal foetuses are so treated, and unless delivery is likely to be easy Caesarean section is indicated, whatever the condition of the foetus.

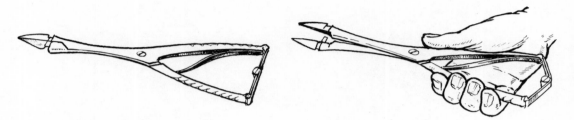

CRANIOTOMY means perforation and extraction of the crushed skull. It is done to-day in cases of hydrocephaly or when there is second stage delay with a dead foetus and apparently a minor degree of disproportion. Simpson's perforator is the best instrument for the purpose, but a Drew-Smythe cannula might serve.

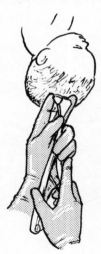

An assistant presses the head downwards through the abdominal wall, and the perforator is passed carefully into the skull, through a suture or fontanelle if possible. The opening is enlarged by closing the handles and rotating the instrument.

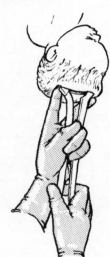

Sometimes it is possible to drain a hydrocephalic skull by passing a catheter up the spinal canal through a meningocoele which is often present, or by cutting across the spine.

DESTRUCTIVE OPERATIONS

Extraction with the Combined Cranioclast and Cephalotribe

    Once perforation has reduced the bulk of the skull, spontaneous delivery or forceps extraction will follow. Very rarely there might be an indication for using the combined cranioclast and cephalotribe, an all-but-obsolete instrument designed to reduce the bulk of the skull so that it might be delivered through the 'chink' of a narrow pelvis. Today it might conceivably be of use in dealing with a dead foetus arrested at the brim or in high cavity because of borderline disproportion. Cephalotripsy can be difficult and dangerous, and in most cases section would be indicated even after perforation.

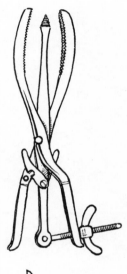

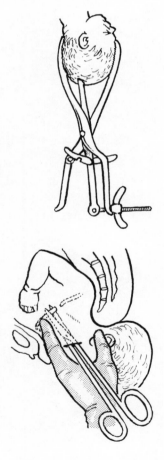

    The middle blade of the cephalotribe is passed through the perforated vault and screwed into the base of the skull, preferably the foramen magnum. The lateral blades are applied in turn and gradually forced in by the butterfly screw until the catch can be applied. The instrument is applied in the transverse diameter of the pelvis and rotation should occur during traction. (Cranioclasm means breaking up the vault of the skull: Cephalotripsy means crushing the whole skull.)

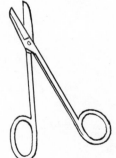

    Cleidotomy. If the shoulder girdle is too large, the clavicle may be divided with cleidotomy scissors. It is easier if the supraclavicular space is pierced by the scissors, but provided they are guarded by the fingers the cut may be made through the skin.

DESTRUCTIVE OPERATIONS

Decapitation

This operation is still indicated in cases of impacted shoulder presentation where the foetus is dead. Version would be dangerous in such circumstances because of the thinning and stretching of the lower segment that accompanies impaction.

Using a Decapitation Hook

The hook is passed with the left hand guarding the maternal tissues. By a combination of swinging and gentle traction the neck is cut through, and the body is delivered by pulling on the arm. The head is hooked out manually or delivered with forceps.

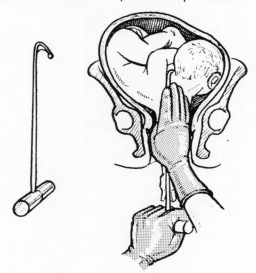

Using the Blond-Heidler Saw

One end of the saw is attached to the thimble and passed round the neck in the manner shown. It may be more difficult to manoeuvre into position than the hook but is superior in action.

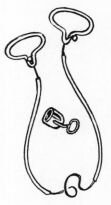
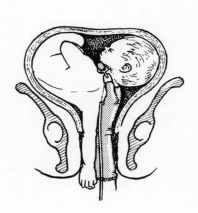
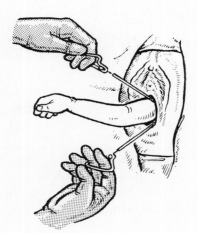

STERILISATION

Sterilisation by Ligation or Division of the Fallopian Tubes

This operation is still technically illegal, and written permission from husband and wife is essential (although permission to commit an illegal act is itself technically meaningless).

In practice sterilisation has for many years been accepted if done to protect the patient's mental or physical health. Today it may be said that multiparity is also an acceptable indication.

The most convenient time for doing the operation (unless at laparotomy for Caesarean section) is in the immediate postpartum period. But as the operation has a slight but recognised association with pulmonary embolism, and as the changes of the early puerperium may themselves also have a similar association, it is probably wiser to delay operation for 2 months. Two other rare sequels are chronic pelvic inflammation, and tubal pregnancy. All techniques of tubal ligation or division carry an exceedingly small risk of failure.

Tubal Occlusion

The tube is crushed with forceps and tied with a non-absorbable silk suture. The object is to occlude the lumen but preserve anatomical continuity so as to avoid the creation of a new ostium.

Tubal Division

The tube is ligated with fine catgut and the distal loop excised. When the catgut is absorbed the ends of the tube are separated and are occluded by exudate and fibrosis.

Tubal Division with Burial of Ends

Two inches or so of tube are excised and the ends of the stumps are buried under the peritoneum.

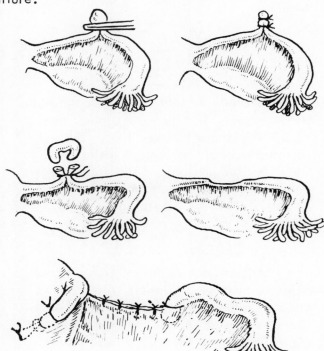

SPINAL ANAESTHESIA

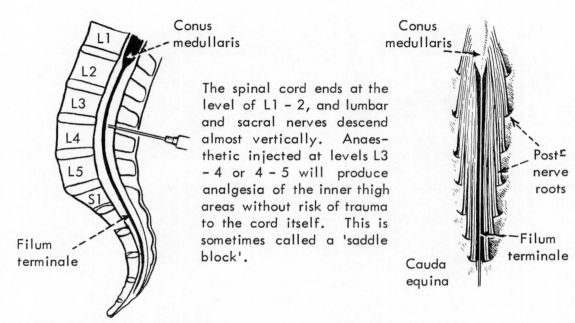

Conus medullaris

The spinal cord ends at the level of L1 – 2, and lumbar and sacral nerves descend almost vertically. Anaesthetic injected at levels L3 – 4 or 4 – 5 will produce analgesia of the inner thigh areas without risk of trauma to the cord itself. This is sometimes called a 'saddle block'.

Filum terminale

Conus medullaris

Post. nerve roots

Filum terminale

Cauda equina

Physiology of Spinal Anaesthesia

The effect is that of 'chemical sympathectomy'. The pre-ganglionic autonomic fibres are blocked first, followed by those serving temperature, pain, touch, motor and proprioceptive function in that order. Skeletal muscle action may still be possible when sensory blockade is complete.

Circulatory Effects

Paralysis of the pre-ganglionic fibres leads to arterial dilatation with a fall in venous return and cardiac output. Blood loss at operation may aggravate this and cause an acute and serious fall in blood pressure.

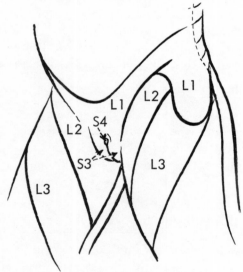

Areas affected by a saddle block

458

EPIDURAL ANAESTHESIA

Epidural Anaesthesia

The epidural space lies between the periosteum of the vertebral canal and the dura mater. It is limited above at the foramen magnum where dura and periosteum fuse, and below by the ligament covering the sacral hiatus. Injection of local anaesthetic into this space which is transversed by the spinal nerves, can be made through the sacral hiatus or between the vertebrae. It is a more difficult and time-consuming procedure than the

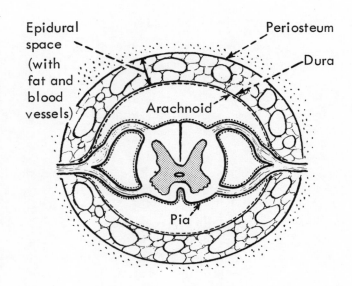

giving of a spinal anaesthetic, but it is virtually free of such post-operative sequelae as headache, meningism or nerve root trauma. The physiological effects are the same as for spinal injection.

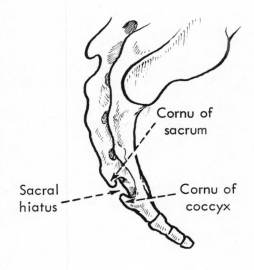

Operative Restrictions

Intra-uterine manipulations are not possible under spinal or epidural anaesthesia. It must be remembered that the vagus is not blocked, and manipulations of the abdominal viscera may cause nausea and vomiting. The obstetrician must not be tempted by the absence of pain-sense in the patient to use excessive force in an attempt to overcome disproportion.

Spinal and epidural anaesthesia should be administered by an experienced anaesthetist, and supervised by him throughout the operation.

ANAESTHESIA IN LABOUR

Paracervical Nerve Block

Autonomic fibres serving the uterus and vagina accompany the vessels and form a plexus lying in the parametrial tissues. This area can be infiltrated by injection of 10 ml of 1% lignocaine with 1:200,000 adrenaline into each lateral vaginal fornix, using a transvaginal guarded needle. Uterine action is unaffected. (See page 435.)

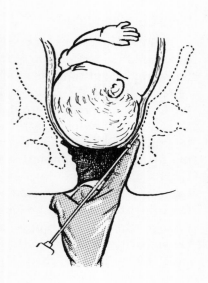

Pain relief lasts for 1 or 2 hours only, but the injection can be repeated. The chief disadvantage is the difficulty that can be experienced in gaining access to the paracervical space in a conscious patient advanced in labour with the head engaged, even when the lithotomy position is used. The area of injection is extremely vascular and it is essential to withdraw the plunger of the syringe before injecting, to make sure that a vessel has not been entered.

Continuous Epidural Anaesthesia

This technique has been used successfully for abolishing the pain of labour, particularly in cases of inco-ordinate uterine action when the pain itself, by increasing psychological tension is contributing to the dystocia. A catheter is passed through a No. 16 spinal needle into the epidural space via the sacral hiatus or an intervertebral space and with aseptic precautions 1% lignocaine with 1:200,000 adrenaline is injected as required to abolish pain.

The physiology of spinal and epidural anaesthesia is referred to on page 458, and as larger amounts are required with continuous administration, a greater risk of hypotension is accepted. In addition increasingly short duration of anaesthesia may be obtained with repeated injections.

Epidural anaesthesia must be administered and supervised by an experienced anaesthetist, and its use in this country is limited because of this. The obstetrician has to remember that the inco-ordinate uterine action may be caused by an unsuspected degree of disproportion, making forceps delivery impossible, no matter how little pain is felt by the patient.

CHAPTER 18

MATERNAL AND FOETAL MORTALITY

MATERNAL MORTALITY

Maternal Mortality – death in childbirth – has for the last 200 years been a recurring tragedy that has caused public energies gradually to be directed towards the research, the legislation, education and administration from which have evolved the high standard of maternal care which exists today. Childbirth is not yet completely safe, but maternal deaths are now so infrequent, that the incidence of foetal mortality has become the indicator of continuing improvement.

The Maternal Mortality Rate (MMR) sometimes called Puerperal Mortality Rate, is calculated as the number of deaths of pregnant women per thousand births live and still.

$$\frac{\text{Number of Maternal Deaths}}{\text{Number of Births (live and still)}} \times 1{,}000 = \text{MMR}$$

Deaths from abortion must also be included, and as they are added to the numerator only, the increase is not quite accurate. The true MMR would be:–

$$\frac{\text{Number of Deaths from Pregnancy}}{\text{Number of Pregnancies}} \times 1{,}000$$

This figure would be lower than the accepted MMR but is obviously unobtainable as neither abortion nor pregnancy itself is notifiable.

Associated Maternal Deaths are deaths during pregnancy or childbirth which are not primarily due to the pregnancy. Nowadays they are commonly the result of cardiac disease or malignancy and there must often be an element of doubt as to the degree to which pregnancy has affected the primary condition.

MATERNAL MORTALITY

Mortality rates are published by the Registrar-General, and the first Report appeared in 1839. Not until 1874 was it compulsory to give the cause of death in a certificate; and in 1857 the Registrar for Birmingham stated that "No-one ever specifies deaths in childbed or from puerperal fever". Births have had to be notified only since 1907 (and stillbirths only since 1915); so 19th century mortality statistics must be accepted as an approximation.

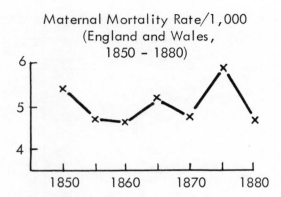

Maternal Mortality Rate/1,000
(England and Wales,
1850 - 1880)

These rates represented between 3 and 5 thousand deaths a year, about 60% from infection.

Some Causes of Death in 1841

Puerperal Fever ⎫
Peritonitis   ⎬ "Metria"
Uterine Phlebitis ⎭
Flooding
Exhaustion
Debility
Convulsions
Mania
 - and simply -
Childbirth

From their inception, the reports of the Registrar-General deplored the deaths of so many women in childbirth - "the deep dark continuous stream of mortality" - and discussed the causes.

"The cases which cause most distress to practitioners ... are undoubtedly those deplorable and rare instances in which they communicate contagious diseases to their patients." (1841).

"A large proportion of the 500,000 English women who lie in every year and have any attendance at all, are attended by midwives who from one cause or another, probably delicacy in the national manners in points of this kind, receive no preliminary instruction in anatomy and other matters." (1841).

"A registered MRCS without any further qualifications has passed no examination in midwifery. Many are in large and successful midwifery practice; others it is to be feared must labour under disqualifications disadvantageous to themselves and to their patients." (1878).

MATERNAL MORTALITY

Maternal Deaths in England and Wales, 1875 (rate 6/1,000)	
Sepsis	2,662
Haemorrhage	1,038
Convulsions	538
Abortion	185
Mania	115
Ruptured uterus	36
Others	36
	4,610

Sepsis (puerperal fever etc.) was the most fatal complication. Spread by the attendants from one patient to another had been described by Alexander Gordon of Aberdeen in 1795. ("It is disagreeable for me to mention that I myself was the means of carrying infection to great numbers of women."). In 1848 Semelweis published his results – a reduction in death rate in his clinic from 12% to 3% by making his students wash their hands in antiseptic before examining patients. Pasteur and Lister published their great discoveries; but the maternal mortality rate remained unaffected.

By the 1870's the mortality in the institutions was being attacked. Florence Nightingale had had to close the lying-in ward in King's College Hospital because of this, and she described in detail designs for an improved maternity unit which would be barred to medical students and the infections they might carry.

The superior results from Liverpool Workhouse shown in this table were correctly attributed to its isolation, absence of visitors, regular 'limestoning' of the wards by the paupers, and rigid segregation of pregnant women at all stages. In Florence Nightingale's recommendations there can be discerned the principles of organisation of present day maternity units at least until the era of antibiotics.

Institution	MMR/1000
King's College Hospital 1862 – 67	33.3
Queen Charlotte's 1828 – 68	25.3
Liverpool Workhouse 1867	9.0
England and Wales 1867	5.1
(from Florence Nightingale)	

MATERNAL MORTALITY

<u>Maternal Mortality in 1910 (England and Wales)</u>. 3,191 deaths
(rate 3.6/1,000)

Sepsis	1,274	Inversion of uterus	8
Placenta praevia and flooding	612	Craniotomy	7
Convulsions	439	Hydrocephaly	4
Thrombo-embolism	334	Administration of	
Abortion	80	chloroform	4
Ectopic gestation	78	Instrumental delivery	3
Mania	48	Adherent placenta	3
Vomiting	38	Prolapsus uteri	2
Contracted pelvis	31	Rigidity of os	2
Ruptured uterus	28	Rupture of vagina	2
Malpresentation	16	Hydramnios	2
Caesarean section	15	Monstrosity	1

It will be seen that the main causes were:-

Sepsis: Haemorrhage: Toxaemia (Convulsions): Thrombo-embolism:
and Trauma.

At the turn of the century a slight improvement occurred, the result probably of several factors: a better understanding and application of 'Listerism'; an improvement in general hygiene and sanitation brought about by Public Health legislation; and the Midwives' Act of 1902, the first of many Acts which regulate the training and practice of midwives.

However a more dramatic and sustained fall was observed at the same time in Infant Mortality Rate; and by the 1920s after the First World War, it became apparent that the risks of childbirth were not much less than they were 80 years before, while the scandal was proportionately greater.

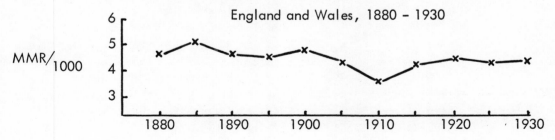

England and Wales, 1880 – 1930

MATERNAL MORTALITY

With the founding of the Ministry of Health in 1919 a period of energetic official enquiry was entered into. Public Health antenatal clinics were instituted largely in the face of the medical profession's opposition, and repeated surveys were made and reported on. Eventually what had long been known was openly asserted; a large number of maternal deaths could be avoided if the standard of obstetric management were higher. A report in 1932 listed four 'Primary Avoidable Factors: -

1. Absence of antenatal care.
2. Errors of management.
3. Lack of reasonable facilities.
4. Negligence by the patient.

Committee on Maternal Mortality England and Wales, 1932		
3,059 Deaths Inquired Into		
Cause	Number	Percent
Sepsis	1,111	36.3
Toxaemia	506	16.4
Haemorrhage	450	14.8
Abortion	410	13.4
Shock and Trauma	319	10.4
Thrombo-embolism	206	6.8
Ectopic gestation	55	1.8

This table shows that the causes of death in 1932 were much the same as in 1910.

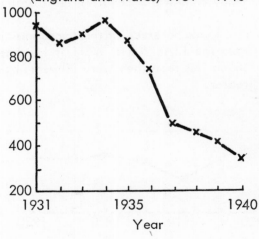

Deaths from Puerperal Infection (England and Wales) 1931 – 1940

In the early thirties the mortality rate appeared static or even rising slightly; until in 1935 the antibacterial action of the sulphonamide Prontosil was demonstrated. It is the action of antibiotics, almost abolishing death from puerperal sepsis, and allowing the obstetrician a freedom of intervention undreamed of 50 years ago that has made childbirth as safe as it is today.

MATERNAL MORTALITY

In 1937 a further Report made a series of recommendations – consultant training and supervision, provision of adequate maternity hospitals and antenatal clinics, flying squads, organisation of the Health Visitor service, and so on – which form the basis of modern practice.

Since then there has been continuous improvement, and maternal deaths are now referred to in actual numbers rather than percentages. There were 223 deaths in England and Wales in 1966 (0.26 per 1,000) and 24 in Scotland (0.24 per 1,000).

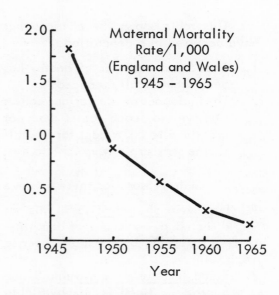

Maternal Mortality Rate/1,000 (England and Wales) 1945 – 1965

Maternal Deaths 1966 (England and Wales)		
Cause	No.	Percent
Abortion	53	24
Toxaemia	38	17
Haemorrhage	27	12.3
Trauma, shock etc.	23	10
Prolonged labour	16	7.2
Thrombo-embolism	11	5
Puerperal sepsis	9	4
Other causes	46	20
Total	223	100

Deaths associated with but not primarily due to pregnancy			
England and Wales, 1966			
Cardiac disease	18	Benign tumours	4
Malignancy	8		
Respiratory disease	5	Cerebral haemorrhage	3
Blood disease	5	Diabetes	2
Accidents	5	Other	6

It will be seen that abortion and toxaemia are the most frequent causes of death, and sepsis the least. Cardiac disease is the main contributor to 'associated deaths'.

MATERNAL MORTALITY

This table shows the changes that have occurred in a generation.

1. The actual number of deaths has been dramatically reduced.
2. The incidence of the various causes relative to each other has not greatly altered except for the fall in the sepsis rate from 25% to 4%.

Cause of Maternal Death	Number 1935	Number 1966	Percent 1935	Percent 1966
Abortion	464	53	18	24
Toxaemia	488	38	19	17
Haemorrhage	292	27	11	12
Trauma etc.	342	39	13	17
Thrombosis	192	11	7	5
Sepsis	647	9	25	4

(England and Wales)

The main reasons for these improvements are:-

1. <u>Discovery of Antibiotics</u>. This has affected every cause of death including toxaemia, by making surgery so much safer.
2. <u>Blood Transfusion and Flying Squad Services</u>. Blood is now available for every patient and can be got to her quickly.
3. <u>Improved Maternity Hospital Services</u>. Severe toxaemia and eclampsia are anticipated by good antenatal supervision and early admission to hospital.

4. <u>Higher Medical Standards</u>. The National Health Service has brought about a great increase in the number and availability of experienced obstetric specialists, and there is close liaison between the specialist, the general practitioner and Local Health Authority.
5. <u>The Social Factor</u>. The last 30 years have seen a steady improvement in health and physique of the population which must tend to reduce abnormalities of pregnancy especially those due to malnutrition.

Avoidable Factors in Maternal Deaths

The number of deaths is now small enough to permit each case to be studied in some detail; and this is done at intervals in a Government publication, 'Report on Confidental Enquiries into Maternal Deaths'. It appears from this study that the risk of death is slightly greater in the following groups of women, who should be seen by a specialist.

1. The woman whose general health is poor.
2. The woman over 35 (or over 30 if a primigravida).

3. The woman pregnant for the fifth or subsequent time.
4. The woman with a bad obstetric history.

FOETAL MORTALITY

Infant mortality has always been a matter of concern to society – in England and Wales in 1839 the mortality rate among children under three was 343 per 1,000 – but the obstetrician understandably feels a greater responsibility for stillbirths and neonatal deaths in the first week of life – the 'perinatal mortality'. This combined death rate is the best index of the standard of practice in institutional obstetrics.

Stillbirth

A stillbirth is a baby that does not breathe or show any other sign of life after being completely separated from its mother. In the United Kingdom the Stillbirth Rate refers to the number of stillbirths per 1,000 total births live and still. Stillbirth has been a notifiable condition since 1915, and registerable since 1927 (1939 in Scotland). The body may not be disposed of until the doctor has issued a Certificate of Stillbirth and the Registrar has issued a Certificate of Registration.

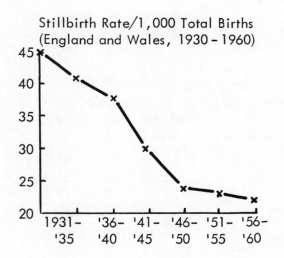

Stillbirth Rate/1,000 Total Births (England and Wales, 1930 – 1960)

The dramatic fall between 1940 and 1946 is attributed to the improvement in the nutrition of working class pregnant women effected by the wartime rationing system.

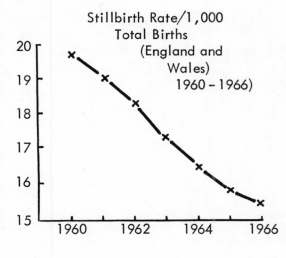

Stillbirth Rate/1,000 Total Births (England and Wales) 1960 – 1966)

The stillbirth rate for 1966 was 15.3 per 1,000 and it will be seen that the rate has fallen slowly since 1960.

469

FOETAL MORTALITY

Deaths of liveborn children are in the first instance included in the Infant Mortality Rate (IMR) which is the number of deaths of all children under a year per 1,000 live births.

The impressive fall in IMR since 1900 has been the result of gradual improvements in domestic sanitation and hygiene, and of great social advances. In addition the fall in birth rate from 29.3 to 16.4 per 1,000 has reduced overcrowding and allowed more attention and care to be given to smaller families.

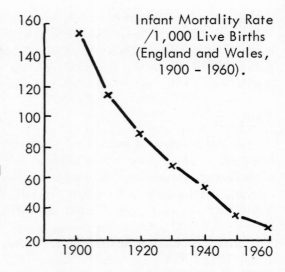

Infant Mortality Rate /1,000 Live Births (England and Wales, 1900 – 1960).

Year	IMR	NND rate	'First Week Death'
1906 – 10	117.1	40.2	24.5 (22% of IMR)
1966	19.0	12.9	11.1 (58% of IMR)

Included in the IMR are the Neonatal Death Rate – all deaths under 4 weeks – and 'First Week Deaths'. These groups now make up more than half the IMR.

The 'First Week' deaths and the perinatal mortality rate (1st week plus still-births) have fallen much more slowly since 1960 and perhaps the irreducible minimum is being approached. Nevertheless avoidable foetal deaths do still occur.

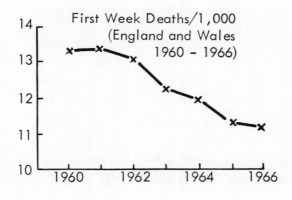

First Week Deaths/1,000 (England and Wales 1960 – 1966)

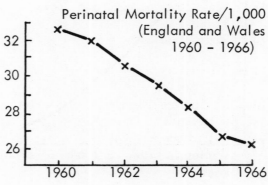

Perinatal Mortality Rate/1,000 (England and Wales 1960 – 1966)

FOETAL MORTALITY

Causes of Perinatal Deaths

The table shows where further improvements must be made. It should be possible to all but eliminate traumatic deaths, but prematurity is largely a social problem dependent on the well-being of the mother. Deaths from asphyxia arise mainly from placental failure which is the subject of much research. Until the aetiology of congenital abnormality is better understood, this cause of death is likely to become proportionately more frequent.

England and Wales, 1966	
17,000 Perinatal Deaths	
Congenital abnormality	29%
Asphyxia	22
Trauma of delivery	22
Prematurity (alone or primary)	22
Erythroblastosis	3
Other	2
	100%

Administrative Factors

A well-equipped and staffed hospital is probably the safest place for delivery; and as modern GP maternity units are established with good specialist liaison, domiciliary confinement must become less and less common.

Scotland, 1966	
Perinatal mortality	29.3
Social Class	
I & II	19.3
III	27.8
IV & V	34.4

Social Factors

Stillbirth, prematurity and multiparity have a marked social gradient which is reflected in this table, in spite of there being a preponderance of younger mothers in the lower social classes.

Illegitimacy always shows a higher rate of foetal mortality.

Regional Differences

These reflect both social and administrative factors. In England and Wales the rate rises as one travels from London and the South-East, much as the level of prosperity tends to fall. This geographical effect is to some extent corrected by the higher rates in urban areas compared with rural ones.

Scotland, 1966. Stillbirth Rate 16.2	
Northern (Highland)	13.2
Southern (Pastoral)	13.9
East Central (Mixed)	14.4
West Central (Glasgow)	18.3

CHAPTER 19

CONTRACEPTION

CONTRACEPTION

This includes all methods used to prevent conception following coitus.

Used by the Male

      1.   Condom or sheath.
      2.   Coitus interruptus.
      3.   Vas deferens ligation.

Used by the Female

      1.   Oral contraceptives.
      2.   Intra-uterine contraceptive devices (IUCD).
      3.   Vaginal diaphragm.
      4.   Spermicidal creams and gels.
      5.   Tubal ligation.

Used by Both Partners

      Rhythm method   ('safe period')

Contraception by the Husband

The Sheath ('Condom'). This is a thin latex rubber sheath (or more exotically a lamb's caecum) which covers the penis and prevents ejaculation into the vagina. It is an extremely efficient method if used properly, and failure is usually due to its being put on too late.

Coitus Interruptus ('Withdrawal'). The husband must withdraw his penis from the vagina before ejaculation. This is so unreliable as hardly to constitute a method of contraception; nevertheless it is widely practised and is what the patient means when she says her husband is 'being careful'.

Vas Deferens Ligation. This operation is simple, safe, effective and in some cases reversible if required. It has been carried out on many millions of men in India and is now being advocated in this country, although there is some doubt about its legality. Its disadvantage is the possibility of unpleasant psychological consequences in the husband, including impotence.

ORAL CONTRACEPTION

Oral Contraceptives (The 'Pill')

These are oestrogen-progestogen combinations which are taken daily and prevent conception by three effects:-

1. Ovulation may be suppressed probably by action of the hypothalamus to inhibit pituitary gonadotrophin secretions from the anterior pituitary gland.

2. The endometrium is altered and becomes unsuitable for implantation.

3. The cervical mucus becomes thick, tacky, and hostile to spermatozoa.

Endometrial Changes

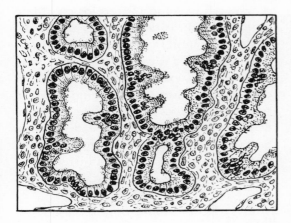

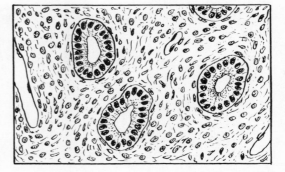

Normal endometrium at the 22nd day, when implantation usually occurs.

The glands are tortuous and serrated with abundant glycogen in their lumina. The stroma is loose, oedematous and vascular.

Endometrium showing the effects of oestrogen-progestogen contraceptive treatment.

The pattern is called 'pseudo-atrophic'. The glands although showing secretory activity are much less numerous and there is little glycogen. The stroma is less oedematous and vascular.

The ovary becomes smaller during prolonged use of oral contraceptives, and histological examination shows a quiescent pattern with atretic follicles and fibrosis in the cortical stroma. This pattern is reversible.

ORAL CONTRACEPTION

Drugs Used for Oral Contraception

Two oestrogenic drugs are in common use, ethinyloestradiol and mestranol which is ethinyloestradiol, 3-methyl ether.

Oestrogens inhibit FSH secretion and by themselves can prevent ovulation.. However when used alone for this purpose fertilisation does occasionally occur, possibly because of forgetfulness by the patient, but also because oestrogens do not bring about the endometrial and cervical mucus changes which have important contraceptive effects.

The optimum dosage is 0.05 - 0.1 mg daily.

Ethinyloestradiol

The progestogens used are a group of powerful synthetic steroids of which norethisterone is an example. The progestogens inhibit LH secretion and produce the desired changes in the endometrium and cervical mucus. They are also necessary for bringing about a regular menstrual cycle. The optimum dose varies with the drug and with the proprietary combination in which it appears. The dose of norethisterone is about 2 mg daily.

Norethisterone

Administration

The patient takes one tablet daily for 21 days, from the 5th to the 25th day of the cycle. Withdrawal bleeding follows at the expected time of the period and tablets are begun again on the next 5th day. The combined oestrogen-progestogen tablet is virtually 100% effective. The 'sequential' schemes of dosage, say 14 days of oestrogen followed by 7 days of the combined tablet, are slightly less reliable, but are claimed to cause fewer side effects and have the long term advantage of reducing the amount of hormone taken. With sequential dosage, ovulation suppression by oestrogen is the sole contraceptive element, the endometrium and cervical mucus following a normal cycle.

Oral contraception with continuous low-dosage progestogens and no oestrogen at all, it still experimental.

476

ORAL CONTRACEPTION—SIDE EFFECTS

Favourable

1. There is usually a regularisation of the menstrual rhythm and reduction in flow, due to the progressive endometrial atrophy. A result of this is often correction of chronic anaemia.
2. Anovulatory cycles give the patient relief from spasmodic dysmenorrhoea if present.
3. There may be an improvement in the skin and hair and acne may be relieved.
4. Sometimes there is an increase in libido and a general feeling of wellbeing, due in part to relief from the fear of pregnancy.

Unfavourable

1. Gastric upset with nausea.
2. Headache of migraine type.
3. Irregular ('breakthrough') bleeding.
4. Fluid retention and weight increase.
5. Appearance of pre-menstrual tension syndrome.
6. Greasiness of skin and hair. (Chloasma is very rare among European women).
7. Loss of libido, depression, irritability, general malaise.

Thromboembolic Disease

There is some statistical evidence of an increased liability to bloodclotting disease in women taking oral contraceptives. It is not related to any particular drug or to length of treatment; and it is estimated that the risk of death from pulmonary embolism during one year of oral contraceptive treatment is equivalent to the risk from one pregnancy.

Management of Side-Effects

Headache, nausea and breakthrough bleeding tend to stop after 2 or 3 cycles. Irregular bleeding sometimes confuses the patient and she should be told to ignore it unless it is so heavy as to represent a period, in which case she should start a new course. If side effects persist a different combination or a sequential dosage should be tried. Gastric upsets and headache suggest too much oestrogen, while too much progestogen causes a greasy skin, pelvic cramps and breast discomfort.

Contraindications

Oral contraceptives should not be given to patients with thromboembolic tendencies, liver disease or breast cancer.

Subsequent Pregnancies

These are unaffected. Cessation after prolonged treatment may be followed by amenorrhoea, and clomiphene should be given to induce ovulation.

INTRA-UTERINE CONTRACEPTIVE DEVICES (IUCD)

A polyethyline spiral or coil is inserted into the uterine cavity and effectively prevents conception although the mode of action is not known. Ovulation is not prevented and no recognisable characteristic changes occur in the endometrium.

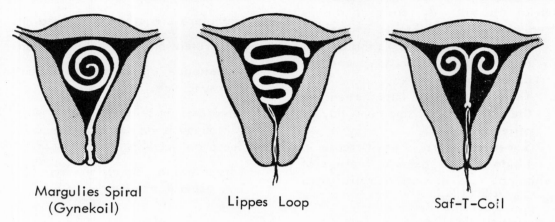

Margulies Spiral
(Gynekoil)

Lippes Loop

Saf-T-Coil

IUCDs are flexible and can be straightened out and held inside a straight cannula for insertion into the uterus. When ejected the coiled shape is resumed, provided the device has not been kept straight for more than 2 or 3 minutes.

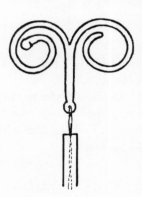

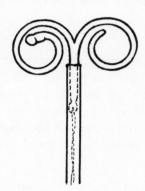

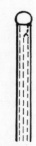

IUCD with nylon thread attached, about to be pulled into introducer.

Halfway into introducer.

Completely inside the introducer. Note how the protruding end of the IUCD acts as an obturator.

INTRA-UTERINE CONTRACEPTIVE DEVICES

Insertion of IUCD

This may be done in the outpatient department or surgery but must be a sterile procedure.

1. Pelvic examination is done to exclude abnormality. The uterus should be anteverted and a uterine sound should be passed if there is any doubt.

2. Insert a bivalve speculum.

3. Grasp the anterior cervical lip with a tenaculum forceps.

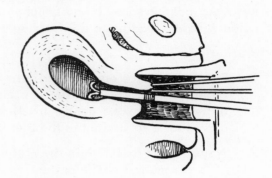

4. Pass the loaded introducer through the cervix as far as the mark indicates.

5. Apply gentle pressure on the plunger and eject the IUCD into the uterine cavity.

6. Remove the introducer and pull gently on the nylon thread to make sure that the device is securely inserted. If there is a plastic tail cut if off level with the cervix.

Complications with IUCD's

1. Irregular sometimes heavy bleeding is the chief disadvantage. As a rule the loss returns to more or less normal after one or two cycles.

2. Insertion is not difficult but occasionally a patient may faint. Cramps may occur for the first 12 hours or so.

3. Pelvic inflammation, unless pre-existing, is rare.

4. An IUCD is best inserted immediately after a period when the uterus is less irritable and pregnancy impossible. Thereafter the patient should be seen at 6 monthly intervals. An IUCD can be left in situ for up to 3 years.

5. The patient must palpate her vagina at regular intervals to feel for the thread or the plastic tail. Expulsion is uncommon but may occur soon after insertion or during a period.

479

INTRA-UTERINE CONTRACEPTIVE DEVICES

Uterine Perforation

This has been seen with all types of device and presumably occurs during insertion. If the operator suspects that it may have happened either because of pain, or because of unusual resistance during insertion, the device should if possible be withdrawn. If not an X-ray with a sound in the uterine cavity will show the position of the IUCD. If it is demonstrated in the peritoneal cavity it should be removed; but there may be no symptoms other than the disappearance later on of the nylon thread, leading to a false diagnosis of expulsion; or a pregnancy may occur.

Precautions

1. Do not use force during insertion. An IUCD should not be inserted into a retro-flexed or acutely anteflexed uterus without special care, and in every case it is helpful to exert gentle traction with the forceps on the anterior lip of the cervix so as to straighten the uterus as much as possible.

2. Never insert an IUCD in the presence of pelvic inflammation or within 12 weeks of a pregnancy. (The patient should know that conception may occur within 6 week of parturition).

3. When inserting the IUCD, the tip of the introducer must be above the internal os but below the fundus and the device must be ejected slowly to allow it to resume its coiled position in the cavity.

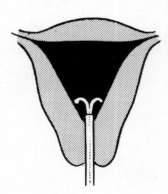 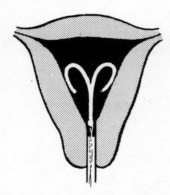 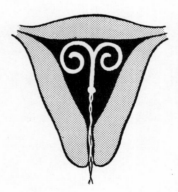

| Correct positioning of introducer. | Slow insertion of plunger and withdrawal of intro-ducer. | Device coils freely in uterine cavity. |

THE VAGINAL DIAPHRAGM

The vaginal diaphragm is a latex diaphragm which prevents sperms from reaching the cervical canal and acts as an applicator to the cervix of a spermicidal cream. It is less efficient than oral contraceptives or the IUCD unless used strictly according to instructions; but it has no side effects.

Diaphragms range in size from 45 to 95 mm diameter. When in the vagina the dome may be up or down, but the spermicidal cream must be applied to the side in contact with the cervix.

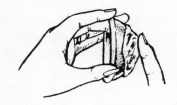

Insertion of the diaphragm by the patient

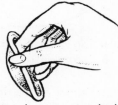

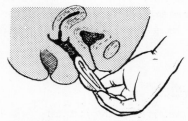

1. The diaphragm is held between thumb and second finger with the index finger inside the rim.

2. With one hand the labia are separated and the diaphragm is guided into the posterior fornix.

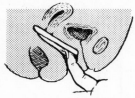

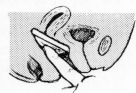

3. The front end is pushed up behind the symphysis.

4. The patient checks position by feeling the cervix through the dome.

Precautions

Spermicidal cream must be spread all round the rim and on the diaphragm itself, and if intercourse is repeated more cream must be injected with an applicator. The diaphragm must not be removed until at least 6 hours after intercourse.

SPERMICIDES AND RHYTHM METHOD

Vaginal Spermicides

Spermicidal agents can be inserted into the vagina in the form of creams, gels, pessaries or aerosols.

Although this method of contraception is not completely reliable it remains popular because of its simplicity, and there are several commercial preparations available. One dose of spermicide will deal only with one ejaculate and if intercourse is repeated more spermicide must first be inserted. It is important when injecting cream with an applicator to deposit it as near the cervix as possible.

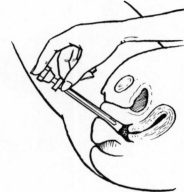

Inserting cream with a
vaginal applicator

Rhythm Method

This means the avoidance of coitus round about the time of ovulation. The woman must take her temperature every morning for several cycles watching for the biphasic response (a slight drop followed by a rise) which indicates ovulation.

Once she has established her normal rhythm she may assume that ovulation occurs between say the 12th and 14th days. Another day must be added if the ovum survives 24 hours. Sperms may live for at least 3 days after insemination; so coitus must be avoided between at least the 9th and the 18th days of the cycle; and the 7th and the 20th would be safer.

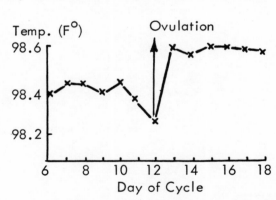

The rhythm method is unreliable because it depends too much on regularity of ovulation; and its effectiveness is in part due to the relative sexual abstinence it imposes.

INDEX

490

Printed in the British Commonwealth